Combating Destructive Thought Processes

To Ronnie Laing, beloved friend, greatly missed

Robert W. Firestone

Combating Destructive Thought Processes

Voice Therapy and Separation Theory

SAGE Publications
International Educational and Professional Publisher
Thousand Oaks   London   New Delhi

For information address:

SAGE Publications, Inc.
2455 Teller Road
Thousand Oaks, California 91320
E-mail: order@sagepub.com

SAGE Publications Ltd.
6 Bonhill Street
London EC2A 4PU
United Kingdom

SAGE Publications India Pvt. Ltd.
M-32 Market
Greater Kailash I
New Delhi 110048 India

Printed in the United States of America

Library of Congress Cataloging-in-Publication Data

Firestone, Robert.
  Combating destructive thought processes: Separation theory and voice therapy/
  author, Robert W. Firestone.
    p. cm.
  Includes bibliographical references and index.
  ISBN 0-7619-0551-0 (pbk. : acid-free paper). — ISBN 0-7619-0550-2
(cloth : acid-free paper)
  1. Psychic trauma. 2. Psychotherapy. 3. Separation
-individuation. 4. Separation (Psychology) 5. Adjustment
(Psychology) I. Title.
BF175.5.P75F57 1996
616.89'14—dc20   96-35618

97 98 99 00 01 02 10 9 8 7 6 5 4 3 2

Acquiring Editor: Jim Nageotte
Editorial Assistant: Nancy Hale
Production Editor: Sanford Robinson
Production Assistant: Denise Santoyo
Typesetter/Designer: Danielle Dillahunt
Indexer: Cristina Haley
Cover Designer: Candice Harman

Contents

ᏝᎶᏮ

Foreword

The morning news carried a story of two Los Angeles teenage girls who tied their wrists together and jumped off a cliff in fulfillment of a suicide pact. This was followed by a detailed account of the murder of an actor who maintained a hidden life as a producer of homosexual pornographic movies, and whose body was found wearing a sign identifying him as a "Gay Basher." Amidst sundry reports of random and impersonal acts of violence, a week ago the news told me that yet another man, frustrated by the loss of a girlfriend, stormed into her place of work and shot her and several coworkers. I am given pause to reflect on the fact that we have just passed the anniversary of the Oklahoma City bombing of the federal building, assumedly by Timothy McVeigh, and that Theodore J. Kaczynski (the Unabomber) is still awaiting trial.

Like most, I look at these violent events with wonder, fear, and awe. I can understand some of these acts more than others. I can "experience the pain" of teenagers in stress, as well as that of frightened, angry people who have been spurned in love—I understand these things because I have known them; I draw upon my own familiarity with these feelings and acts of hopelessness. But when I read of the acts of those who commit random violence, my professional and personal experiences fail me in finding the empathy that I consider to be a cornerstone of human survival. My inner search for empathy was not helped recently as I watched a major network anchorman interview Magied Youssef Al-molqi, the terrorist who stormed the *Achille Lauro* and killed aging and physically impaired Leon Klinghoffer. As I watched, the terrorist became the victim, pleading for understanding of his group—"We are people too—we have families and loved ones, just like you." Rather than raising my empathy, this plea stimulated my anger; I wonder how one can believe that merely sharing the confusion of the world justifies such crimes. I marvel at the helplessness that I feel in mending the ills of isolation and abandonment that pervade this society.

In the midst of this chaos, I am writing the Foreword to a misleading book—but misleading in a most productive and interesting way. But I digress . . .

In this book, Dr. Robert Firestone places the nucleus of societal aggression within the disturbing influences of dysfunctional family life. He identifies two major processes that account for the violence and self-destructiveness of modern society, the joint workings of which lead to the inevitable conclusion that ultimately societal violence can only be understood at the level of the individual. And it also is at the level of the individual that the hope for peace and change lies.

The first process to which Firestone directs our attention is that of identifying with the aggressor (Chapter 5). In taking on the role of victimizer, the child attempts to reclaim the power that has been denied him or her by an aggressive other. The child unhappily takes on the guilt, fear, and neurosis of the aggressor as well. And, as he notes, in this process the child incorporates into him- or herself the method of treatment that he or she has been exposed to. In a sense, we parent ourselves and conceptualize ourselves in the way we were treated because of this internalization process.

The second process that he identifies as a root of societal aggression is the development of the fantasy bond (Chapter 6), a relationship with a wish-driven image of a support object. This fantasy of the person with whom the child develops an attachment differs from the real person in several ways, not the least of which is that it is not imbued with the shades of gray that are an inevitable part of real people. However, a fantasy bond is simplified and offers clarity to issues that a more realistic and complex perception may obscure; it also offers acceptance, nurturance, and love when reality denies it; and it provides the illusion of constancy that stands in contrast to an unstable reality.

Relying on a fantasy bond propels the object of this infatuation (or deinfatu-ation) to be injected into other ongoing relationships. The implications of this process exceed those of either simple transference or the repetition compulsion in which one relates to others in a patterned and recurring way. They also reflect the way in which one recalls and conceptualizes one's parents and one's own personal worth. One comes to seek, in the object of the fantasy bond, the nurturance needed to sustain life. The futility of this search commits the child to live in a virtual reality environment. Virtual reality may allow one to experience what it is like to eat, drink, and engage in the other tasks of living, but it is unlikely to provide much physical protection against starvation. The discrepancy between the fantasized and the actual attachment object can do no less than produce a life of confusion, unfulfillment, and emotional starvation.

A corollary but very important consequence of the discrepancy between what one imagines and what is, is the "inner voice." It is this aspect of the fantasy bond to which Firestone rightly devotes the preponderance of this volume. Indeed, identifying and understanding the dynamics of this inner behavior is his unique and most intriguing contribution. That is not to say that inner voices, even critical and unrealistic inner voices, have not been identified by other theorists and other psychotherapies. They have. But both the nature of the inner voice with which Bob Firestone deals, as well as its treatment, are quite different from those conceptualized by others. The inner voice of Voice Therapy is not the practical, misguided but irrational voice that misattributes cause and over-generalizes consequences, which is the target of work during cognitive therapy. It is not one that debates the locus of cause. It is one whose objectives are to attack, punish, and destroy (Chapter 9).

Neither is this voice the mere expression of a negative self-image, as in various theories of "self." It is "antiself"; it is antithetical to the very survival of a self system. It is critical, destructive, punitive, and external, but these words are insufficient to describe it; it is a primitive introjection that long precedes the development of the executive functions of problem analysis. Its language and form are primitive, and its existence is a constant and explicit attack on one's very existence and one's fundamental value. Through it, one not only filters the experiences of intimacy but directly prevents and destroys the potential for truly intimate relationships (Chapter 11).

One's search for equivalents in other theories may lead to the conviction that the "voice" that Firestone describes is most similar to the hostile and rejecting "top dog" described by Gestalt therapy. However, there are logical reasons to believe that one is not well served to treat it in the fashion of Gestalt therapy. This is not a voice that one might be helped to accept or "own" by changing its form from the third to the first person (Chapter 9). Coming to own this voice might easily produce psychopathology rather than alleviating it. Because it is based on an unrealistic and destructive fantasy, far removed from a semblance of reality, owning such a voice even part of the time is an unsatisfying objective of treatment. This voice is managed by identifying its form, confronting it, reflecting on its genesis, and reconfiguring the relationships from which it arose—breaking through the fantasy bond (Chapters 10 and 11). Firestone asserts that it is not until this is done that one becomes free to develop a more kindly and realistic alternative in a manner reminiscent of the objectives of cognitive therapy.

Seldom do we see in clinical literature the articulation of a differential hypothesis that is so clear, so testable, and so socially significant as Firestone's conceptualization of treating the inner voice. Which treatment produces the most significant reduction in aggressive and suicidal potential, an intervention that emphasizes patient ownership of negative and critical voices or one that disowns and reconfigures them?

Even more highly than I value my identity as a clinician, I value my status as a scientist. To me, the description of a new theory, even one as intriguing and moving as this, is of little value unless it is founded on sound empiricism. Theories are easy to come by, they are all persuasive, and few theorists look for truth beyond the demonstration of face validity—it is true if it makes sense. But there are far too many bad theories that "make sense" and far too little research to support most of them. Yet this book has the refreshing characteristic of reporting a theory that is devoted to empirical test. Firestone has taken what is an all too often missing step among those whose professions are maintained outside of major universities and research centers. He advocates a step beyond theory, even beyond advocating for sound empirical evidence or relating theory to extant research. He has created innovative research studies to provide prospective tests of the fundamental premises. This step illustrates that his commitment is to truth rather than simply to personal recognition, and represents one of the best illustrations of the successful working of the scientific-professional tradition.

True to the author's intent, this volume clearly illustrates the integrative nature of Voice Therapy. This approach is integrative even beyond the blending of the psychoanalytic and existential views to which it most obviously owes homage. It views people as being innately innocent rather than destructive or corrupt, and thereby it rejects Id Psychology in favor of an existential view of humankind. Its ties to existentialism and humanism are in its acceptance of the viability of the emerging "self," its observation of the preoccupation of humans with death (Chapter 16), its assertion that people must transcend desires for immediate gratification, and its view that there is an inevitable drive of the organism to become a differentiated system. In Firestone's concept of defense, moreover, one sees the influence of psychoanalysis, and in the descriptions of the fantasy bond and separation fears, one sees a similarity to object relations theory. But in Voice Therapy, one also sees the influence of cognitive psychology and experiential therapy.

The empirical status of the theory and practice of Voice Therapy is still difficult to judge. However, at least three of the major theoretical tenets of Voice Therapy are grounded in contemporary, empirical research within the traditions of developmental psychopathology, cognitive science, social biology, and psychotherapy outcome. The "self" has been an object of scientific study for five decades, for example. Research from Carl Rogers to Albert Bandura has supported the vitality of various self-conceptions, their importance in change, and their roles in personal development. Likewise as a fundamental developmental process, attachment formation has not lacked for supportive empirical evidence. Permutations of "Self" and "Attachment" can be reliably measured; they are predictive and their presence follows a normal as well as a pathological developmental process.

Still further, research on thoughts, schema, and self-talk has bridged the traditions of cognitive psychology, developmental psychology, Gestalt therapy, and Transactional Analysis. Characteristic internal dialogues have been identified among those who are habitually impulsive, ineffective problem solvers, suffering from low self-esteem, depressed, and anxious. Firestone and colleagues have identified the introjected aspect of these self-destructive and life-threatening voices and have developed a method for studying their presence. Using traditional empirical methods, the rejecting (second person) injunctions identified by Voice Therapy have been found to dominate the mentation of those who are at risk for suicide (Chapter 12), and are being explored in many other problems (Chapters 14 and 17). The qualitative and observational methods, those that are more highly valued by the author and most clinicians and that form most of the work reported in this volume, however, go beyond the quantitative evidence, even suggesting that these critical voices may be universal phenomena. The suggestion that we all have limiting, hostile, and self-rejecting internal voices, apparently modeled from parental and societal efforts to maintain control over children, is very disconcerting. Although the idea that self-hostility is universal and inevitably limits one's growth may raise the eyebrows of many empiricists, the presence, form, and content of these "antiself" voices strike a resonant chord among those who seek help for personal distress.

Although promising, Voice Therapy, itself, has not yet undergone the empirical tests needed to fully assert its unique effectiveness. Clinical experience, while positive, can take us only so far toward validating the therapeutic power of the principles of intervention that Firestone outlines. As an empirically committed psychotherapy researcher, I reserve the concern that the conceptual similarity with experimental and developmental psychopathology research is insufficient grounds to assume that the treatment effects reported for this method are more than placebo responses. Yet, as a practitioner, I'm moved and tempted to say about its effectiveness, as did a well-known Supreme Court Justice say of pornography, "I know it when I see it."

Collectively, this book (a) offers an integrative view of psychopathology and intervention, (b) identifies in the pathology of the fantasy bond some of the major destructive forces that infect Western societies, and (c) outlines a method for correcting these ills. You may wonder, in the face of these accomplishments, is it not therefore unfair to represent this book as misleading? And I would retort that it is misleading, not by what it says but by what it does not reveal about the power of Firestone's views—it errs by an act of omission rather than of commission.

What this book provides would be enough if the true but undisclosed experiment of its validity were not so much more. It is misleading to see only this critical but passive analysis of how individual disturbance is transported across generations. There is another message to be found here—one of immense importance—and it is to be found in the life of its author. A glimpse of the promise is revealed in Chapter 18, but only a glimpse. Words are weak representations of the most important contribution Firestone makes—his experiment with and of life, his test of validity. The validity experiment is the life of Robert Firestone, and the complexity of this life experiment cannot be fully captured in this medium.

I met Bob Firestone through his daughter Lisa, a clinical psychologist who expressed some interest in collaborating with my training and research programs at the University of California, Santa Barbara. I confess that I had not previously been aware of Bob's writings, his development of a parent education program, or of his close relationship with R. D. Laing. And my becoming aware of these is not what has drawn me to him. I first saw Bob on a videotape that was initially aired on PBS some years ago. On the surface, this tape is a travelogue of an around-the-world trip by sailboat. It is a novel trip, however, in that it was initiated, undertaken, and led by a group of adolescents (Lisa among them). They planned the trip, elected their captain, and battled the physical elements and psychological obstacles during 17 months, living within a closed social system, supported but not directed by loving adults, and held together by commitment and a common objective. The most important message is not to be found in this trip, however interesting in and of itself, but in what has happened since.

The voyage was conceptualized by Bob Firestone and several of his friends who had come to form a close "friendship circle." The young crew came from several families who shared their concern with the problems of their emerging adolescents. Largely in the interests of protecting their children from the drug abuse prominent in the neighborhood, the families purchased a partially completed 85-foot wooden schooner to involve them in wholesome activities. Initially intended as a way of sharing a common friendship, the project developed into a world cruise and an experiment in communication, trust, and self-sufficiency. The 11 "kids" who made that trip became fast friends and eventually business partners, marital partners, and colleagues. These friends and families have continued to share their time, their resources, and their expertise with one another and with their children, to ensure that the spirit of that adventure is passed on to each succeeding generation. Bob describes some of the evolution of this circle of friends in Chapter 1, noting that since 1979, he has assumed the full-time task of observing and documenting the evolution and growth of this truly remarkable group. During this time, the "friendship circle" has expanded, propelled to do so by an enthusiasm for life that has been fostered by the mutual love that characterizes these people. This enthusiasm drives them to understand the workings of every "interesting" person with whom they come in contact. By virtue of what they have learned about listening, respecting, sharing, and loving, in the process of living, working, and reasoning together, the friendship circle has been a magnet to which people, from all walks of life, many diverse belief systems, and three continents, have been drawn. These friends have participated and succeeded in business and have become financially successful. They work together, vacation together, and share in open communication. Many have taken part in the making of over 30 documentary films used for professional training by sharing their personal insights, which evolved from years of talking together. These people live each day in a manner commensurate with the principles discussed as a therapy in this book. It is a way of living that I've come to appreciate, respect, envy, and enjoy, from a "safe" distance.

The most important thing to come of Bob's life work is not the model of attachment or the model of psychotherapy presented in this book—it is an alternative and healing way of living. It is a lifestyle of hope! It is a dawning confirmation, tested through the crucible of a multitude of daily lives, that we do not need to settle for a society of violence and abandonment. I resonate to R. D. Laing's urging of Bob a decade ago: "Preach what you practice." But what Bob practices can only partially be captured in a two-dimensional medium such as this book. His is not an office practice; this is not a therapy alone, although it is practiced by professionals in the mental health field and probably is therapeutic; it is an experiment in human living and relating—a demonstration of the value of life. It is captured in the continuity and optimism of the "friendship circle."

One should hear in the words of this volume not only a tertiary treatment of societal and personal ills but a surprising and optimistic statement of how the self-destructiveness of society can be aborted and prevented. Although couched in descriptions of the frustration that attends destructive family environments, the lifestyle view that is behind this book offers hope, both of defining what goes wrong in the formation of human attachments and in proposing how to prevent or reduce the harm. The solution is in the formation of a loving, sharing, and respectful way of living, not simply of relating to a psychotherapist. This is a book of theory, application of tertiary care, and hope for primary prevention. It is a book about failures of bonding and the reversible, destructive forces of the family. But most important, it is about a way of life that Bob Firestone and his "friendship circle" have both pioneered and lived—it is not a method of mere therapy, it is a way of living decently with other people.

LARRY E. BEUTLER
Professor and Director of Training
Counseling/Clinical/School Psychology Program
University of California–Santa Barbara

Preface

The individual faces an enormous struggle against overwhelming odds to retain a unique selfhood. In this postmodern era, we exist in a restrictive social[1] structure that largely deprives us of important human qualities, among them the capacity for maintaining personal feelings, the drive to search for meaning, and the ability to live in harmony with others. Demands for uniformity and conformity lead to a life of dishonesty, self-deception, deadening habit patterns, and addictive relationships. Most people fall by the wayside in an attempt to numb their pain and anxiety with habit patterns that offer the illusion of security at the price of integrity and individuality.

People are damaged early in their lives in the incidental process of being socialized (Briere, 1992) (Endnote 1). Children are first exposed to the idiosyncratic programming of the microculture of the family in which they are raised. As they expand their boundaries into the neighborhood, the school, and the larger society, they encounter new programming and social pressures. The cultural complex in our society represents a serious assault on the self, placing

---

1 I conceptualize society and social mores as a pooling of combined defenses of all its members. Conventionality and conformity support the individual's defense system. Both act in concert to oppose the natural striving of the individual (R. Firestone, 1985).

value on role-playing and image over real experience, data in place of wisdom, spectatorship in place of participation. This cultural pathology reinforces the familial and individual pathologies and they, in turn, act to support it in a complex feedback system (Endnote 2).

As a result of training and acculturation within the context of the nuclear family, an individual cannot easily escape early imprinting. Even when exposed to psychosocial contexts where there is more freedom, love, and respect than in the home environment, there is difficulty in making the necessary adjustment in the defensive posture. Indeed, most adults remain prisoners of their internal conditioning. My position, however, is not that the nuclear family is inherently detrimental to human growth and development, but that in many ways it has developed into a destructive institution. The way family practices have evolved and the resulting psychopathology are evident in the increased rate of drug addiction, violence, and suicide among our youth. It is important to state that I am not opposed to families in any sense; indeed, the close, harmonious, loving relationship with my wife and nine children is my highest value. However, I favor an extended family atmosphere where the input of significant others is not only valued and respected but considered to be of major importance.

The therapeutic task is to modify the harmful patterns of interactions within the family. A concerted effort needs to be made to offset the perpetuation of these damaging patterns in future generations. However, if one maintains an idealized picture of the family, it constitutes a serious resistance to exposing and correcting the deleterious aspects of family relationships. Only by focusing our understanding on the unique nature of human beings can we begin to ascertain what modes of parenting constitute an affront to the true nature of the child.

The psychotherapy process must enable the individual to recognize and break with negative parental prescriptions, emancipate him- or herself from early programming, and learn to embrace more successful, life-enhancing ways of satisfying his or her needs and priorities. Because of these challenges, any effective therapeutic system needs to be a courageous, risk-taking endeavor. This is the ethos for which Voice Therapy, described in the chapters that follow, aims. My goal in writing this book is to provide insight and perspective on treatment methods that challenge the insidious forces that affect the individual both from within and without.

I was persuaded to embark on this writing project because of the numerous requests I have received from clinicians, academicians, researchers, and students asking for a comprehensive volume that explains my theoretical approach. In this work, I present a holistic overview of Voice Therapy theory and methodology and include findings from recent empirical studies based on the conceptualization of the "voice."

The Glendon Association, a nonprofit organization, has supported my work since its founding in 1982. During those years, the association produced and disseminated a large body of resource material, including books, articles, video documentaries, a parent education program, and a suicide identification and treatment methodology. According to psychologists, psychiatrists, and other mental health professionals, their clients and students have made extensive use of these materials and have benefited from our orientation. The Glendon Association's publications of my theoretical position address the subjects of couples and parent-child relations, suicide, addiction, sexuality, and existential issues related to death anxiety. As of this date, our parent education program has been adopted by 30 agencies in six states, British Columbia, and Costa Rica. The association's workshops on suicide prevention and risk assessment have disseminated vital information to therapists, counselors, and teachers.

The materials, the training workshops, and, more recently, the results of our empirical research have attracted the attention of many workers in the mental health field. They exhorted me to write a theoretical volume where they could find a collection of my major ideas in one place. I agreed because I felt that my overall theory had been valued only in bits and pieces that corresponded to the broad and varied subject matter. The positive response to my work has encouraged me to make a concerted effort to distinguish my ideas from other theoretical systems, particularly those formulations that appear to overlap, that is, Gestalt, object relations theory, and cognitive approaches. By bringing together the different facets of my theory in this work, I hope to provide a more comprehensive view of my concepts and methods than is currently available, one that may be more fully grasped as a whole by the reader.

My theoretical position represents a synthesis of psychoanalytic and existential ideas in that it emphasizes defenses formed early in life, while at the same time explaining the impact of existential issues, particularly death anxiety, on these defenses. The basic tenets and concepts on which it rests are closely related to clients' everyday experience. Understanding the voice process has predictive value in understanding personal relationships and defensive lifestyles. The system of thought presented here provides a cogent explanation of resistance in psychotherapy and insight into the psychodynamics operating in varied forms of psychopathology. It has proven to be of significant value in understanding fantasy, addiction, and self-destructive behavior.

Although theorists have touched on aspects of these ideas in their work, and many clients have reported that the concepts resonate with "something I've known all along, but I've never been able to articulate," this system of thought, when understood in its entirety, is different from the majority of contemporary theoretical systems, and my associates and I feel that it represents an advance on current ideology and practice in the field of psychotherapy.

My approach to psychotherapy is very different from attempting to adjust people to a society or social system. If anything, I am interested in adjusting the social process to enhance the individual's development. I am deeply concerned with answering a vital question: Whose life is the client really living? Is he or she truly following his or her own destiny or recapitulating the life of parents or caretakers? Is he or she a programmed robot or a fully vital human being? Voice Therapy supports individuation as a primary goal, and the efforts of my associates and I are directed toward helping human beings develop their own priorities and their own search for meaning.

ENDNOTES

1. A key theme in John Briere's (1992) book, *Child Abuse Trauma*, is that "the majority of adults raised in North America, regardless of gender, age, race, or social class, probably experienced some level of maltreatment as children" (p. xvii). In his chapter on the long-term effects of abuse, Briere cited research findings supporting correlations between child maltreatment and intimacy disturbance, altered sexuality, tendencies toward victimization due to impaired self-reference, and/or aggression in later relationships, adversariality and "manipulation," use of substances, suicidality, tension-reducing behaviors such as self-mutilation, compulsive sexual behavior, binging and purging, codependency, and borderline personality disorders.

2. Social theorists have noted "cultural pathology" in modern societies. Erich Fromm (1962) emphasized the effects of society on the individual mediated through "the social unconscious." Fromm defined the "social unconscious" as

> those areas of repression which are common to most members of a society; these commonly repressed elements are those contents which a given society cannot permit its members to be aware of if the society with its specific contradictions is to operate successfully. (p. 88)

Herbert Marcuse (1955/1966), in *Eros and Civilization*, stated, "The methodological sacrifice of libido, its rigidly enforced deflection to socially useful activities and expressions, *is* culture" (p. 3). Later, he went on to write about the subtle pathology inherent in modern society:

> Civilization has to defend itself against the specter of a world which could be free. If society cannot use its growing productivity for reducing repression (because such usage would upset the hierarchy of the *status quo*), productivity must be turned *against* the individuals; it becomes itself an instrument of universal control. (p. 93)

Marcuse's thesis represents an elaboration on the critical theory of the Frankfurt School (Adorno, Frenkel-Brunswik, Levinson, & Sanford, 1950; Fromm, 1941; Horkheimer, 1936). Marcuse's more trenchant critique is congenial with that of Norman O. Brown (1959).

R. D. Laing (1967), in *The Politics of Experience*, challenged the "normalcy" of culture:

> What we call "normal" is a product of repression, denial, splitting, projection, introjection, and other forms of destructive action on experience.... Society highly values its normal man. It educates children to lose themselves and to become absurd, and thus to be normal. Normal men have killed perhaps 100,000,000 of their fellow normal men in the last fifty years. (pp. 27-28)

Acknowledgments

I would like to express my appreciation to Joyce Catlett, M.A., associate and collaborative writer, for her help in completing this project, and to Tamsen Firestone, loving wife and editor, for her interest, encouragement, and guidance.

I want to thank Jo Barrington and Marty Zamir for reviewing the material and Lisa Firestone, Ph.D., my daughter, for pressuring me to compile my ideas under one cover.

Thanks to the Glendon Association, especially Anne Baker, Jerome Nathan, Ph.D., Catherine Cagan, Ana Blix, Irma Catlett, and Jina Carvalho, for helping with the manuscript, supporting our work, and disseminating my ideas.

I would like to express my gratitude to Stuart Boyd, Ph.D., Jean-Pierre Soubrier, M.D., Richard Seiden, Ph.D., M.P.H., Deryl Goldenberg, Ph.D., Susan Short, M.A., and Dan Staso, Ph.D., for their ongoing interest, commentary, and representation of my theoretical work.

I am grateful to Larry Beutler, Ph.D., for challenging me to articulate my ideas in a form that can be applied to sound empirical research, and for raising important questions for psychotherapy theory and practice.

1

The Self Under Siege

The psychotherapeutic alliance is a unique human relationship, wherein a devoted and trained person attempts to render assistance to another person by both suspending and extending himself. Nowhere in life is a person listened to, felt, and experienced with such concentrated sharing and emphasis on every aspect of personal communication. As in any other human relationship, this interaction may be fulfilling or damaging to either individual. To the extent that a new fantasy bond or illusion of connection is formed (for example, doctor-patient, therapist-client, parent-child), the relationship will be detrimental; whereas in a situation that is characterized by equality, openness, and true compassion, there will be movement toward individuation in both parties.

R. Firestone (1990d, p. 68)[1]

M y therapeutic orientation helps a person to expose and challenge depend-ency bonds and destructive "voices," remnants of negative childhood experiences that seriously impair his or her sense of self, spirit, and individuality.

This theoretical approach represents a broadly based, coherent system of concepts and hypotheses that integrate psychoanalytic and existential views, yet should not be considered eclectic. I explain how early trauma leads to defense

---

1 This statement is excerpted from *What Is Psychotherapy? Contemporary Perspectives* (Zeig & Munion, 1990), a volume consisting of invited contributions from theorists and practitioners in the field of psychotherapy. Used with permission.

formation and how these original defenses are reinforced as the developing child gradually becomes aware of his or her own mortality. My orientation focuses on an individual's search for self and personal meaning in the face of internalized inimical processes and ontological anxiety.

The self is under siege in almost every aspect of a person's daily life. It is vital at this stage of man's evolution to develop a new perspective and alternative modes of thinking to transcend these destructive environmental and cultural influences. My goal in writing this book is to provide such a perspective, an uncompromising and illuminating view of the myriad forces existing within the family and social system that contribute significantly to people's distress. I intend to outline a methodology for countering this destructive process.

This book is addressed to my colleagues who cope repeatedly with psychological pain in an attempt to minimize or alleviate human suffering, and to all people truly concerned with humanity. My intention is to share data and hypotheses generated during 35 years of clinical experience in several psychotherapy settings, particularly emphasizing the results of studying a group of high-functioning individuals in a unique psychological laboratory.

In this regard, I will draw from a compendium of resource material including books, articles, and transcripts of filmed documentaries that represent the broad spectrum of my work. One of my primary objectives is to describe the concept of a better way of living, that is, a more constructive form of communicating and affiliating with others than is currently practiced in the larger culture.

In exploring the concepts set forth in this book, the reader may encounter ideas that are threatening to his or her customary ways of thinking or theoretical approach. However, despite the painful issues raised throughout this work, the perspective does provide a realistic basis for leading an honest, richer, more rewarding life, with internal consistency and integrity.

I will delineate an insidious process of defensive inwardness[2] that limits the lives of all people to varying degrees. Readers will better understand why so many marital relationships fail; why often those that remain intact do so at great expense to the individuality of each partner; why symbols of love come to mean more to the beloved than real acknowledgment; why couples' sexual relationships generally deteriorate or become routinized; and why men and women manipulate each other so that they become unlovable in their lover's eyes and actually become intimate enemies.

You will learn why parents unintentionally damage their children and seriously affect their human experience, leaving them with a compelling need to relive their parents' lives. The reader will come to understand why parents

---

2 Inwardness should not be confused with introspection, sensitive time alone, and creative thought. It refers to a defended, depersonalized state of mind manifested in self-protective, self-limiting behaviors and lifestyles.

inadvertently attempt to take back the gift of life they gave. You will become aware of the reasons both children and adults become duplicitous and hide behind social roles, and why they build a false self and obliterate the true self.

In comprehending how the power of the imagination is both a creative and a destructive force in human life, the reader will perceive how individuals use abstract symbols, fantasy, illusion, and self-deception as attempted survival mechanisms in relation to their mortality. After all, *Homo sapiens* is the only species cursed with the conscious awareness of its own death. I will reveal how fantasy processes become addictive because they alleviate separation and death anxiety. These illusions partially satisfy primitive needs at the expense of real experience. Defensive modes and actions are analogous to drug addiction and alcoholism in that they are partially gratifying and initially ego-syntonic and yet ultimately have a negative effect on a person's adjustment in life.

The findings that have contributed to my understanding of human behavior were derived from two principal sources: (a) data gathered from adult patients, ranging from hospitalized schizophrenic patients to neurotic and "normal" clients in an office setting, and (b) individuals in a unique social milieu who were motivated by an interest in psychological ideas with a focus on their own development.

This psychological laboratory began more than 20 years ago, formed out of a small group of professional associates and friends of long standing and has since expanded to include over 100 persons. These people enjoy discussing philosophical and psychological issues and are concerned with child rearing and humanistic pursuits. They are dedicated to minimizing or eliminating toxic influences in their important personal relationships.

In 1979, these men and women asked me to relinquish my private practice and involve myself full-time as a participant-observer in their discussions and talks. Despite some initial feelings of trepidation in terms of giving up an extensive psychotherapy practice, I was moved by their request and I agreed to commit myself to the endeavor.

For more than two decades, I have had the opportunity to view the larger society from this vantage point, one that, as noted earlier, has been a valuable source of hypotheses. In the course of participating in this group process, I became involved in a longitudinal study of these people and their families. Because of this extraordinary setting, a new window from which to view the "normal" psychopathology of everyday life was made available, permitting me access to material not usually seen or heard by therapists working within the confines of the 50-minute hour. I was provided with an unusual opportunity to match internal dynamics, exposed through honest self-disclosure, with observations of the participants' interactions with their mates, their original families, and their children. For example, if a man were passive, I could observe all the dimensions of his passivity—in his work, in sports and other activities, and in his personal interactions. This exposure to the key dynamics of interpersonal relationships over three generations enabled me to extend my insight into the problems of "normal" living as well as psychopathological phenomena.

ASSUMPTIONS AND BIASES

My theory reflects a personal bias toward integrity and self-fulfillment and a humanistic view of people as innocent rather than inherently bad or corrupt. Human beings are not innately destructive or self-destructive; they become aggressive, violent, or even harmful to the self only in response to emotional pain, fear, rejection, and deprivation. Aggressiveness aroused in early interpersonal relationships is reinforced by frustration and anguish brought about by the child's growing awareness of the concept of his or her personal death. The corollary to this basic assumption about human nature is my belief that no child is born troublesome, bad, sinful, or evil. I have found that the defenses that the child forms are appropriate to actual situations that threaten his or her emerging self. In this sense, people come by their defenses and limitations honestly and, indeed, many should be congratulated on surviving their early programming. My belief has always been that an individual's unnecessary torment, as contrasted with ontological suffering, had a definitive cause in his or her early relationships.

My approach emphasizes the exposure of destructive fantasy bonds (imagined connections) as externalized in interpersonal associations or internalized in the form of object representation (parental introjects). Dissolution of these bonds and movement toward separation and individuation is essential for the realization of one's destiny as a fully autonomous human being.

I refer to my approach as Separation Theory because it focuses on breaking with parental introjects and moving toward individuation. The theoretical position represents an ultimate challenge to the defense system. It is my contention that psychological defenses are maladaptive because they cut deeply into an individual's life experience, and when they persist into adult life, they eventually become the essential psychopathology. The reality of one's experiences and emotions is primary; anything that fragments or denies that reality or deprives a person of his or her experience is, in my opinion, clearly destructive. As noted, however, these defenses were originally formed under conditions of stress, where annihilation anxiety and overwhelming terror forced the child to develop various self-protective mechanisms.

From an evolutionary perspective, defenses can be seen as serving a functional purpose during the child's early years. (a) Defenses protect the infant and young child against complete ego disintegration or even physical death under conditions of stress. (b) Defenses diminish or eliminate the experience of excessive emotional pain, anxiety, sadness, grief, shame, and other emotions that, when they reach a certain level of intensity, can interfere with effective coping behaviors. In that sense, the formation of psychological defenses increases the probability that the individual will attain sexual maturity, reproduce, and contribute to the gene pool. As Paul Gilbert (1989) pointed out, "All life forms are equipped to defend against threat and also to advance their own life form" (p. 79) (Endnote 1). For example, the psychological defense of symbiosis, or the formation of a *fantasy bond* under conditions of tension and anxiety, is the only solution available, because the child is helpless and completely dependent on the family system. Nevertheless, defended individuals' lives are limited and restricted, and need to be challenged or modified for them to fulfill their destiny (Endnote 2).

VOICE THERAPY THEORY

Voice Therapy theory involves a process of individuation and separation from internalized parental introjects and addictive attachments. Separation as conceptualized here is very different from isolation, defense, or retreat; rather, it involves the maintenance of a strong identity and distinct boundaries at close quarters with others. Indeed, without a well-developed self system or personal identity, people find it necessary to distort, lash out at, or withdraw from intimacy in interpersonal relationships.

An inward, defended life characterized by imagined fusion with another or others acts to limit a person's capacity for self-expression and self-fulfillment. A merged identity or diminished sense of self is a microsuicidal[3] or even suicidal manifestation, as one no longer lives a committed feelingful existence, and life seems empty, meaningless, and without direction.

My theory contrasts fantasy life and illusion with goal-directed lifestyles and points out that people largely relate to themselves as objects, that is, they treat themselves the way their parent or primary caretaker treated them. I emphasize that there are conflicted choices in life between defending oneself by cutting off painful emotional experiences and moving toward the fulfillment of one's potentialities. At each moment in time, one is either capitulating to one's internal programming or moving toward individuation.

My philosophy places primary importance on the individual as a unique entity. Efforts toward preserving the life within each person are given priority over supporting any group or system, whether the couple, the family system,

---

3 *Microsuicide* refers to behaviors, communications, attitudes, or lifestyles that are self-induced and threatening, limiting, or antithetical to an individual's physical health, emotional well-being, or personal goals (R. Firestone & Seiden, 1987).

ethnic or political groups, nationality, or religion. Another singular aspect of the theory is implied in my description of a lifestyle that involves moving toward separation and independence, toward compassion and transcendent goals. This focus on transcendent goals is not a moral issue; rather, it represents a sound mental health principle. By involving themselves in goals that have a deeper meaning than immediate gratifications, people increase their capacity for joy as well as pain and expand their life space.

The emphasis on experience and preserving every aspect of it is central. Feeling one's true sadness frees one to know exhilaration. I agree with Viktor Frankl's (1946/1959) assertion that the pursuit of happiness in itself is doomed to failure. Happiness can only be a by-product of facing the tragic dimensions of life and investing oneself in the pursuit of goals that go beyond the narrow confines of one's self and family.

In contrast to many conceptual frameworks, my theory offers no solace in that it provides no "loopholes." It offers no illusions, no means of escaping existential despair or the inevitable vicissitudes of life; however, it shows that people can choose a brave new world in which honesty is paramount and adventure and awareness are truly valued.

It is important to recognize that this book deals primarily with psychological or environmental factors that affect personality development. However, it does not deny or minimize other influences on the psyche of the child or adult. Biological tendencies, inherited temperamental differences, and hereditary predispositions combine with personal environmental influences to form unique and complex phenomena. Indeed, all human experiences are psychosomatic, that is, inclusive of mind and body. In addition, there is no single cause of specific symptoms or mental aberrations, as all psychological functions are multidetermined. Brain activity, physical impairment, and psychological disturbance always coexist, just as some form of rational thought always exists in conjunction with feeling bodily sensations.

VOICE THERAPY METHODOLOGY

My specific orientation and approach to psychotherapy has come to be known as "Voice Therapy." Voice Therapy techniques bring internalized negative thought processes to the surface with accompanying affect in a dialogue format such that a person can confront alien components of the personality. It is so named because it is a process of giving language or spoken words to negative thought patterns that are at the core of an individual's maladaptive or self-destructive behavior. The methods of Voice Therapy are complex and varied; however, one technique that is used is to ask patients to verbalize their negative thoughts *toward* themselves in the second person, "you," as though they were talking to themselves, instead of "I" statements *about* themselves. Statements such as "I'm a failure, I can't succeed" become *"You're* a failure. *You're* never going to make it." As soon as this method is employed, strong affect is released as patients give vent to thoughts and feelings indicating an intensity of self-contempt and animosity toward self of which they were previously unaware.[4] This procedure exposes the enemy within, and the sources of one's animosity toward self become obvious. Voice Therapy has provided a valuable mechanism for elucidating the division of the mind. It is beneficial in that it is nonintrusive and it allows for the rapid achievement of insight, independent of therapist interpretation. The methods are applicable to individual and group psychotherapy. In the latter setting, when one person expresses self-attacks that reflect core issues in his or her life, strong feelings are often aroused in the other participants.

Voice Therapy is not a panacea; instead, it points out the dilemma in psychotherapy, which is the fact that no therapy can eliminate existential pain and despair. I concur with Freud's statement regarding the limitations of psychoanalysis, that curing the patient of his or her neurosis opens the patient up to the miseries of everyday life.

Although the methods uncover elements of the personality antithetical to self, they do not imply a simple solution; the process of working through and risk-taking is essential for expanding one's life. Voice Therapy is not a didactic instructional procedure or a rigid system with structured intervention strategies. The techniques have been applied to a wide range of emotional disorders and diverse populations.

My therapeutic approach is not based on a moral position, although it implies an ethical choice. The decision to break away from early conditioning, restrictive bonds, and deadening habit patterns is partially an ethical one, given the inherent damage caused by defenses that limit not only a person's life and feeling but also those of his or her loved ones. The theory and methodology have value in revealing the core of resistance to any form of psychotherapeutic movement or constructive behavioral change. The therapeutic venture, by counteracting the dictates of the negative voice and disrupting fantasies of connection, offers people a unique opportunity to fulfill their human potential, thereby giving life its special meaning.

---

4 One has to witness a Voice Therapy session, either on film or as a direct experience, to fully appreciate the incredible division within the self and the aggression toward self that is part of the makeup of "normal" people. Individuals manifest emotions in the sessions in a manner that is very different from what they experience in their everyday lives.

BASIC CONCEPTS OF
VOICE THERAPY THEORY

Voice Therapy theory differs from psychoanalysis and object relations theory because it defines and explains the existential issues involved in defense formation and focuses not only on transference distortions and transference acting out but on how the individual reacts to and treats him- or herself. People both nurture and restrict themselves in a manner similar to the way they were nurtured and/or restricted by their parents. I am concerned not only with transference distortions that are introduced into interpersonal relationships, but also in helping the patient to develop an incisive awareness of forces that are an integral part of the personality, yet alien to the self.

In integrating psychoanalytic and existential systems of thought, the approach sets forth several important concepts that have been hitherto neglected or unexplained in neopsychoanalytic, object relations, and self psychology paradigms.

1. Voice Therapy theory provides in-depth understanding of the internal voice process operating within the psyche that is antithetical to self and hostile toward others. The theory explains the methodology that my associates and I employ to bring these partly conscious and unconscious thoughts and their associated affect into conscious awareness. Individuals are essentially divided within themselves. They possess conflicting points of view about themselves, others, and events in the world. One point of view is rational and objective, while the other is made up of a negative thought process opposed to the ongoing development, or even survival, of the self.

I have developed the procedures of Voice Therapy that access elements of the antiself system, thereby advancing our knowledge of humans' self-destructiveness. In Voice Therapy sessions, aggression toward self comes out clearly, powerfully, and in a way that is psychodynamically important. I feel that the material that is elicited, that is, the voices that are uncovered, are a valuable tool in predicting behavior because all forms of self-limitation and self-destructive behavior are related to these internalized attitudes and prescriptions. Empirical research has already demonstrated the predictive power of the concept of the voice in suicide. The process also operates in reverse; when we become familiar with an individual's dysfunctional behavior as contrasted with his or her stated goals and desires, we can also deduce the underlying voices.

2. The theory explains the role of *death anxiety* as a primary factor in the formation and maintenance of maladaptive defenses that play an important part in human self-destructiveness. As noted, defenses formed during the pre-Oedipal phases are critically reinforced when the child becomes aware of death.

Existential issues continue to have an enormous impact, generally negative, on individuals throughout their lives. Although the response to existential trauma usually acts to support the maladaptive defensive process, an individual might choose to brave the real world and remain vulnerable to the feelings of sadness and anxiety associated with the inescapable facts of separation, aloneness, and the terminal nature of life.

In addition, on a societal level, conventional institutionalized defenses against death anxiety (religious dogma, political systems, and "isms") support the denial of death and accommodations to death anxiety through negative social pressure. In contrast to much of object relations theory (as criticized by Marcuse (1955/1966) [Endnote 3]), my theory retains the important focus on society's active destructive interference with the individual and his or her project of becoming an authentic self. It also takes into account a suicidal potential existing within the personality (the antiself system). The incorporated aggression toward others is *not* derived from a death instinct or innate aggression turned back against the self; rather, the antiself system represents the internalization of negative parental attitudes and hostility, destructive forces in society, and painful existential realities.

3. Voice Therapy explains the core defense (the *fantasy bond* or *self-parenting process*) and the fact that internal gratification through self-nourishing fantasies and habit patterns comes to be preferred over real relationships or the pursuit of goals in the interpersonal environment. The *fantasy bond* may be defined as an imagined connection, formed originally with the parent or primary caretaker, that arises in response to emotional deprivation and separation trauma in early childhood. Internalized, idealized parental images, in conjunction with primitive self-nurturing habits, provide the child with an illusion of self-sufficiency or pseudoindependence, because they partially gratify basic needs and reduce tension.

As adults, most individuals develop an addictive attachment, that is, a fantasy of love and connection in place of the deterioration that often occurs in relationships. Moving toward closeness and mature sexuality is tantamount to separation from the illusory connection with the mother or primary caretaker. The increase in death anxiety aroused by one's sense of vulnerability in loving and being loved is the driving force underlying men and women's retreat from intimacy. In insulating and distancing themselves to protect against separation experiences and death anxiety, they often give up their real lives together for an illusion of connectedness and immortality.

The self-parenting process contributes to the etiology of the "addictive personality" and is the basis of all addictive behaviors. The concepts of the fantasy bond and the voice process have broadened our understanding of resistance in terms of patients' tenacity in holding on to fantasized connections because they are part of an addictive process of self-parenting.

4. The theoretical approach elucidates the concept of *parental ambivalence.* All people are divided within themselves in the sense that they have feelings of warm self-regard as well as feelings of self-depreciation and self-hatred. Much as parents have positive and negative feelings toward themselves, they exhibit both tender, nurturing impulses and covert aggression toward their children. The fact that parents want to love and gratify their children does not negate the possibility of critical or hostile feelings toward them. Conversely, the fact that they have angry (destructive) feelings toward their children does not negate their love or concern for them. These conflicting responses have far-reaching significance for child rearing.

5. The developmental theory emphasizes the distinction between parents' genuine love, nurturance, and concern for the child and *emotional hunger,* which is a strong *need* caused by deprivation in the parents' own childhood. These two emotional states and the associated behaviors have not been sufficiently differentiated from each other by developmental theorists, but making this distinction is vital for an understanding of one of the major factors that contribute to secure attachment versus anxious or avoidant attachment patterns described by attachment theorists Bowlby (1969, 1973), Ainsworth (1963), Ainsworth, Blehar, Waters, and Wall (1978), Ainsworth, Bell, and Stayton (1972), Main (1990), Main, Kaplan, and Cassidy (1985), and Shaver and Clark (1994) (Endnote 4).

On a more personal note, my inspiration for compiling this work came partly from a comment that R. D. Laing made to me in 1989 shortly before his death. At that time he was working on the Foreword to my book, *Compassionate Child-Rearing* (R. Firestone, 1990b). While visiting with me in the environment I described earlier, Laing affectionately challenged me, saying, "You should take a chance on preaching what you practice." The remark was complimentary, though ironic, in the sense that both he and I disapprove of preaching. But I knew what he meant.

Laing was referring to his observation that my colleagues and friends and I were living a reflective, active, and meaningful life and that our companionship was adventurous, congenial, and affectionate. He recognized that people were operating on an implicit value system based on openness and integrity, with deep concern for children as real people and with sensitivity and genuine feeling for others. He was affected by an underlying philosophy of individuals learning to bear their own pain rather than acting out on each other, and by their dedication to helping ameliorate the suffering of others.

Laing saw people who were involved in a way of life that challenges each dimension of a defensive, self-protective, inward lifestyle. His appraisal implied that he had witnessed a genuine democratic social process in action, one that was protective of individual rights and personal freedom, between people and within the person. It is just as serious and reprehensible to hurt oneself as it is to mistreat another.

I was deeply touched by what Laing said to me. It strengthened my conviction that I should make a comprehensive statement regarding my ideas and describe those aspects of theory that differentiate my approach from traditional psychological thought and practice. Laing's acknowledgment led me to a deeper realization that an individual's natural striving toward growth and individuation emerges within the context of a particular social process, whose dimensions can be delineated.

Recognizing this, I began to outline the parameters of an "ideal" lifestyle, showing how each dimension exemplifies the principles of sound mental hygiene as well as a basic philosophical outlook concerning human rights. My desire is to share these insights about mental health and psychopathology forthrightly in a manner that appeals to the emotions of the reader as well as to his or her intellect.

In summary, although many points in this book are controversial, it is essential that mental health professionals, social theorists, and other members of the general public carefully weigh the issues discussed here. I would be pleased if this volume not only would shed new light on people's lives and their relationships but would also lead to the development of important empirical research. We have already used a voice scale to determine individuals' self-destructive potential. This project involved testing over 1,300 subjects, and the results indicated significant correlations with established and respected scales already in existence. In addition, we were better able to predict the threat of actual suicide than these other measures. Pilot studies investigating the connection between critical voices and violence are now being conducted and preliminary results are being analyzed.

It is my hope that this work might be a step toward questioning and challenging traditional modes of thought. Perhaps we can stimulate an urgently needed movement toward the creation of a sane, humanistic, less pathogenic society that would foster personal growth and individuation.

ENDNOTES

1. Gilbert (1989), in his book *Human Nature and Suffering*, described three systems of defense: (a) antipredator, (b) territorial breeding, and (c) group living. Gilbert delineated the various coping responses to stress and the underlying neurochemical changes that occur during both the fear state and the helplessness stage in confronting uncontrollable events. In his chapter "Psychobiology of Some Basic Mechanisms," he stated,

By understanding the different subsystems of the defence system . . . [listed above] we can advance our understanding of "neuroticism" in terms of sensitivity in threat (defensive) systems. Furthermore, we are better placed to understand why sociability is positively correlated with well being . . . why social support works (by increasing safety, activating hedonic modes and reducing arousal in the defence system). (p. 90)

2. However, Ernest Becker (1973) and Gregory Zilboorg (1943), among others, have also noted that some form of defense mechanism is almost mandatory to allow people to function in their everyday lives without being overwhelmed by the affects of intense anxiety and dread about their anticipated end.

3. Herbert Marcuse (1955/1966) criticized object relations theory and especially the social revisionists, Erich Fromm, Karen Horney, and Harry Stack Sullivan, for dispensing with Freud's instinctual theory in constructing their models of "the whole person." According to Roazen (1973), Marcuse's arguments are based on his belief that instinct theory is necessary to make a "case for the possibilities of a nonrepressive society" (p. 15). Marcuse (1955/1966) argued that modern societies, including capitalistic democracies, consist of "the emergence of new forms of civilization: [in which] repressiveness is perhaps the more vigorously maintained the more unnecessary it becomes" (p. 4). According to Marcuse, in dispensing with biological givens within the psyche, post-Freudian theorists have defused, covered over, or watered down concepts explaining the real tension that necessarily exists between instinctual forces within the personality and powerful antagonistic elements in society.

Marcuse is troubled that the neopsychoanalysts have blurred the destructive effects of society. As a social theorist, he believes that if one takes away the death instinct, and with it the understanding of the division between the death instinct and the life force, one will not deal sufficiently with the oppressive forces in society. Marcuse is correct in his analysis of society as oppressive but wrong in stating that the revisionists have watered down Freud's theory. In my opinion, Fromm, Horney, Erikson, and object relations theorists did not take away from this issue but instead understood aggression as a function of malparenting rather than an instinctual drive. Manifestations of individual psychopathology become the building blocks of corrupt and maladaptive societies, and these societies have a negative impact on their members.

4. The literature on attachment theory delineating differential patterns of attachment is extensive and includes, among others, John Bowlby's books, *Attachment and Loss: Volume I, Attachment* (1969) and *Volume II, Separation: Anxiety and Anger* (1973), and Mary Ainsworth's (1963) initial studies on attachment patterns in a naturalistic setting ("The Development of Infant-Mother Interaction Among the Ganda") as well as her discussion of research differentiating patterns of secure, anxious/avoidant, and anxious/resistant attachment between infant and care-taker (Ainsworth et al., 1978).

Recent developments in attachment research can be found in Mary Main's (1990) chapter "Parental Aversion to Infant-Initiated Contact Is Correlated With the Parent's Own Rejecting During Childhood: The Effects of Experience on Signals of Security With Respect to Attachment." Main et al. (1985) developed the Adult Attachment Interview that evaluates the attachment history and, by inference, internal working models in parents of young children assessed as securely or insecurely attached.

Finally, Philip Shaver and his associates (Brennan & Shaver, 1995; Kunce & Shaver, 1994; Shaver & Clark, 1994; Shaver & Hazan, 1993) have investigated correlations between adult styles of relating and early patterns of attachment.

PART I

Developmental Perspective

2

The Reality of Childhood Trauma

To grow up at all is to conceal the mass of internal scar tissue that throbs in our dreams.

Ernest Becker (1973, p. 29)

To be able to see anybody as abusive, I had to acknowledge that the woman who gave me life also devalued it, demeaned it and nearly destroyed it.

Barbara Dolan (1991, p. 47)

A disease that is kept hidden behind closed doors and shuttered windows, whose existence is ignored or denied, can never be cured. . . . At that time, we had no statistics; we only had our gut reactions to personal experiences. It was difficult for those of us who believed child maltreatment to be a major disease to convince those who did not.

Vincent Fontana (1983, pp. 30-31)

AUTHOR'S NOTE: Material in this chapter and the next two chapters is taken from a paper, *The Universality of Emotional Child Abuse,* presented at the Twentieth Annual Child Abuse and Neglect Symposium, Keystone, Colorado (May 1992), and the Ninth International Congress on Child Abuse and Neglect, Chicago (August 1992).

15

Unfortunately, the trauma of birth does not end with the last contractions. Every child experiences varying degrees of emotional pain in his or her development. Even in an ideal parenting situation, there is inevitable frustration, and, furthermore, environmental conditions are usually less than ideal. The emotional climate in the nuclear family in our society often predisposes maladaptive patterns of adjustment. In some important ways, the statistical norm has become pathogenic (Gil, 1987) (Endnote 1).

This fact is underscored by the alarming increase in adolescent suicide rates, the hatred and violence of young people necessitating children arming themselves for protection in school, the widespread use of drugs and painkillers, and the general deterioration of mental health in our communities (Hewlett, 1991; Kozol, 1995). In short, we have produced a generation of young people filled with cynicism, cut off from feeling, devoid of hope and dreams, and with little regard for their human heritage (Endnote 2). For example, the Centers for Disease Control (1993) reports that during 1991, up to 26% of students in Grades 9-12 reported carrying a weapon. In 1992, homicide became the leading cause of death among New York City youth aged 15-19 years (Centers for Disease Control, 1993).

Aside from these shocking figures, the media bombards us with reports of teenagers engaging in risk-taking activities that threaten their lives as well as the lives of others. The other day, a friend related a frightening story: While driving on a freeway through Detroit, he narrowly escaped death when teenagers dropped bricks from an overpass and one hit his car. This dangerous practice has become a popular pastime for adolescents in many cities.

THE UNIVERSALITY OF EMOTIONAL PAIN

There are two major sources of psychological pain and anxiety, interpersonal and existential, that impinge on the child and disturb the individuation process: (a) deprivation, rejection, and overt or covert aggression on the part of parents, family members, and significant others, particularly during the formative years, and (b) basic existential problems of aloneness, aging, illness, death, and other facts of existence that have a negative effect on a person's life experience: social pressure, racism, crime, economic fluctuations, political tyranny, and the threat of nuclear holocaust.

Interpersonal pain refers to the frustration, aggression, and mistreatment one experiences in relationships, whereas issues of aloneness, inevitable separation experiences, crime, poverty, and contemplating death's inevitability fall into the existential category. Historically, in their efforts to understand psychological pain, a number of theorists have investigated the effects of interpersonal trauma, while others have directed their attention to philosophical and existential concerns (Endnote 3). Neither system deals sufficiently with the important concerns of the other, however, and to ignore either seriously impairs an understanding of psychological functioning.

Both systems of thought, psychoanalytic and existential, must be integrated to fully understand the individual. One must consider both the "down and dirty" issues dealt with by the psychoanalysts as well as the "higher level" or ontological concerns of the existentialists. To develop a more comprehensive picture of our struggle to be human, one must understand that defenses formed in early childhood are critically reinforced as the child develops a growing awareness of death. No one gets through life unscathed; the existential anguish inherent in the human condition and interpersonal distress are both operant. Some pain is inevitable in growing up, as in routine separation experiences, but much personal torment is unnecessary. Indeed, suffering in relation to interpersonal sources plays the most significant part in the life of the adult.

The long-lasting effects of the painful experiences children endured can be observed in their adult reactions to parents and family members. Why are so many family reunions marred by disharmony and disillusionment? What really happened between the time the infant gazed with innocent love and trust into mother's eyes, and the time this now grown child regards his or her parents as an unpleasant obligation and feels awkward in their company? What transpired in the intervening years to erase the bright smile from the face of the toddler who once leaped joyfully into his or her father's arms?

THE ESSENTIAL NATURE OF THE CHILD

The prolonged dependence of the human infant on his or her parents for physical and psychological survival provides the first condition for the development of neurosis. The infant's need for "reliable maternal support" is absolute, and failure to provide it is so nearly universal that "varying degrees of neurotic instability . . . are the rule rather than the exception" (Guntrip, 1961, p. 385). Parents feel, and are very much aware of, the responsibility implied by their child's utter dependence on them. At the same time, they are awed by the unique capacity for human response in their baby.

From the neonate's first smile of recognition, parents sense the capability for deep feeling. Later, they become aware of the child's potential for imagination and creativity in his or her underdeveloped mind. These latent qualities make the child especially precious, and they inspire unusually strong and tender feeling responses from parents.

However, the child is not born into a neutral atmosphere because so many parents have difficulty handling these emotions. Due to their own defensive limitations, most find it necessary to transform this extraordinary creature into an ordinary creature. They offer the gift of life and then unintentionally retract it. In attempting to structure and socialize their children according to their own defensive, self-protective prescriptions for living, they unwittingly deprive their children of their human heritage. Once human beings are "processed" in this way and divested of their individuality, they are reduced to a subhuman level of existence. Children retain their capacity to suffer, however, and their condition is now worse than that of an animal; they have been stripped of their humanity, yet still retain their exquisite sensitivity to negative experiences.

THE DISCREPANCY BETWEEN PARENTS' INTERNAL FEELINGS AND ACTUAL BEHAVIOR

Most mothers and fathers honestly *believe* that they love their children even when an objective observer would view their behavior patterns as indifferent, neglectful, or even abusive. They tend to imagine closeness and form a fantasy bond. In that way, they preserve an illusion of positive feeling while, at the same time, maintaining emotional distance. Parents readily acknowledge their affectionate feelings toward their children yet strongly resist recognizing negative or hostile elements because these feelings are socially unacceptable. To understand parent-child interactions and their effect on child rearing, however, the observer must take into account the obvious discrepancy between feelings and attitudes on the part of parents and their actual behavior. Indeed, mixed messages create havoc with the child's sense of reality and play an important part in neuroses and psychoses. The anthropologist Gregory Bateson (1972), who directed his energy to observing patterns of behavior in mental illness, considered mixed messages, "the double bind," to be the central issue in the schizophrenic process (Bateson, 1972; Bateson, Jackson, Haley, & Weakland, 1956/1972; Wynne, 1972).

Emotional Hunger and Love

One explanation for this duplicity is related to the mistaken notions that many people have about love. Almost everybody takes for granted that parents, especially mothers, have an innate propensity to love their children (Badinter, 1980/1981). Unfortunately, this assumption is not necessarily reliable. Many parents confuse intense feelings of need and the subsequent anxious attachment to their offspring with feelings of genuine affection. They don't distinguish emotional hunger, an unsatisfied longing for love and care caused by deprivation in their own childhood, from real warmth and concern. They imagine that they love their children, while their behavior tells a different story.

To illustrate the case in point, after her daughter's serious suicide attempt, a mother complained about the inconvenience and annoyance caused by the desperate act. Pained by her self-centeredness and the obvious disregard for her daughter's well-being, members of her therapy group questioned her feelings toward her daughter. The mother said, "How can you question my love for my daughter when I feel this burning sensation inside of me?" This mother mistook her deep sense of emptiness and hurt as proof of love for her child.

Feelings of emotional hunger and imagined connection to the child are experienced by parents as deep internal sensations that range in intensity from a dull ache to a sharp nostalgia. Quite often, they express physical affection with ostensibly loving gestures in an attempt to dull their own hurt. They offer affection and love when they feel the need for it themselves and inadvertently take *from* their children rather than give to them. Sustained contact with an emotionally hungry parent is damaging to the child's well-being. In this type of situation, the more extensive the contact, the more detrimental. Needy parents tend to drain the child of his or her emotional resources (Levy, 1943; A. Miller, 1979/1981; G. Parker, 1983; Rutter, 1981).

In my work, I have pointed out the fundamental differences in parents' emotional states that predispose the development of an anxious/avoidant attachment as compared with a secure attachment between parent and infant (Ainsworth et al., 1978). Many children raised by immature parents develop a reciprocal hunger toward their parents (Khan, 1963; Searles, 1962/1965a). This is frequently observed in the child who clings desperately to the mother and who is afraid to venture out on his or her own. Other children are refractive to affection and resist being held or cuddled by their parents, and stiffen their bodies when they are picked up.

With few exceptions (Endnote 4), the concept of emotional hunger has not been sufficiently investigated in the psychological literature. Yet it is one of the principal factors affecting hurtful child-rearing practices. In summary, parents' desperation expressed as a need to fulfill themselves through their children has powerful negative effects on the child's development and subsequent adjustment.

EMOTIONAL CHILD ABUSE

Emotional child abuse refers to damage to the child's psychological development and emerging personal identity, primarily caused by parents' or primary caretakers' immaturity, defended lifestyle, and conscious or unconscious aggression toward the child. We must consider it an abuse when imprinting from early interactions with family members has long-term debilitating effects on a person's conception of self and personal relationships, leads to a condition of general unhappiness, causes pain and anxiety in one's sexual life, and interferes with and stifles development of career and vocational pursuits. Although personal deficiencies and limitations in adult functioning are at times a result of biological or hereditary factors, in our experience they have been more closely related to, even overdetermined by, abuses suffered in the process of growing up.

In commenting on the increasing normalization of psychopathology in the Western world, R. D. Laing (1990) stated, "Pathology has, or has almost, taken over, and has become the norm, the standard that sets the tone for the society . . . [we] live in" (p. xi). As one example, Kaufman and Zigler (1987) reported a national survey of disciplinary practices that showed 97% of all children in the United States have been physically punished. Parents who administered daily or weekly spankings were more reflective of a cultural norm than a deviation (Straus, 1994). In Germany, destructive child-rearing practices became so widespread that legislation against *Kinderunfreundlichkeit* (antagonism and sadistic behavior toward children) was instituted in an effort to control these unconscionable actions (M. Meyer, 1991).

Physical, sexual, and emotional abuses experienced by children in the course of a so-called normal upbringing are far more common and the effects are far more damaging and long-lasting than most people recognize (Blumberg, 1974; Conte & Schuerman, 1987; Emerson & McBride, 1986; Garbarino, Guttmann, & Seeley, 1986; Shearer & Herbert, 1987; Shengold, 1989; Steele, 1990) (Endnote 5). Indeed, no child enters adulthood without sustaining injuries in basic areas of personality development that disturb psychological functioning and yet leave no visible scars (Briere, 1992; Hassler, 1994; A. Miller, 1980/1984).

Although harmful child-rearing practices are virtually omnipresent in some form, the degree of insensitivity, abuse, and neglect varies considerably. The more parents were deprived, rejected, or misunderstood during their own formative years, the greater the impairment of their parental functions, regardless of their stated commitment to or concern for their children. The majority of mental health practitioners are aware that children who are physically maltreated more often than not become parents who compulsively act out similar abuses on their offspring.[1] It is logical that emotionally abused children will unconsciously reenact these practices on their own children (Endnote 6).

It is important to emphasize that many of the behaviors that hurt children occur on the periphery of parents' consciousness. There are many reasons that parents are seemingly insensitive or oblivious to the ways they damage their

---

1 Straus (1994) concluded, on the basis of three studies, that "the more the parents themselves were corporally punished as adolescents, the greater the percentage who went beyond ordinary corporal punishment with their own children and engaged in attacks severe enough to be classified as physical abuse" (p. 85).

children; however, two reasons are relevant here: (a) Most parents have forgotten or rationalized their own parents' mistreatment of *them* (Ensink, 1992; A. Miller, 1980/1984), and (b) the majority of people are insensitive to *themselves,* relating to, mistreating, and punishing themselves in much the same style that they were treated as children.

ARGUMENTS THAT SUPPORT THE REALITY OF CHILDHOOD TRAUMA

Observations of Family Interactions

In observing and investigating families in public settings, patients in psychotherapy, and the long-term effects of family life in our longitudinal study, my associates and I found that, in general, parental responses were *not* consistent with a reasonable or responsible operational definition of love.

Loving behavioral responses would include genuine warmth, tenderness, physical affection, pleasure in the child's company, respect for the child's boundaries, responsible and sensitive care, and a willingness to be a real person with the child rather than simply act the role of "mother" or "father." When parental actions contradict these criteria and are disrespectful, overprotective, intrusive, neglectful, or overtly hostile, they cannot be considered to be loving operations, regardless of the subjective inner feeling described by parents. Parents' behaviors must coincide with their internal feeling state for their love to have a beneficial effect on the child (Endnote 7).

Dysfunctional Adults

The majority of individuals in our culture have been adversely affected by their early experiences in their self-confidence, overall sense of self, and personal relationships (Loring, 1994) (Endnote 8). Their attitudes are contaminated by feelings of self-hatred and self-critical voices concerning performance. These negative thoughts and feelings also affect people's capacity to function in the workplace. For example, fear or rage toward authority, withholding, and other forms of passive-aggression are indicators of early trauma.

The consequences of faulty or harsh child-rearing practices are evident in the statistics related to dysfunctional adults, such as the increase in the divorce rate and the breakdown of the family. Surveys show that the lifetime prevalence for depression is 20.4% of the population and for emotional disturbance in general, 37.1% (Lewinsohn, 1991). The effects of abuse are visible early on, as evidenced by the fact that over 20% of school-age children exhibit some form of serious (diagnosable) emotional disturbance or learning disability requiring intervention (Freiberg, 1991). In the United States, a recent survey indicated that in 1 year over *a million young people attempted suicide, with more than 250,000 requiring medical treatment* (Cimons, 1991). Toth (1992) reported that "the last major study, conducted by the department [U.S. Department of Health and Human Services] about a decade ago, estimated that 1 million youths run away from home each year" (p. A5). A more recent study by the National Association of Social Workers (cited by Toth) found that "two-thirds of all runaways who seek shelter have been physically or sexually abused by a parent" (p. A5).

Antisocial children and juveniles arrested for crimes (over 2.3 million in 1986) exhibit patterns of behavior that begin early in life. In tracing the etiology of antisocial behavior, Patterson, DeBaryshe, and Ramsey (1989) found that "harsh discipline and lack of supervision [are] evidence for disrupted parent-child bonding. Poor bonding implies a failure to identify with parental and societal values regarding conformity and work. These omissions leave the child lacking internal control" (p. 329).

Most people rely on shopworn explanations blaming social upheaval and personal suffering on the breakdown of religion and the dissolution of the family; however, the reverse is true. The deterioration in family relationships and social structure is largely a by-product of harmful practices within the family unit, rather than the result (deMause, 1974; A. Miller, 1980/1984).

One significant indicator of childhood distress resulting in the formation of self-protective defenses is the subsequent damage to adults in the quality of their *interpersonal relationships.* Most people's personal interactions are characterized by a general distrust of others, fear of involvement and vulnerability, a toughness or hardness of men and women in relation to each other, and a good deal of generalized hostility. It is logical that distress and unhappiness in adult relationships are a direct consequence of painful experiences in people's early associations. Distrustful attitudes and fear experienced in family relationships are later extended to others.

Adverse Reactions to Parental Contacts

Regression in schizophrenic and psychosomatic patients following parents' hospital visits is an important indication of negative parental influences. At the National Jewish Center for Immunology and Respiratory Medicine, my associates and I observed the impact of separation from parents on young patients suffering from intractable asthma. Their symptoms considerably improved or virtually disappeared during a 2-year separation period or "parentectomy." This change was not due to geographic relocation, as some of the recovered children came from the same region. In addition, there was increased symptomatology preceding, during, and immediately after parental visits. In a large number of cases, when these children returned to their homes, the asthmatic symptomatology recurred (Endnote 9).

In regard to schizophrenia, many therapists work with patients for months to achieve minimal progress, only to have this progress reversed in a matter of an hour or two in the course of a seemingly harmless family visit. This is a common experience in residential treatment centers and mental hospitals (Lidz, 1969/1972).

Many "normal" children appear more agitated, tense, and antisocial in the presence of their parents than in the company of other children and adults. This is particularly true of young children. In addition, in our reference population, we often noted that there was a lack of genuine eye contact and regression to more infantile behaviors in children after they spent extended periods of time with their parents.

Our observations are supported by other studies, including the work of Anna Freud and Dorothy Burlingham (1944), who described the reactions of children separated from their parents in wartime England. They observed varying degrees of emotional upset and regression in children following reunions with their families and upon their subsequent return to the Hampstead Residential Nursery (Endnote 10).

John Bowlby (1973) described behavior typical of 199 children between the ages of 2 and 8 who had been separated from their mothers for 1-day visits to a research center and reunited with them at the end of the day: "At the sight of mother . . . [the child's] needs for autonomy and independence vanished, and he reverted to the degree of babyishness he had overcome early in the morning" (p. 35).

Educators aware of the effects of parent-child interactions often adjust their classes accordingly. For example, instructors who teach skiing, swimming, and other sports frequently make it a prerequisite that parents not accompany even very young children to class or practice.

In adult patients, negative attitudes toward self appeared to be reinforced by parental contacts, and patients reported a deterioration in mood, a mounting tension, and marital disputes after family visits. One common occurrence involved the situation where the new mother's own mother arrived to help out with the infant. Instead of having a positive effect, it complicated the caretaking of the baby and led to increased stress in the home.

It is interesting that grown children's attitudes toward parents reflect a good deal of conscious and unconscious hostility and a desire for distance. Parents constantly complain that their children don't write or visit. Why, if family life is so constructive and personally rewarding, must grown children be coerced or be made to feel guilty to maintain contact? Why wouldn't it be a powerful choice for them to maintain close relationships with their parents over the span of life (Endnote 11)?

Findings From Investigations Using Voice Therapy

Further evidence of the validity of harsh, abusive child-rearing patterns in our culture can be seen in abusive attitudes and inner voices that people direct toward themselves. We were able to bring these attitudes to the surface using the specialized techniques of Voice Therapy (R. Firestone, 1988, 1990c). As noted, self-critical, self-attacking thoughts and attitudes exist to varying degrees in every person, undermining self-confidence and influencing maladaptive behavior. Without any encouragement or prior suggestion, participants in our study directly related the tone, style of communication, and content of their self-attacks and voices to experiences in early family interactions. People remembered personal attacks leveled against them and recalled examples of abusive attitudes and behavior they had endured.

Parents' Admission, in Parenting Groups and Individual Psychotherapy, of Abusive Feelings and Actions

In recent years, considerable controversy has been generated surrounding the validity of adults' recollections of being mistreated as children. The most convincing evidence in opposition to those who claim that these memories are merely fantasies or distortions has come from parents in psychotherapy or group process who openly admitted the abuses they inflicted on their children. Their self-disclosures validated and often added to the accounts of their adult children's recollections of being mistreated while growing up. For example, one mother contributed more details surrounding an incident that her adult son recalled from childhood in which he had been severely punished for a minor transgression:

> I remember once or twice I lashed out angrily at Bill when he was really small. I don't recall exactly what provoked me, but one time, I think he walked through a wading pool with new shoes on, and I had such a fury that I kept on hitting him on the legs. I didn't beat him, but I *did* hit him over and over again on his legs. I also remember, so clearly, that it felt as if someone were standing behind me telling me that it was a good thing to do, that I should punish him.

Participants in a specialized parenting group have observed the transmission of abusive attitudes and behaviors through three generations, beginning with their parents, perpetuated through themselves, and subsequently directed toward their offspring. In our reference population, we found that (a) parents' admission of abusive treatment of their children coincided with reports of their grown children, and (b) abuses were closely related to their children's personal limitations and later suffering. If their grown children's reports were fabricated or were merely fantasies, parents' disclosures would have failed to confirm them.

The reason child abuse in *all* forms has been minimized or denied in our society is that this dismissal is a basic part of a core defense to maintain an idealized image of parents and family members. Becoming cognizant of parents' inadequacies is extremely threatening to the ego of the child. Therefore, as a survival mechanism, children prefer to fantasize that parents are "good" and that they themselves are "bad" rather than face the painful truth of their experience (Arieti, 1974; R. Firestone, 1985, 1990b). This defense is generalized in adult life and has become a social norm.

Unfortunately, in supporting the sanctity of the nuclear family and in protecting parents' rights over their children, our society indirectly condones the harm done to children. Worse yet, many professionals and experts in child development have moved in the direction of deemphasizing or even negating the important link between early childhood trauma and subsequent maladaptive behavior in adult patients (A. Miller, 1981/1984, 1990/1991; Plomin, 1989; Rosenfeld, 1978). This trend has contributed to the atmosphere of doubt and controversy surrounding the validity of adults' recollections of being sexually, physically, and psychologically abused as children (Conte, 1994; Masson, 1984; Whitfield, 1995) (Endnote 12).

CONCLUSION

Years of clinical experience with patients and their families convinced me of certain unavoidable and painful truths about family life and its adverse effect on both children and parents. Originally my attention was directed toward families of schizophrenics, later toward families that produced neuroses, and, finally, I began to investigate the effects of the structure of the nuclear family on "normal" individuals. My abiding interest was an attempt to understand the causes of personal suffering, limitation, and maladjustment. In the course of this effort to fathom the meaning of symptoms and pain and determine the underlying causality, I had to gradually relinquish my own inclination to idealize the family. I was forced to look at parental attitudes and responses that were injurious to people's well-being. I discovered that the origins of self-defeating behavior and a good deal of personal misery were directly traceable to harmful operations within the traditional family structure.

My position, however, is not that the nuclear family is inherently detrimental to human growth and development, but that it has degenerated into an institution hurtful to parents and children alike. Only by recognizing this fact and dealing with the issues that make families dysfunctional can we modify or change family life so that it has a more constructive effect on future generations of children.

My approach, while accounting for and understanding the roots of psycho-pathology, is opposed to focusing blame on parents and families. Parents who were damaged themselves in their upbringing will inadvertently pass on this damage to their children. In any case, both parent and child should be viewed with compassion.

In summary, we have noted the universality of childhood pain, the impressionable nature of the child, and the prevalence of emotional child abuse, and we have introduced the concepts of parental ambivalence and emotional hunger so often directed toward children. The following chapters will delineate the varied patterns of emotional abuse and explain the underlying dynamics—the reasons why well-meaning parents act out destructive machinations.

ENDNOTES

1. In a chapter titled "Maltreatment as a Function of the Structure of Social Systems," David Gil (1987) contended that institutional abuse is an intrinsic aspect of the social order of the United States, including its socialization and child care facilities. He suggested that "reductions of inequalities should result in corresponding reductions of violence and abuse" (p. 170).

In *Slaughter of the Innocents,* David Bakan (1971) declared that "child abuse is a problem central to the larger question of how a generation of adults cares for its children" (p. 20). For indicators of the social "pathology" of neglect and inequality, see *When the Bough Breaks* (Hewlett, 1991) and "Parenting in the Promised Land" (Pinar, 1996).

2. Pamela Cantor (1989) lists the factors most frequently cited as related to feelings of hopelessness and the rising suicide rate in our young people, including the following: the violence that children and adolescents are exposed to, that is, real violence such as rape, murder, and child abuse and created violence in the media; the disappearance of the extended family; the pressures put on kids to grow up too quickly; the special sensitivity of many kids to social isolation; the lack of socially acceptable ways for youngsters to express anger; and a high level of social and academic competition and pressure.

3. The early psychoanalysts theorized about the trauma and psychological conflict experienced in successive stages of psychosexual development, particularly the Oedipal phase. In a more recent evolution to object relations theory and ego psychology, psychoanalysts concentrated on problems arising during pre-Oedipal phases (Balint, 1952/1985; Blanck & Blanck, 1974; Bowlby, 1973; Fairbairn, 1952; Guntrip, 1961; Hartmann, 1964; E. Jacobson, 1964; Kernberg, 1980; M. Klein, 1948/1964; Kohut, 1971; Mahler, 1961/1979; and Rank, 1936/1972 [who was, according to Kramer, 1995, the first object relations theorist]).

The European existentialists described man's despair and the predicament posed by the discrepancy between human aspirations and human limitation. Existential/humanistic psychologists (J. Bugental, 1965, 1976; Frankl, 1946/1959; Laing, 1960/1969; Maslow, 1968; R. May, 1958; Yalom, 1980) emphasized the importance of subjective experience (phenomenology) in the search for identity, authenticity, and meaning in life. See Ernest Becker's (1973) synthesis of Otto Rank's, Freud's, and Kierkegaard's theoretical concepts.

4. Belsky, Taylor, and Rovine (1984), Levy (1943), G. Parker (1983), and Tronick, Cohn, and Shea (1986) have discussed manifestations of emotional hunger, including parental overprotectiveness and the notion of affective hunger. D. N. Stern (1985) notes an "overattunement" on the part of some mothers, which he sees as the clinical "counterpart of physical intrusiveness. Maternal

psyche hovering, when complied with on the infant's part, may slow down the infant's moves toward independence" (p. 219). See also a more recent review and study by K. S. Rosen and F. Rothbaum (1993) on the subject. Manifestations of "father hunger" have been studied by Herzog (1982). He defined father hunger as an affective state of considerable tenacity and force, in which there is "fear of the loss of control of aggressive impulses" (p. 163) in children and adolescents without fathers.

5. In 1995, over 3 million (3,111,000) children were reported for child abuse and neglect to Child Protective Service agencies in the United States. Nearly a million (996,000) children were found to be victims of child maltreatment by CPS. This represents 15 out of every 1,000 children in the United States. In 1995, an estimated 1,215 child abuse and neglect related fatalities were confirmed by CPS agencies. More than three children die each day as a result of child abuse and neglect; 82% of these children are less than 5 years old at the time of their death, with 41% under 1 year of age (Lung & Daro, 1996).

6. On the basis of cross-cultural studies encompassing 35 cultures, Rohner (1991) concluded that parental rejection has a universal effect on children. Parental rejection can be measured *intergenerationally* (in both parent and child). The patterns measured included hostility and aggression, dependency, emotional unresponsiveness, negative self-evaluation (negative self-esteem and negative self-adequacy), and emotional instability as well as a negative worldview.

The Psychologically Battered Child (Garbarino et al., 1986) and *Understanding Abusive Families* (Garbarino & Gilliam, 1980) contain in-depth discussions of the effects of emotional child abuse and neglect and its multigenerational nature.

7. Experimental studies have shown that children have adverse reactions or are unresponsive to adults when the adults' affective expressions do not match their internal state or are inhibited. For example, D. Bugental (1986) found that children (age 7 to 12) were unresponsive to adults who communicated with duplicitous affect, "the polite smile," and other unnatural expressions. The children reduced the frequency of their communications and nonverbal responses to these adults, whereas they maintained a certain level of responsiveness to adults who communicated with sincerity and authenticity. Other studies demonstrated that children are able to detect deception in facial expression by the third grade (Feldman, Devin-Sheehan, & Allen, 1978). Tronick (1980) reported that "when mothers held a frozen posture and a still face while looking toward their infants, the babies looked away and eventually slumped away with a hopeless facial expression" (p. 7).

8. In her discussion of patterns of emotional abuse prevalent in society, M. T. Loring (1994) drew attention to the effects of "traumatic bonding," a form of attachment also referred to as the "Stockholm Syndrome." The effects include the loss of self, an increased vulnerability to abuse as an adult, and the inability to detach from the abuser. The model is

> based on the paradoxical psychosocial responses of hostages to their captors. It was found that hostages develop a genuine fondness for their captors when the latter use a method of control that alternates terror with kindness. This mixture results in a power imbalance . . . that renders hostages dependent on their captors for emotional as well as physical needs. (p. 45)

Citing the case of Patty Hearst and the SLA as an example of this phenomenon, Loring referred to the explanation provided by Symonds (1975): "Overwhelming terror in a victim causes clinging, nonthinking behavior; he clings to the very person who has placed him in danger" (p. 22).

9. Seiden (1965) reported on "parentectomy" treatment in a residential treatment center (the National Jewish Center for Respiratory Disease and Immunology):

> During their two-year stay, their health improves so rapidly and significantly that hospitalization [referring to the above-mentioned treatment program] is often considered a life-saving experience. . . . Ruling out improvements in specific medical or psychological care, workers in this field have concluded that separation itself is the key factor in improvement. (p. 27)

In a more recent case-controlled study, Strunk, Mrazek, Fuhrmann, and LaBrecque (1985) described individual and family characteristics of 21 children with severe asthma who died of asthma sometime following discharge from the National Jewish Center for Immunology and Respiratory Medicine. These children were matched with 21 control asthmatic cases. A stepwise discriminate analysis revealed eight variables that discriminated the two groups. Two variables are relevant to our discussion: (a) "conflicts between the patient's parents and hospital staff regarding medical management of the patient" and (b) "increased asthmatic symptoms during the week preceding discharge" (p. 1193). The authors noted,

> Severe psychological and social characteristics also helped to differentiate the two groups. . . . Patient-parent conflict reflected longstanding parent-child problems that were identified in the medical record, or persistent or severe arguments and clashes that were noted during parental visits or telephone calls. These negative and uncooperative behaviors were common in the interactions of families of children who subsequently died, but occurred in only about 25% of the control families. (p. 1196)

10. In their book, *Infants Without Families,* Anna Freud and Dorothy Burlingham (1944) reported their observations of parents' behavior during children's home visits:

> Every one of our mothers, except those who are completely indifferent and neglectful, will fondle the child, usually beyond the infant's momentary desire; she will handle it, far beyond the necessities of bodily care. . . . Some mothers certainly treat the child's body with possessiveness. They cannot leave it alone, kiss the child one minute, slap it the next, and continually interfere with its movements or its handling of its own body. . . . But all the bodily stimulation which the mother interferes with on the one hand, is given to the child on the other hand through this incessant handling by the mother herself. We may assume on the basis of much evidence, that the child's feeling of oneness with the mother's body has a parallel in the mother's feeling that the child's body belongs to her. . . .
>
> We are at the present moment not discussing whether this mother-child relationship is helpful or harmful to the infant, or what consequences these early experiences will have for later life. (p. 70)

11. See *Mother Love, Mother Hate* (Grizzle, 1988) and *When You and Your Mother Can't Be Friends* (Secunda, 1990) for cogent discussions of the reasons many adults are reluctant to maintain close emotional contact with their parents.

12. In his book, *Memory and Abuse,* Charles L. Whitfield (1995) addressed the controversy over recovered memories and declared,

> After Freud's retraction of the seduction-trauma theory, with few exceptions—such as psychoanalyst Sandor Ferenczi—we continued to deny the abuse. For most of the 20th century we also maintained the myth of "The Family" as being always ideal, private and sacrosanct, even in the face of the obvious abuse of millions of children and adults. (p. 56)

3

Patterns of
Emotional Mistreatment

☙❧

One does not need to rely on statistics to understand the universality of children's suffering. Personal observations as well as the media continually remind one that the mistreatment of children is far more widespread than was previously recognized. In addition, clinical investigations using data from an intense feeling release therapy support the hypothesis regarding the pervasiveness of painful trauma in childhood.

Several years ago, my associates and I found that many patients were blocked or stuck at a certain level of therapeutic development, and we sought new methods to help them get closer to their feelings. We eventually settled on a method similar to Arthur Janov's (1970) technique for eliciting primal emotions. In this endeavor, we instructed our clients to get into a comfortable position, breathe deeply, and let out sounds when they exhaled. We encouraged them to express their emotions freely with suggestions, "Say it louder, let go, just let go." Within a short period of time, their sounds became loud and impassioned, and people tended to relive traumatic incidents from their childhood. We were so impressed with the therapeutic results that we extended our research to associates and volunteers who were fascinated with the work in progress.

In applying the technique to over 200 patients and normal subjects, we found that, without exception, each person expressed deep-seated pain that he or she had previously suppressed. Indeed, the widespread fantasy of a "happy childhood" is made possible only by the magic of repression. I agree with Janov's hypothesis that people maintain a defensive posture and bend their lives out of shape in an effort to avoid any intrusions or reminders in their adult lives of this psychic pain. We conjectured that at critical points in their past, people were forced to cut off the distress that they now allowed themselves to experience in the trusting atmosphere of the sessions. The majority made lucid connections between events that tormented them in their childhood and their problems in later life.

From observing the feeling release sessions, my associates and I came to recognize two major categories of mistreatment of children. One is best characterized as aggression, the other as neglect. *Aggression* refers to degradation, physical or sexual mistreatment, verbal abuse, and a lack of respect for the child's boundaries, and so on, whereas *neglect* refers to lack of nurturance, insensitivity to the child's needs, and a paucity of physical affection, interest, and concern.

During the sessions, patients in the former instance, aggression, shouted statements such as the following: "Get away from me!" "I'm scared of you!" "I'm not crazy!" "Leave me alone!" In relation to neglect, however, they cried out: "Hold me!" "Touch me!" "You don't see me!" "Look at me!" "You don't love me!" "Don't go away!" "Don't leave me!" These emotional expressions were accompanied by intense affect and a flood of insight.

There are a number of specific forms of maltreatment that have lasting effects on the personalities of children. The following patterns of emotional or psychological abuse may be delineated: those based on (a) conscious or unconscious parental hostility, (b) parental indifference or neglect, (c) a generalized ignorance or misunderstanding of children, (d) overly restrictive or harsh moral codes and value systems, and (e) parents' negative character traits and defended lifestyles. These maladaptive patterns are identified with and incorporated by children to their own detriment.[1]

---

1 In stressing the profound negative effects of emotional or psychological abuse, Garbarino et al. (1986) stated, "Rather than casting psychological maltreatment as an ancillary issue, subordinate to other forms of abuse and neglect, we should place it as the centerpiece of efforts to understand family functioning and to protect children" (p. 7).

BEHAVIORS BASED ON
PARENTAL HOSTILITY

Verbal Abuse

Parental hostility is often communicated to a child through sarcastic, derisive, or condescending commentary. Parents are considered verbally aggressive when their spoken words are characteristically negative, overly critical, or severe. Constant derogatory statements directed toward children about their basic appearance, performance, and mannerisms are debilitating. In addition, many parents repeatedly make unfavorable comparisons with siblings or peers. Children have no way to combat parents who maliciously tease them or humiliate them. Their feelings of embarrassment and shame are generally ignored, discounted, or even laughed at. Insinuations and sneering questions—"Why are you so sensitive?" "Can't you take a joke?" "Why are you so quiet and shy?"—intensify children's hurt feelings and sense of shame.

Often children are ridiculed in situations where they are particularly vulnerable. Many are teased, criticized, or put off when they express spontaneous affection. Parents remind them: "You're too old for such things," or taunt them with such statements like the following: "Isn't she the sexy one?" or "Isn't he cute?" Many women in our study recalled being rejected or pushed away while being affectionate with their fathers.

One woman remembered a particular evening when she was 11 years old and was out to dinner with her family. She was wearing a new dress and her father commented that she looked pretty. She ran over to her father and gave him a kiss. Her mother pulled her aside and whispered a sharp reprimand, "Nice girls don't act like that."

Adult patients report numerous incidents of feeling shamed when parents and relatives made derisive, belittling remarks about their early romantic inclinations. They remember being teased about their nudity and sexual nature and responding adversely to parents' anxiety in relation to sexual issues. Indeed, some parents mistakenly associate physical affection with unacceptable sexual impulses and retreat from and withhold affection from their offspring. In more serious cases, parents actually punish or beat their children because of repressed sexual feelings toward them (R. Firestone, 1988).

Condescending attitudes are manifested by many parents toward children in other areas, for example, parents, teachers, and doctors who characteristically treat children as inferiors and talk down to them: "Now it's time to take 'our' bath," or "How are 'we' doing?"

Many adults see children in the diminutive, as being less competent or knowledgeable than they really are. They caution children about the "dangers" of the world in tones that reflect this attitude: "You're too young to understand" or "You don't know what I'm talking about now, but one of these days you'll thank me."

Lecturing and moral lessons by parents delivered in a pedantic, syrupy, or disrespectful style infantilize children and increase their feelings of unworthiness. Statements implying that children are bad and must learn how to be good are detrimental to a child's self-esteem. Children treated in this manner start out with a negative image of themselves and maintain a sense of guilt throughout their lives.

Parents' tendencies to classify children are comparable to clinicians' overreliance on diagnostic labeling, which dehumanizes and detracts from an overall view of the person. Harsh, judgmental attitudes, expressed through categorizing and name-calling, undermine children's self-esteem. Parents tend to pigeonhole a particular child as "the shy one," "the beautiful one," "the plain one," or "the defiant one," and refer to children in pejorative terms, telling them that they are "lazy," "inconsiderate," or "selfish." Name-calling or addressing a child with a nickname that has a strong negative connotation robs him or her of dignity and a positive sense of identity.

Harsh Mistreatment During Socialization of the Child

Mistreatment of children during the socialization process can range from minor irritability and disrespect to sadism and brutality. Many parents believe that children must be made to submit to parental authority "for their own good" to be properly socialized. They feel justified in angrily punishing the child when he or she refuses to comply immediately with their directives or demands. In direct confrontation or showdown, parents manifest fierce, punitive attitudes and, at times, violent rage, which stand out from their usual behavior. Explosive outbursts intimidate and terrify children, who perceive the adults as out of control. This type of parental response in regard to discipline is weak and ineffectual and is threatening to the child's sense of security. Situations that require authority often provide an outlet for parents' repressed hostility or sadistic tendencies. It is incredibly destructive and totally unnecessary to enter into a "battle of wills" where complete submission or subversion of self is required of the child. Parents invariably ask me how to handle the issue where a child is obstinate and directly refuses an order. It is difficult to explain that this type of showdown need never arise with a mature, self-possessed parent. It takes two infantile people to battle it out on this level.

Many parents equate discipline with punishment and feel prideful and righteous in using forceful measures. This faulty approach to discipline tends to be supported legally in our society (Endnote 1). Even in the absence of physical force, psychological coercion, thought control, and angry threats of future punishment constitute a serious misuse of parental power. In one example, a mother threatened her young daughter several times a day with statements such as the following: "I'd like to break your neck, you little brat!" "Get out of my sight, you make me sick!" "You're driving me crazy!"

In another case, a 10-year-old girl had been invited by her best friend's father to go miniature golfing. Her mother seemed to take vicarious pleasure in helping her daughter get ready for the outing by selecting her daughter's dress and putting makeup on her face. Returning home, the young girl enthusiastically described her happy afternoon and showed her mother pictures she and the neighbor had taken at a photo booth.

Her mother flew into a rage and grabbed the photographs from her daughter's hands. Paralyzed with fear, she watched her mother tear them up. Then her mother turned on her, ripping her blouse open and smearing the lipstick across her face. Dragging her daughter to the hall mirror, she screamed, "Look at yourself! You look like a little slut! Don't you ever let me see you looking like that again!"

Years later, in therapy, she recalled, "At that minute I swore that I would never feel the way I had felt toward a man again."

The event had a significant impact on the girl's choice of sex objects. In the years that followed, she directed the rage she had incorporated during the incident toward other girls and developed an ambivalent homosexual pattern that persisted into her adult life. Years of therapy helped her to change her angry orientation toward men, but her close heterosexual relationships were still stormy.

Another form of indirect hostility toward the child is manifest in parental withholding, where parents hold back praise or rewards and inhibit positive emotional responses to children. This is not an unusual pattern, but it is difficult to pinpoint.

Generally, there are mean feelings underlying parents' negativity or withholding behavior. They tend to withhold from their children particularly at those times when their offspring are the most wanting and enthusiastic. They seem to take delight in saying "no," even though they may later give in and grant the child's request. As a consequence, many children are discouraged from asking directly for what they want and eventually turn against their desires and priorities. The majority of adults in our culture are indirect and duplicitous and frequently conceal their feelings about important and meaningful personal issues. Alan, 37, is a case in point.

He is congenial, successful in his career as a computer programmer, and has within his means the resources to lead a fulfilling, happy life. He has enjoyed an active life, especially sailing and pitching hardball with friends. Over the years, however, he has increasingly avoided activities, feelings, and personal relationships that he previously valued. He constantly punishes himself by saying "no" to himself (and to his friends) in much the same way his parents took pleasure in saying "no" to him as a child.

He lives alone and has become more and more inward and miserable. He rationalizes his self-limiting and self-destructive choices with statements such as the following: "I'm too busy at work to play baseball every weekend. I just don't have the energy for sailing trips or social activities. My time is all taken up." These rationalizations directly contradict other statements Alan has made about his love of travel and adventure, that "those voyages were the happiest times of my life."

Alan has gradually submitted to a parental voice that negates his aspirations in life, and he has progressively sided against himself. In this case, I was familiar with this man's background and had often observed his parents' tightness in denying Alan gratifications. The sadistic smile that was noticeable on his father's face as he denied Alan freedom and pleasurable activity now appears on Alan's face when he puts his friends off and denies their benign request for fun and companionship.

Often, negative treatment and incidental acts of cruelty against children go unnoticed as a part of normal child-rearing practices. Some mothers always manage to get soap in their child's eyes when bathing them, and some fathers think nothing of throwing a terrified youngster into a pool, rationalizing this behavior as a benevolent attempt to help the child conquer his or her fear. There are many instances where indirect hostility is manifested in subtle behaviors; for example, the way a child is handled, dressed, fed, and changed, can be rough and insensitive.

Lack of Respect for the
Child's Personal Boundaries

Parents who believe that their children "belong" to them, in the proprietary sense, tend to speak *for* their children, take over their child's productions as their own, brag excessively about their child's accomplishments, and, in general, live vicariously through their children.

For example, one man told of a time when he was 6 years old, and he drew a picture of a rocket in school that he was proud of. When he brought it home, his mother raved about it, praising him and showing it off to all of her friends, relatives, and neighbors. He ended up hating the picture and felt that it belonged to her, not him. Later he found he was unable to draw or paint, despite a strong interest in art. This response generalized to other areas of functioning as the boy matured, and he was unable to sustain interest or enthusiasm in any project because he feared it would somehow be taken away from him. Often, patterns of passive-aggressive withholding, procrastination, and nonproductivity in the workplace can be traced to this particular type of emotional maltreatment.

Many parents who are unable to feel for their children offer them flattery and special praise as a substitute for affection and love. This exaggerated buildup leads to irrational feelings of omnipotence and vanity in the child and contributes to performance anxiety. False reassurances that the child is pretty or smart do not counteract or diminish his or her feelings of inferiority or unlovability.

Parents overstep the personal boundaries of their offspring by inappropriately touching them, invading their privacy, going through their belongings, reading their mail, and requiring them to perform for friends and relatives. An extreme violation of a child's rights is manifested in many parents' insistence that their child reveal his or her innermost thoughts and emotions. This form of inquisition and demand for an immediate personal response closely resembles procedures used in brainwashing.

Studies have conclusively shown that exploitation of the child as a sexual object constitutes a severe infringement on the child's boundaries, leading to ego fragmentation and later to addictive behavior and dissociative disorders (Briere & Runtz, 1987; Chu & Dill, 1990; Sanders & Giolas, 1991) and multiple personality disorders (Putnam, Guroff, Silberman, Barban, & Post, 1986; Ross et al., 1990). One must consider that general disregard for a child's personal boundaries can be equally as harmful; in some cases, the effects are more insidious and pathogenic. Children who are intruded on and used for a parent's narcissistic needs grow up feeling as though they don't belong to themselves but exist only as an object for others.

Threats of Abandonment or Loss of Love

Threats of being sent away (to boarding school, hospital, or jail) are far more common than one might think and frighten children unnecessarily. John Bowlby (1973) reported that threats of this sort are widely used by parents as disciplinary measures and frequently lead to serious school phobias, psychosomatic illness, and other symptoms in children. Warnings or threats that a parent might leave or desert the family, run away and abandon the child, or commit suicide are even more terrifying and, in addition, impose an enormous burden of guilt on the child.

Stifling or Punishing a Child's Aliveness, Spontaneity, and Curiosity

The spontaneous action, liveliness, noise, and lack of shame typical of young children often arouse tension, embarrassment, guilt, and anger in many parents, who then feel compelled to control and restrict their children. Statements such as "What are you getting so excited for?" "Stop asking so many questions!" suppress children's natural expressions of enthusiasm, curiosity, and freedom of movement. Children are also admonished: "Don't be so proud of yourself!" "Don't be conceited." They eventually stop taking pride in their accomplishments and have difficulty acknowledging their self-worth.

DESTRUCTIVE PRACTICES BASED ON INDIFFERENCE AND NEGLECT

Deprivation and Outright Rejection

Neglect is a passive form of abuse. According to Garbarino and Gilliam (1980), "Most estimates figure the rate of neglect at three to four times the rate for physical abuse, and it probably accounts for more deaths" (p. 14). Many so-called accidental drownings of infants and younger children and some incidents of sudden infant death syndrome (SIDS) are attributable to parental neglect (Endnote 2).

Injuries are the leading killer of children, causing more deaths than all diseases combined. "In 1993, unintentional injuries (car accidents, drowning, mishaps) and intentional injuries (homicide, suicide, child abuse) took the lives of 20,636 children and adolescents under 19 years of age" (National Center for Health Statistics, 1996).

During infancy and early childhood, *emotional* deprivation and neglect can lead to death. Spitz's (1945, 1946a, 1946b) studies of children raised in an orphanage who were cared for in every bodily respect but deprived of affectionate handling showed, in a sample of 91 orphans, an infant mortality rate of *over 33%.*

Some parents fail to take even the minimum precautions for their child's physical health and safety (Endnote 3). I am aware of cases where neglect led to death. Children who are not provided with the necessary supervision, who are not watched carefully, are involved in more accidents and sustain more injuries, burns, broken bones, and so on than other children. Later, as adolescents and adults, they tend to be more accident-prone and self-destructive (Endnote 4).

Similarly, children raised by "psychologically unavailable" parents often exhibit symptoms of "nonorganic failure to thrive" such as apathy, lethargy, developmental delays, and even a failure to grow, a phenomenon known as "deprivation dwarfism" (Altemeier et al., 1979; Drotar, 1985; Drotar, Eckerle, Satola, Pallotta, & Wyatt, 1990; Gardner, 1972; Kotelchuck, 1980; Pollitt, Gilmore, & Valcarcel, 1978).

Emotional neglect is manifested in parents who reject or ignore their children, refuse to speak to them for extended time periods, or are unconcerned with their whereabouts (Endnote 5). These children tend to take on a rejected, pathetic appearance. Their unappealing demeanor, combined with clinging, dependent, or negativistic behaviors, provoke rejection by others, thereby diminishing any chance for corrective experiences.

Lack of Genuine Physical Affection, Interest, or Concern

Parents who have been deprived of love during their formative years often lack the emotional resources to offer love and affection to a needy child. Some rationalize their lack of response as an attempt to avoid spoiling the child by giving him or her "too much" affection or attention.

Other parents reassure their offspring with statements like this: "Your father really loves you, he just doesn't know how to show it." They assume that their inner thoughts and feelings about loving their children are comparable with outward expressions. They imagine that they care deeply while, in fact, they make very little real meaningful contact with their children.[2] When there is no outward expression of physical warmth, children feel unacceptable or unlovable. On the other hand, the type of intrusive touching and nervous caressing manifested by an emotionally hungry parent attempting to fill his or her dependency needs through the child must be distinguished from genuine physical affection that nurtures the child.

As their children grow older, uninterested parents often remain ignorant, indifferent to, and unaware of their children's lives and emotional well-being. An insidious, disguised example of neglect can be observed in parents who maintain excellent standards of physical care (their offspring are meticulously cared for, clean, and well-groomed) yet remain emotionally cold, unfeeling, and distant. Children who are handled insensitively by people who lack warmth grow up with much unhappiness and an exaggerated hunger and desperation for love. Ironically, this desperation limits their possibility of ever attaining love in future relationships.

Lack of Sensitivity to a Child's Needs

Parents who have closed off aspects of their own personalities and are cut off from their feelings are necessarily insensitive to the needs of their children. Some parents are incapable of feeding and caring for an infant without arousing undue anxiety or frustration in the child. They are inappropriate in the scheduling of feedings, delay their responses to their child's cries of hunger, and at times overfeed or force-feed the child. Others tend to overstimulate their baby at times, responding to their own inner agenda rather than adjusting their responses to the

---

2 Szalai (1972) showed that the average parent spends only 5.4 minutes per day talking with his or her child.

infant's mood. At the same time, they can often remain oblivious to their toddler's smiles of delight and enthusiasm and fail to respond in kind. Indeed, many fathers and mothers appear unable to empathically attune their caretaking responses to the child's signals and behavioral cues (Brazelton & Cramer, 1990; D. N. Stern, 1985).

Excessive Permissiveness

Overpermissiveness is a form of neglect because the child fails to develop appropriate inner controls over acting-out behavior. Immature parents are remiss in failing to provide sufficient direction and control for their offspring. If children are not properly socialized, in the best sense of the word (for example, if they fail to learn to control their aggressive impulses), they become anxious as adults because of their inability to manage their emotions. As a result, they tend to act out irresponsibly, develop negative attitudes toward themselves, and manifest a high degree of self-hatred (Shengold, 1991). Indeed, when children fail to receive either affection or regulation, both of which are basic needs, they grow up feeling unloved and unlovable.

Parental Inconsistency

Parental inconsistency is often more damaging than consistent ill treatment, which the child can more readily identify. It sets up a pattern of anxiety and distrust. Parents tend to respond to the child more in terms of their own moods (which vary considerably), rather than reacting appropriately to the child's behavior. Often, outbursts of anger and abuse are followed by feelings of contrition and apologetic behavior. One particularly destructive pattern of inconsistency is exemplified by parents who, following close personal interactions with their children, react negatively by becoming especially withholding or punishing toward them. This vacillating pattern confuses the child and leads to a defensive process of inwardness, distrust, and emotional tightness.

BEHAVIORS BASED ON
GENERALIZED IGNORANCE

Parental Role-Playing and Dishonesty

It is always detrimental for parents to role-play (act out so-called proper responses) or respond in a manner different from their true feeling state. The majority of "how-to" child-rearing books inadvertently encourage parents to offer children mixed messages, a form of abuse characterized by discrepancy between spoken words and actual feelings that distorts the child's sense of reality. Children suffer from the lack of a real person in their lives. What they need most is a parent who is an emotionally responsive human being, willing to relate to them directly with genuine feeling, not a robot reacting with pro-grammed, socially acceptable, or role-determined emotions.

Parental Overprotection

Overprotective behavior limits a child's experience and ability to cope with life and indirectly teaches him or her an abnormal form of dependency. Parents who lack an understanding of a child's need to grow and individuate tend to restrict their youngster's freedom of movement, discourage or even prevent the child's independent interests and pursuits, or become overly concerned with his or her physical health. In overidentifying with their child's pain, they soothe, reassure, coddle, or oversympathize, which limits his or her development of ego strength and independence. There appear to be two factors underlying overprotective tendencies in parents: (a) a benevolent, albeit inappropriate and destructive, desperation to spare the child pain, and (b) disguised hostility or aggression toward the child.

Isolation

Isolating children and adolescents from social contacts, including peers or extrafamilial influences that would offer a different point of view from that of the parents, is detrimental to a child's personal development and future mental health. Many parents, assuming that children are easily influenced (adversely) by "outsiders," strictly limit their child's or adolescent's contact with other people.

Physically abusive parents, in particular, attempt to prevent their offspring from forming other relationships that could possibly facilitate a healing process for the trauma they suffer. Joseph Richman (1986) describes the destructiveness of a closed family system in which the child "is alienated and isolated both outside the family and within it. It is that combination that often produces the particular pattern that is fundamental to a suicidal resolution" (p. 133). With respect to prevention, the importance of an extended family situation or support network cannot be overemphasized. Recent studies have shown that certain resilient children who experienced severe abuse and neglect, yet failed to develop symptoms as adults, usually had a significant other—a relative, family friend, or teacher—who took an interest in them and provided them with support (Cohler, 1987).

OVERLY RESTRICTIVE OR
HARSH MORAL CODES AND VALUES

Parents' negative attitudes and defenses are transmitted to their offspring through direct teaching and through unconscious modeling or imitation. There are two principal methods of explicit training or teaching used by parents in the socialization process: (a) verbal instruction and (b) differential rewards and punishment (R. Firestone, 1990b).

Virtually every adult in our society grew up in a family in which he or she was taught distorted views about sex. Then, as parents, they go on to indicate, both directly and subtly, that sex is bad, that masturbation is harmful, that the subject of sexuality is taboo, and that sex should be confined to a separate sphere of life (Berke, 1988; Calderone, 1974/1977). In spite of the so-called sexual revolution of the 1960s, many still refuse to allow their teenagers to attend sex education classes. Negative views held by parents in relation to nudity and the human body cause children to develop a deep sense of shame about their bodies and guilt in relation to sexual feelings (Gunderson & McCary, 1979).

Although attitudes toward masturbation appear to have changed from punitive to tolerant over the past several decades, many parents still react severely when they discover their child masturbating. The guilt engendered by these overreactions can have serious consequences.

The typical introduction to sexuality (implicit attitudes and training) encountered in family life actually constitutes a form of sexual abuse, as the majority of adults in our society are eventually impaired to varying degrees in their sexual feelings, attitudes, and capacity to enjoy mature sexual relationships (Vergote, 1978/1988).

Closely related to distorted views of sexuality are parental beliefs derived from the concept of "original sin." Some people believe that children are born sinful or basically evil. Statements and clichés such as "Children should be seen and not heard" and "Spare the rod and spoil the child" are representative of this point of view. Moralistic and restrictive training procedures based on this supposition produce children who perceive themselves as innately bad and behave accordingly. For example, it is harmful to teach children that certain thoughts or feelings, such as anger, envy, or competitiveness, are unacceptable. Children need to learn that any thought or feeling is acceptable while, at the same time, they must learn to evaluate and control their behavior. Because actions have external consequences, they must be governed by a value system, whereas freedom of thought and feeling are necessary for children to understand themselves and come up with creative solutions.

PARENTS' NEGATIVE CHARACTER
TRAITS AND DEFENDED LIFESTYLES

The process of imitation has been shown to be more powerful than direct learning (Bandura & Walters, 1963). Even infants of 2 to 3 weeks have the ability to imitate the actions of a model (Kumin, 1996). As role models, many parents exhibit toxic personality traits, behaviors, and lifestyles that are passed on to succeeding generations.

In passing on these defenses, often they're teaching their children aspects of their own personality that are maladaptive. For example, they are teaching them to be suspicious of other people, to be afraid to be open in their expression of feeling, and *not* to be vulnerable, whereas being connected to one's feelings for self and others and being vulnerable are basic human qualities.

Children incorporate and imitate parents' maladaptive approaches to life. Parents who are suspicious and paranoid will pass on to their children a paranoid orientation to life. Similarly, parents who are perfectionistic or rigid will transmit this posture to their offspring.

Parents' prejudices toward women or men or toward people of other races or religions, and other ideas that predispose alienation, are taken on by children as part of their belief system. These negative attitudes cause distrust among people and support an isolated self-protective lifestyle.

Children imitate their parents' self-denying posture and assimilate their belief that personal wants are "selfish" or undesirable. The result is that most children progressively turn their backs on their wants and priorities, which is tantamount to surrendering a basic part of their identity.

In a group discussion,[3] Lee, former systems analyst and currently director of a growing real estate business, described how he learned from both parents to stifle his natural curiosity and deny his wants and personal freedom, and substituted a compulsive work neurosis:

> There's a recurring dream of when I was a little toddler of running and exploring and sensing life and touching and smelling and sensing things, and then this vise or being picked up by my mother, who was very depressed, who stayed in bed, and she wanted me to stay out of trouble. So she put me in the crib in the dark room with her while she took her nap, while she slept, while she whiled away

---

3 This excerpt was taken from a video documentary (Parr, 1995a), *Invisible Child Abuse.*

the daytime with the shades drawn. And you could see the light outside, but I had to stay in this crib in this room to stay out of trouble.

My father took over then as I got older but it was the same thing. I had to report for work after school. I had jobs to do. There's work to be done! One day I went to the soda shop where all the rest of the kids went after school for just a few minutes and my father came in raging like a bull and he grabbed me by the collar and dragged me out literally by the scruff of the neck.

"Don't you dare not report to work like you're supposed to! What are you doing here?"

So there was always this creation of demands on me that a life is not for me. I was thinking of the recurrence of this throughout my life, that I did it to myself after that. I got my girlfriend pregnant and had three children before I was 23. I was working and carrying 25 hours of engineering because I had this demand to support my family and to finish school.

Then my career in engineering was a succession of going into a job, creating a grandiose scheme—and I would wallow in it, I would wallow in it to the point of where it was consuming, always consuming, always consuming.

I started a career in real estate and development and I enjoyed it. I loved it. But once again it's become a consuming nightmare for me, the financial pressure, pressures of the times. It's devoured me for the past couple of years.

The creation of these consuming problems in my life has kept me from having a life over and over again.

Lee's adult daughter, Sara, exhibits work patterns similar to those of her father. Although her compulsivity may have played a positive role in her accomplishments as president of a successful corporation, she finds it increasingly difficult to strike a balance between her work and her personal life. Responding to her father in the group discussion, she said,

I know the way you were with me and the way that you were with yourself really affected me. I feel that I'm only good if I'm really driving myself, and I get really scared any time I start to balance it the other way. When I start to think about love and about people I care about, about my children, I get really scared and I run back to your way of being.

It's a much more comfortable way for me to live, to have that attitude and to give myself just little dribs and pieces of affection. It has to be balanced the other way, though, where I'm "good" only when I'm working hard and I'm driven.

Sara's statements indicate that she assimilated her father's belief that working compulsively was "good," whereas simply enjoying life and her relationships with family and friends was "bad." One can see here the pattern through the generations. Many people, like Lee's parents, teach their children to be selfless, to give up their own point of view and strivings to meet certain obligations. They teach the children, in effect, to give up themselves, and yet if they give up themselves, they have little to offer.

Generally speaking, people treat themselves emotionally the way they were parented. As children, they incorporated their parents' defensive way of living. As adults, they conduct their lives in a manner similar to the way they were treated; that is, they deprive themselves, punish themselves, and nurture themselves (addictively).

Addictive parents transmit their addictive behaviors and lifestyles to their children. Researchers who have studied the etiology of substance abuse and other addictions have noted the intergenerational cycle of these negative patterns. Studies show that there are at least 22 million adults in this country who have lived with an alcoholic parent (Seixas & Youcha, 1985). The National Council on Alcoholism estimates that 3 million teenagers are problem drinkers (Macdonald, 1987). Claudia Black (1981) reports that "fifty to sixty percent of all alcoholics (a low estimate) have, or had, at least one alcoholic parent. Alcoholism is a generational disease" (p. 4).

Children learn to be dishonest by observing and imitating their parents' dishonesty. Paradoxically, parents who wish their children to develop into moral, honest adults often lack personal integrity, engage in corrupt business practices, or are deceptive in their own relationships. The dishonesty and deception inherent in most couple relationships, in which partners' actions toward each other contradict their words, make children suspicious in their own relationships.

Finally, children imitate their parents' repression and denial by suppressing unacceptable feelings such as anger and fear. Because of their intolerance of certain emotions, parents not only damage their children but also unknowingly prevent their recovery. To recover from initial trauma, it is necessary to express oneself. Failure to create an environment where children can cry, vent anger, or talk about their feelings perpetuates their misery and suffering (M. Lewis & Michalson, 1984).

In summary, we have described various forms of parental mistreatment that affect the lives of children. Now it is important to consider the dynamics underlying parental abuses.

ENDNOTES

1. Garbarino and Gilliam (1980) noted that

there is clear legal sanction for the use of physical force against children. The Texas legislature, for example, in 1974 enacted legislation containing the following statement: "The use of force, but not deadly force, against a child younger than 18 years is justified: (1) if the actor is the child's parent or stepparent . . . (2) when and to the degree the actor believes the force is necessary to discipline the child." This law reflects the historical role of violence in our civilization. (p. 32)

Other cultures do not necessarily conform to Western conventions regarding the sanctity of family versus protecting the rights of children. See Norma Feshbach (1980), "Corporal Punishment in the Schools: Some Paradoxes, Some Facts, Some Possible Directions," and Jill Korbin (1981) for documentation of legal and ethical standards in Sweden that support children's rights. Straus and Gelles (1986) reported that spanking, slapping, and hitting a child with an object are legally considered "abuse" in Sweden and several other countries.

2. Studies documenting accidental deaths and SIDS that may be attributable to parental neglect include those of Jason, Carpenter, and Tyler (1983), Luke (1978), Newlands and Emery (1991), and T. Rosen and Johnson (1988).

3. Recent court decisions (e.g., Indiana Supreme Court decision revoking the "religious defense" argument in the deaths of two children) may help prevent some future deaths from this form of neglect. These decisions are relevant in cases where parents refuse medical treatment for a sick child because of religious beliefs, and where the resulting neglect caused unnecessary death (Hughes, 1990).

4. Margolin and Teicher (1968) found a history of maternal deprivation during the first year of life in a group of *suicidal* adolescent boys. A study by Schneer, Kay, and Brozovsky (1961) showed parental loss or separation experiences among 84 suicidal adolescents; this was accompanied by a large number of instances of neglect by the mother. Israel Orbach (1988), summarizing the research on neglect, stated, "Neglect appears to amplify the destructive impact of abuse. The parents' apathy creates a feeling of superfluity in the child. At the most simple and direct level, the child learns that she is an unwanted burden" (p. 93).

5. Schakel (1987) cited a 1981 report by the Office of Human Development Services showing that "of the six major categories of maltreatment they identified, emotional neglect had the highest proportion (74%) of demonstrably serious impairments such as attempted suicides, drug overdose, and severe medical problems" (p. 104).

Egeland and Sroufe (1981) found that

the outcomes for the psychologically unavailable group seem severely malignant, pervasive, and pernicious. Having a mother who is chronically unavailable and unresponsive has devastating consequences on the child that touch every aspect of early functioning. . . . This pattern of maltreatment seems to have a greater effect than any other form of maltreatment on emotional functioning. (p. 89)

These authors found that by 18 months of age, none of the infants in the psychologically unavailable group were securely attached.

4

Psychodynamics Involved in the Intergenerational Cycle of Child Abuse

M any theorists have dealt with the issue of emotional child abuse and described its manifestations (Garbarino & Gilliam, 1980; Kempe & Kempe, 1984; Laing, 1969/1972; Rohner, 1986; Shengold, 1989). Alice Miller (1979/1981, 1980/1984) has written magnificent works expressing the various forms of torment children are exposed to. Although it is necessary and important to deal with child maltreatment on a phenomenological level, it is not sufficient to merely point out the problem and document its extent and pervasiveness. It is most important to understand the psychodynamics involved in the intergenerational cycle of child abuse. Emotional damage to children is a complex phenomenon (Belsky, 1980) and no single pattern is explanatory; however, several significant factors that bear on this issue can be delineated.

PARENTAL AMBIVALENCE

To understand the basic problem involved in the mistreatment of children, we need to recognize that all people are divided in the sense that they have feelings of warm self-regard as well as self-hatred and self-depreciation. Therefore, it is not surprising that parents would exhibit contradictory attitudes toward their offspring. Indeed, they act out aggression as well as tenderness and caring. Everyone expresses *both* tendencies in their close relationships. These conflicting responses have far-reaching significance regarding child development.

In addition, children are finely tuned to their parents' self-image; they feel comfortable and are able to relax and feel secure when their parents manifest positive regard for themselves. However, if parents exhibit strong feelings of inferiority and are predominantly self-critical or self-hating, children sense an implicit threat to their own security. They experience heightened anxiety and tend to have anticipatory fears of loss.

Parental attitudes toward their children are a by-product of their fundamental conflicts and ambivalence toward themselves. Only through developing compassion for themselves, and insight into their ambivalent feelings, can parents provide the necessary ingredients for their children's well-being. By the same token, to the extent that they fail to recognize these contradictory attitudes toward themselves and their children, they will act out insensitively, causing much unnecessary damage to their offspring.

THREATS TO PARENTS' DEFENSE SYSTEMS

As noted, children threaten the parents' defense system by reawakening suppressed feelings from the past. Consequently, parents maintain a certain distance and relate to the child primarily in terms of role-determined emotions and behaviors.

R. D. Laing (1990) has eloquently described the threat posed by the infant to the parents' defense system and parents' reactions to this threat:

> *Diaphobia: The fear of being affected, of being directly influenced by the other.*
> Babies, and infants, before they have become normalized (dulled and deadened, etc.) have to be defended against. They are tiny foci who emit signals genetically programmed to elicit reciprocity from adults. The schizoid, narcissistic, autistic, paranoid adult who is diaphobic is terrified of spontaneous reciprocity. The baby's genetic programmed devices to evoke responses which are cultured out of the normal adult pose a paranoid danger therefore to the normal adult.

However, the normal adult may still be "soft." The smiles, eyes, the out-stretched arms of the still healthy baby "demand." Their genetically programmed evocative qualities, programmed to elicit happy, effortless, complimentary, return-ing, reciprocal responses in the adult, are experienced by the normal schizoid, narcissistic, autistic, paranoid parent as assaultive, demanding, draining.

The normal adult has had his/her genetic own responses either completely cultured out, *or,* has learned at least to be suspicious, very, very ashamed, or guilty of them. He/she senses those of the baby as a threat, a danger, a manipu-lation, a demand, a pull, a tug, a *drain,* a trap. If the normalized adult gives into them, he/she will invite catastrophe. One has to resist them.

For example, it is necessary to avoid the eye contact. That eye "contact" is more than mere "contact." "Contact" is just the opening of the vertical barrier, the letting down of the barrier. . . .

Those outstretched arms open up a well of loneliness. The resistance to being drawn into the sphere of the *horizontal* reciprocal influence out of the stable isolation across the *vertical* dividing line, the *invisible wall,* brings up *gushes* of "bad" feelings—physical feelings, horrible feelings, feelings one has never felt before. But in these feelings, mixed up in them at once physical smells new and stale of ghosts of awakened sensations in oneself, are evoked, by that dead *me,* that me that was me, I see in the baby. . . .

I can't distinguish me from the baby. I see my feelings in his-her-your/its eyes. I tell myself that that baby is not-yet a you, a him, or a her, much less another me. It is just an it. But I "know" emotionally that is not true. This is another paranoid *danger.* I am in danger of seeing *it* as a him, or as a her. The baby is still appealing to me with the language of the heart, the language I have learned to forget and to mistrust with all my "heart." I can go in different directions. I can hate the baby for making me feel bad. I can envy the baby for still being human. I can feel bad/guilty/for feeling bad. I can feel a terrible burden of responsibility because I feel incapable to respond spontaneously. (pp. ix-x)

THE IMPLICIT PAIN OF
SENSITIVE CHILD REARING

When parents treat their children tenderly and in ways they themselves were not treated as children, they experience a certain amount of discomfort. Being sensitive to the child tends to reawaken primal feelings of sadness and pain related to the love and tender care that may have been lacking in their own childhood. For example, a father described feeling awkward and self-conscious when his 6-year-old son expressed affection toward him.

Father (in parent group): Mark was sitting on my lap at the movies and two or three times, he reached up to hug me and looked me straight in the eyes. I felt very uncomfortable, but I tried not to do anything to stop his affection. I instinctively understood that it would be a bad thing. I just sat there and felt sad and really pained for some strange reason, which I didn't understand at the time. Later, I realized that my father was rarely affectionate with me when I was a kid and that's what caused my discomfort.

Being loved and valued by their offspring induces in many parents a poignant, painful sadness that they find difficult to endure. Many pull away from their child after close contact. *The unwillingness of defended parents to allow repressed emotions to reemerge during tender moments with their children is a major reason they find it difficult to sustain loving, affectionate relationships with their children.*

NEGATIVE ATTITUDES TOWARD
SELF EXTENDED TO THE CHILD

Many parents dispose of their self-hatred and the qualities they dislike in themselves by projecting them onto their child. In this process of projection, the child is basically used as a waste receptacle or dumping ground (Bowen, 1978; Brazelton & Cramer, 1990; Kerr & Bowen, 1988). Many parents disown weaknesses and unpleasant characteristics in themselves, perceiving and punishing them instead in the child.

In one example, a mother with a rigid, prudish view about sex disowned any sexual feelings in herself and constantly worried about her daughter's emerging sexuality. Fearing the girl would become promiscuous when she reached adolescence, she intruded into her daughter's privacy by opening letters from her boyfriend and searching her belongings and schoolwork for clues indicating misconduct. Later, when she attended college, the girl fulfilled her mother's predictions by becoming promiscuously involved with many men and by deceiving her parents about her sexual activities.

In general, children accept parental attributions and take on the assigned negative identity while maintaining an idealized image of their parents. They become imprisoned for life in the narrow, restrictive labeling system that formed their identity within the family.

THE STYLE OF RELATING WITHIN THE COUPLE

The emotional climate into which a child is born is largely determined by the nature of the relationship that has already evolved between the parents, based on their own defense systems. Traditional coupling fosters dependence and exclusivity in the parents' relationship that has a detrimental effect on the child.

In forming a fantasy bond or illusion of connection, each partner has been diminished in his or her vitality, individuality, and sense of self through the use of the other for purposes of security. Parents in this situation have little energy to offer affection or direction to their children.

THE DEPENDENCY LOAD IMPLIED IN ASSUMING FULL RESPONSIBILITY FOR A CHILD

Parenthood symbolizes the end of childhood, and, to many, this signifies separation from parental support systems and the assumption of a role for which they are not emotionally equipped. This separation anxiety experienced by the parents, together with the needy demands of the infant, often arouses feelings of resentment toward the child.

Many expectant mothers and fathers entertain idealistic fantasies of what life will be like after their baby arrives. Reality quickly intrudes when new parents face the responsibilities of 24-hour care for their infant. Reactions to having such fantasies disrupted are varied. Many parents express disappointment, anxiety, resentment, disillusionment, and feelings of being burdened by the care of a new baby.

My associates and I have found that the infant is often perceived as an intrusion by his or her parents because the newborn makes them aware of their responsibilities for another person. Many people find it difficult to take this significant step into adulthood and feel insecure and self-doubting. Parents who were deprived or neglected as children discover they have trouble offering security and guidance to their own children, particularly during times of stress. In a parents' talk, a mother connected her fears about being a parent to her own parents' immaturity:

> When Chuck was small, as long as things were running smoothly and there were no ups and downs, I more or less provided for his needs, but if anything happened which disturbed the routine, not even a crisis, but simply changing schools or joining a club, then my whole mood changed. My anxiety became so intense that I didn't know how to deal with it, and I became almost paralyzed, like a child myself.
>
> I also remember when I was a child and didn't have any mature person around for guidance. Sometimes my anxiety was aroused to the point that I didn't even know my name; I couldn't think clearly at all. When I had to go to a new school, I felt totally lost.

Immature parents often perceive their child as getting the care and attention that they desire for themselves, and they have strong angry reactions. Childlike, undeveloped parents actually respond to the child as a competitor for affection and love. In some cases, new mothers and fathers show significant signs of jealousy toward the needy infant because the baby requires the undivided attention of their partner.

REASONS PARENTS HAVE CHILDREN

One interesting existential issue often overlooked is that most parents have children for the wrong reason—as a defense against death anxiety, a bid for immortality. They believe their children are extensions of them and experience feelings of exclusivity, connectedness, and possessiveness in relation to their progeny. To the extent that children closely resemble their parents in appearance, personality characteristics, behavior, and style of defense, they are the parents' legacy to be left in the world after the parents' death as evidence that their lives were meaningful. Parents imagine, on some level, that this "belonging" or merger imbues them with immortality.

However, this defense "works" only to the extent that the child is essentially the *same* as the parents in the qualities noted above. The more the child is *different* from the parents, the more he or she poses a threat to their illusions of immortality. Nonconformity and individuation are judged or perceived as "bad," while sameness with, or submission to, one's parents is seen as good.

In using the child as a symbol of immortality, parents feel both the need and the obligation to impose their own standards, beliefs, and value systems on their children. They feel duty-bound to teach their own self-protective coping mechanisms, although they may be distorted, crippling, and maladaptive. They transmit their defenses, beliefs, and values to children *both implicitly and explicitly,* that is, by example and direct instruction. Having been "processed," most children grow up feeling alienated from themselves, as though they have no inherent right to their own point of view as separate human beings.

SOCIAL PRESSURE TO OFFER
UNCONDITIONAL LOVE TO CHILDREN

The myth of unconditional love has become a fundamental part of our morality and leads to guilt reactions in parents who have a limited ability to sustain loving interactions with their offspring. The fact that parents are *supposed* to love their children, all the time, unconditionally, creates considerable pressure. Parents find it difficult to live up to this ideal; however, it serves no constructive purpose for them to conceal their limitations or weaknesses from themselves and their children.

MANY CHILDREN BECOME UNLIKABLE

Another reason parents find it difficult to sustain affectionate responses toward their offspring is that hurt children often develop unpleasant, undesirable personality traits; they become unlikable. Damage to children early in life tends to have negative effects on their character, making them difficult to like and love. Many deprived or rejected children become desperate, spiteful, unattractive, hard to be with, and inspire further rejection by parents and other people as well (Endnote 1).

Defenses and bad habits are formed very early in life. A cycle of rejection is set in motion. By the time children are 2 or 3 years old, they no longer are the naive, innocent, pure creatures they once were. By then, they have begun to withhold their capabilities, to act out passive or active aggression, to whine and complain, and to embarrass and manipulate their parents through "learned helplessness" (Endnote 2). Contrary to popular opinion, children are not just "going through a phase" when they display these regressive behaviors or act "bad" or unpleasant. Unless interrupted, the obnoxious habits children form at an early age will persist and develop into more sophisticated negative behavior patterns and deep character defenses when they are adults.

PARENTING GROUPS:
A PREVENTIVE PSYCHOTHERAPY

In the unique psychological laboratory described in Chapter 1, my associates and I started parenting talks to help people develop better relationships with their children.[1] This became a topic of major concern as more and more children were born into the friendship circle. The parents in the reference population have participated in these specialized parenting groups for a period of many years. They observed the transmission of faulty child-rearing practices through three generations, beginning with grandparents, perpetuated through parents themselves, and subsequently directed toward their offspring. In these talks, people were able to challenge their negative attitudes and behaviors, thereby interrupting the cycle of maltreatment.

The dual focus of our specialized parenting groups was (a) to allow parents to expose negative attitudes and behavior toward children in a supportive environment and (b) to encourage parents to remember painful incidents they experienced in their own upbringing (Endnote 3). As these talks progressed, a systemized approach to parenting groups evolved that was later extended to the general public.

---

1 Material in this section is taken from a (1989) article, "Parenting Groups Based on Voice Therapy," *Psychotherapy, 26*, 524-529. Used with permission.

The steps in the therapeutic process included parents (a) opening up and working through ambivalent feelings and attitudes toward themselves and their children; (b) recalling painful events from their own childhoods; (c) releasing the repressed affect associated with negative experiences in growing up; (d) exposing deficiencies in their families, thereby breaking the idealization of their own parents; (e) understanding the connection between their present-day limitations and the defensive patterns set up to cope with early trauma; and (f) developing more compassionate child-rearing practices based on constructive attitude change.

When parents discussed their ambivalent feelings, especially negative attitudes toward themselves, they used Voice Therapy techniques to bring out the content of their self-critical thoughts. We asked parents to state their self-attacks in the second person—"You never do anything right!" "You're not a good mother (father)"—as though they were being addressed or spoken to by another person. Through this method, parents developed considerable insight into their own childhoods and became aware of how they projected their negative attitudes and qualities onto their children.

In one group discussion, Mario revealed his negative attitudes toward himself in relation to women:

> The main attack I make on myself is: "You're not really a man! What kind of a man do you think you are? You can't do anything. You are worse than a kid! You have never grown up. Yeah, you had a son, so it just happened [*Snide, sarcastic tone*]. Big thing! By mistake. You're still a kid. Don't you know that a kid can't have sexuality?"

In a separate meeting, Mario's 20-year-old son exposed self-attacks similar to those expressed by his father: " 'What makes you think a woman could be attracted to you? [*Baiting, derisive tone*] You have no features that could be attractive to a woman. You're ugly. You're short. You're small! You're just like a kid!' " (Later, in a pilot study, we found that children's self-critical thoughts or voices closely corresponded to those of their parents in terms of core issues in their lives and significant areas of conflict.)

In this unusual forum, mothers and fathers came to understand their destructive behavior and developed a sense of compassion for themselves and their children. Regaining feeling about their own childhood experiences was the key element in the therapeutic process that enabled them to alter their child-rearing practices in a positive direction.

Although it is true that increasing parental awareness can foster guilt reactions, when this awareness was carried to a more complete understanding of the cycle, parents' guilt was actually diminished. One woman who had been afraid of acting out internalized rage toward her children, spoke of important changes that had taken place in her life over the course of the meetings:

Since I've been talking about these abusive feelings in the parents' talks, I've felt different. I don't feel so afraid. Before we talked about these feelings, I felt terrified almost all the time to be around children, and particularly my own children. Now that I've told the "truth" about how I really feel, it's not like I'm a bad person, so I think that I relate better to children in general, but especially to my daughter, Carol. I relate to her more as a person.

Another parent, who described verbally abusing his son, subsequently recalled being the recipient of similar treatment as a youngster.

I remember yelling at my son, telling him that he had no right to think or behave a certain way, that he had no right to feel a certain way, yelling at him in a way that took away his right to think or feel something.

But then, I remembered, and I think it was for the first time, my father furiously yelling at me, screaming, "You *won't* feel that way! I won't have you thinking such things! You can't act that way!"

First I was able to recall incidents about my son, and then I could remember being treated exactly the same way by my father. I feel like I've gained some kind of understanding about why I punished my son, and this has made me feel compassion for myself and how *I* was hurt as a kid.

The format of the specialized parenting groups described here has been extended to parent education programs attended by mothers and fathers from diverse ethnic groups and populations throughout the country. Early findings from pilot studies evaluating this program indicate that it is an effective prevention methodology in that it helps alter parents' attitudes toward themselves and their children in a positive direction (Endnote 4).

Apologists, or those who deemphasize parental influences, tend to base their explanations regarding the etiology of psychological disturbance on biological or hereditary factors. As stated previously, I feel that the harm done to children is overdetermined by environmental factors—actual abuses that injure the child's psyche. People who subscribe to the former explanations rely heavily on the concept of temperamental differences, which detracts from the significance of parents' impact on a child and lessens their accountability for responsible child-rearing practices. However, even temperamental differences can be modified in a healthy environment.

John Bowlby in 1984[2] commented on the issue of temperamental differences in a videotaped interview:

---

2 Dr. Bowlby's statements were transcribed from a videotape titled *Theoretical Aspects of Attachment* (David Scott May, M.D., and Marion Solomon, Ph.D., Producers), Division of Child Psychiatry, UCLA Neuropsychiatric Institute and Hospital (1984).

An awful lot has been talked about in temperament. Now, temperament is a rubbish bin; if you can't understand something, you put it down to temperament. . . .

There's no reliable way of measuring infant temperament, which doesn't mean to say that there aren't temperamental differences, but simply that we don't know how to measure them. One important finding has been this: that, with few exceptions, the way an infant behaves in the first week or two of life, he's responsive or unresponsive, or he's hypersensitive or he's less sensitive, or whatever he might be, does *not* correlate with the pattern of attachment as seen at twelve months.

In other words, sensitive, responsive mothers are capable of enabling an infant who is, by any standards, rather touchy or difficult in the early days, to become a securely attached child by twelve months. That's very heartening! So the notion, oh well of course, these patterns of attachment correlate with temperament, does not stand up.

My clinical experience agrees with and tends to confirm Bowlby's statements. In a number of cases, I have observed the relief of serious symptoms and significant improvement in disturbed children raised by substitute or foster parents. With two cases in particular, my colleagues and I conjectured that the youngsters' disturbances were caused by a constitutional weakness or biological propensity because of the early onset of symptomatology. However, when the children's symptoms became so severe that the parents asked for help from friends in the reference population, there was immediate improvement following separation from the parents. In these cases, it was clear that we were wrong in our original thinking. It became obvious that the parental environment had been the major contributing factor in early symptom formation.

I am reminded of a woman whose family I knew as she was growing up. As a teenager, she was described by her parents as cold, hateful, and capable of aggressive or even violent behavior. In the 40 years I have known her, however, she has never exhibited a trace of the hostile nature attributed to her by her parents; to the contrary, she is a warm, even-tempered person, who is known for her friendliness and congeniality.

CONCLUSION

I have demonstrated that the psychological mistreatment of children is widespread in our culture and its effects are long-lasting. I have outlined the form that these abuses take in the child's development. To elucidate these problems, my associates and I have developed a series of documentary films, articles, and books that illustrate the phenomena. In terms of preventive mental health, it is vital to recognize the core issues involved in breaking the chain of emotional child abuse and to intervene, whenever possible, in cases where infants and children are experiencing serious emotional problems and psychological disturbance. I concur with the statement made by Gregory Zilboorg (1932) in a speech delivered at the 1931 conference of the American Orthopsychiatric Association:

> I should like to say in conclusion not only that the hostile trends operating in the unconscious of the parents present a universal phenomenon which deserves to awaken the curiosity of the practical psychopathologist, but that they are potent, dynamic factors which we must know in considerable detail if we are to deal with neurotic maladjustment, delinquency, and other related problems in children. (pp. 41-42)

To help future generations of children, we must try to overcome our prejudices, develop an objective view of dynamics in the nuclear family, and critically evaluate dehumanizing child-rearing practices that are an extensive part of our culture.

My optimism in writing about childhood suffering stems from my belief that some people, by *not* surrendering to their internal processing and their parents' fears and anxieties, can break the chain of pain and neurosis that is passed from generation to generation. Perhaps, over the generations, there could be movement toward a better environmental picture in relation to child rearing. Perhaps, in future generations, parents will no longer be "the lost children."

ENDNOTES

1. Schakel (1987) reported results from a study of diagnosed failure-to-thrive infants:

> These infants, if placed in a hospital or with foster parents, become cheerful and active. Eventually, however, they are likely to begin to seek attention and they will become "shallowly affectionate." Later, unpleasant traits such as spitefulness or selfishness appear. Stealing is reported to be common among such children. . . . Their anxious emptiness becomes hidden behind a shield of brittle, hostile defiance; in other words, they "turn mean." (pp. 104-105)

2. Children who are psychologically mistreated form "the expectation that events are uncontrollable" (Seligman, 1975, p. 60). They tend to believe that their actions are also uncontrollable, as do their parents. Seligman, who developed the concept of "learned helplessness," contended that maternal deprivation as well as a lack of provision of resolvable frustration and conflict on the part of parents leads to the child's lack of self-control and feelings of hopelessness.

3. In their classic article, "Ghosts in the Nursery," Fraiberg, Adelson, and Shapiro (1975/1980) discussed methods for dealing with these "intruders from the past." They wrote,

Our hypothesis is that access to childhood pain becomes a powerful deterrent against repetition in parenting, while repression and isolation of painful affect provide the psychological requirements for identification with the betrayers and the aggressors. (p. 195)

4. Instruments to assess changes in parents' feelings of self-esteem and positive attitudes toward their children are administered prior to, immediately following, and 6 months after participants complete classes in *The Compassionate Child-Rearing Parent Education Program.* The self-report questionnaires include two Rohner Parental Acceptance/Rejection measures, the Mother PARQ and Adult PAQ (Rohner, 1991), the Coopersmith Inventory (Coopersmith, 1975), the Parenting Satisfaction Scale (Guidubaldi & Cleminshaw, 1994), and the Parental Attitude subscale of the Human Sexuality Questionnaire (Zuckerman, 1959).

5

Identification With
the Aggressor

The weak and undeveloped personality reacts to sudden unpleasure not
by defence, but by anxiety-ridden identification and by introjection of
the menacing person or aggressor.

Sandor Ferenczi (1933/1955, p. 163)

In the face of emotional pain or intolerable anxiety, the child attempts to preserve some level of rationality and sense of unity. Efforts to maintain logic and systematic thought under unusual, stressful conditions lead to the specific defense of identifying with the aggressor. Rather than suffer complete ego disintegration, children make a strong identification with the same forces that produce the torment they are trying to escape.

In situations where there are deficiencies in the parental environment or where parents are punitive or abusive, the child ceases to identify with him- or herself as the helpless victim and assumes the characteristics of the powerful, hurtful, or punishing parent. This maneuver of splitting from the self partially alleviates the child's terror and provides a sense of relief. In the process,

AUTHOR'S NOTE: The substance of this chapter is taken primarily from an article titled, "A New Perspective on the Oedipal Complex: A Voice Therapy Session," *Psychotherapy, 31* (1994), pp. 342-351. Used with permission.

however, he or she takes on not only the parent's animosity and the aggression directed toward him or her, but the guilt, the fear, indeed, the total complex of the parent's defensive adaptation. Once incorporated, the process lends itself to a feeling of being invaded or possessed by an internal enemy. Feelings of demonic possession as demonstrated in films and other accounts are symbolic exaggerations of this phenomenon. Furthermore, this complex of internalized parental voices represents an integrated point of view, a systematic organization of feelings and attitudes toward the self that are inflexible and become the core resistance to change and the opportunity for a better life (Endnote 1).

R. D. Laing (1960/1969) has described this form of splitting or depersonalization:

> The splitting is not simply a temporary reaction to a specific situation of great danger, which is reversible when the danger is past. It is, on the contrary, a basic orientation to life, and if it is followed back through their [patients'] lives one usually finds that they seem, in fact, to have emerged from the early months of infancy with this split already under way. (p. 79)

In the circumstances that Laing describes, the hurt child incorporates a negative thought process at a very young age and develops a point of view opposed to his or her own priorities. It is my conjecture that covert or unspoken parental aggression or rage may be more threatening to the child than rage expressed in punitive or explosive actions.[1] The child sensing unconscious or covert malevolence in his or her parent or parents experiences intense anticipatory fear or terror without insight into its source. The child's tendency is to split off from the identity of the powerless "victim," identify with the powerful parent or aggressor, and later act out parents' destructive attitudes against him- or herself. In situations where parental death wishes were extreme and pervasive, some people eventually mutilate or physically destroy themselves.

In his analysis of patients who manifested serious self-destructive behaviors, Bruno Bettelheim (1983) posed the question: "Why should we incorporate into the essence of our being the desire of those who (at least once) wished to destroy us?" (p. 302). Bettelheim answers by noting that

> the parent-child bond is powerful. . . . The younger we are, the more we respond to what we feel are the most powerful emotions of the person who is most important to us, and it does not matter what the nature of these emotions is. (p. 302)

---

1 This statement does not deny the damage caused by overt physical and sexual abuse. For example, several studies have demonstrated correlations between physical abuse in childhood and later suicide attempts (Frederick, 1985; Sabbath, 1969).

The identification with the parental power structure is strong, whether or not the situation is punitive; the more children feel powerless and victimized, the stronger the identification. The use of the phrase *parental power* does not connote power in the positive sense, that is, intelligence, resourcefulness, personal or physical strength, or greater understanding. It pertains more to control, and, ironically, the most controlling and intimidating person in the family will often be the weakest, most self-destructive, or the most disturbed. Under these circumstances, other family members tend to give up their power and defer to this individual out of fear or guilt. In identifying with this type of controlling individual, the helpless child, facing painful circumstances with an uncertain outcome, internalizes the characteristics of the disturbed person to his or her own detriment. In this manner, he or she achieves an illusion of security and mastery, which, to varying degrees, relieves his or her anxiety. Thereafter, a strong sense of pseudoindependence and denial of external need develops within the child.

Even when the prevailing family attitudes are positive, elements of parental insensitivity are introjected during infrequent stressful situations. When parents become excessively anxious, irrational, or angry, destructive attitudes are incorporated that become part of the individual's personality as he or she develops into maturity. R. D. Laing (1960/1969) has depicted this "takeover" of an individual's personality by the internalized parent as follows:

> A most curious phenomenon of the personality, one which has been observed for centuries, but which has not yet received its full explanation, is that in which the individual seems to be the vehicle of a personality that is not his own. Someone else's personality seems to "possess" him and to be finding expression through his words and actions, whereas the individual's own personality is temporarily "lost" or "gone." This happens with all degrees of malignancy. There seems to be all degrees of the same basic process from the simple, benign observation that so-and-so "takes after his father," or "that's her mother's temper coming out in her," to the extreme distress of the person who finds himself under a compulsion to take on the characteristics of a personality he may hate and/or feel to be entirely alien to his own. (p. 58)

For example, a woman noted that whenever she wanted to say something positive or sweet to her husband, she found herself saying something angry or argumentative in place of her original feelings. Instead of acting loving and vulnerable, she acted tough and defining in a manner that was reminiscent of her mother's style. Her mother was hateful and critical of men and thought of them as inept. The woman treated her husband in that way even though she was aware that he was capable. In free-associating about the situation, she reported a feeling that if she gave in and trusted her husband, "her spirit would have been broken." It was difficult for her to break this defense and experience her softness as a woman.

Anna Freud (1966) asserted that the mechanism of identification or introjection combines with imitation to "form one of the ego's most potent weapons in its dealings with external objects which arouse its anxiety" (p. 110). "By impersonating the aggressor, assuming his attributes or imitating his aggression, the child transforms himself from the person threatened into the person who makes the threat" (p. 113).

Bruno Bettelheim (1943/1979) applied the concept of identification with the aggressor (in a limited sense) to his interpretation of the behavior of "old prisoners" (prisoners who had undergone years of torture and deprivation) in Nazi Germany's concentration camps.

> Old prisoners who identified themselves with the SS did so not only in respect to aggressive behavior. They would try to acquire old pieces of SS uniforms. . . . Old prisoners accepted Nazi goals and values, too, even when these seemed opposed to their own interests. (p. 79)

In summary, when faced with covert or overt parental aggression, children make the best adaptation possible to preserve some form of rationality and sanity, no matter how primitive (Noyes, Hoenk, Kuperman, & Slymen, 1977) (Endnote 2). When conditions are miserable or terrifying, elements of an observing, punishing, parental self combine with parts of the hurt, frightened child-self to form the antiself system, as depicted in Figure 5.1, "Division of the Mind." Ironically, the child's desperate struggle to preserve intactness and wholeness produces fragmentation and disintegration.

ORIGINS OF PARENTAL AGGRESSION IN RELATION TO THE OEDIPAL COMPLEX

In the course of our study, my associates and I uncovered a number of reasons parents feel angry and resentful toward their children and at times wish to get rid of them. As noted previously, parents' defenses are threatened by their children. The helplessness and vulnerability of the child remind parents of their own weaknesses and fears, qualities that many parents find unacceptable in themselves. In addition, children represent a dependency burden that threatens immature parents. Finally, the child is perceived as a rival by the parent of the same sex.

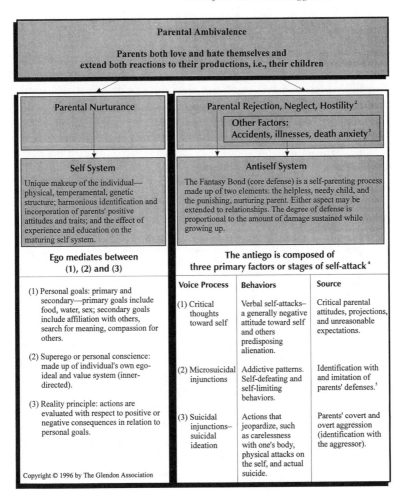

Figure 5.1. Division of the Mind[1]

1. Division as indicated on the chart is oversimplified with abrupt boundaries for purposes of elucidation. Psychological functions are more complex, and mental events and internal conflict are always multidetermined.

2. I feel that psychological factors are more significant in emotional disorders than other factors, that is, inherited characteristics, biological states, and accidents, illness, and so on affecting the human condition. Also, negative experiences in the family contribute most directly to human suffering. For example, in times of war, the suicide rate decreases, and in times of tragedy, there is not a corresponding increase in mental illness.

3. Despair is inherent in the human condition in relation to the fact of death. People feel scared of the unknown and vulnerable. Death anxiety supports the defense system, particularly at the point in the developmental sequence when the child first becomes aware of death.

4. The three factors correspond to the patterns of negative thoughts accessed by the Firestone Assessment of Self-Destructive Thoughts (1996) developed in collaboration with L. Firestone.

5. The imitation of parents' attitudes and defenses is inevitable; it has a powerful survival function on a primitive level, as in the animal kingdom.

Sexual Rivalry in the Family System

Despite the fact that incestuous and competitive feelings toward one's children are unacceptable to most parents, they do exist and are capable of arousing intense jealousy and aggression in insecure parents. In many families, the child is seen as a threat to the security of the couple and an intrusion into the fantasy bond they have formed. Couples whose relationships are characterized by exclusivity, possessiveness, and excessive dependency experience considerable jealousy in relation to rivals or competitors. However, most men and women find it difficult to admit feelings of anger, jealousy, and sexual rivalry in relation to their children.

The Incest Taboo

The formation of a fantasy bond in long-term relationships is based on an attempt to attain security, safety, and immortality by assuring sexual fidelity. The marriage ceremony, monogamy, and restrictive or exclusive coupling are attempts to prevent threats from competitors to the security of the couple. However, the birth of a child brings a new rival into the picture, disturbing the sense of equilibrium and security within the couple. Historically, the incest taboo, which existed even in most primitive cultures, is an attempt to avert threats from a rival *within the family system*. In fact, the taboo evolved because there is a basic competition between same-sex family members, indeed, between all individuals living in close quarters. However, incestuous feelings and the resultant rivalry are not eliminated by prohibitive or restrictive codes. These rivalrous feelings exist within families and are exceptionally strong in parents who are narcissistic, jealous, and overly possessive. As noted, immature parents are threatened not only by the child as a sexual rival but also by his or her demands for attention from the other partner as well as the partner's response to such demands.

Thus insecure parents often feel considerable resentment and hatred toward their children, but suppress their wish to get rid of them. Nevertheless, children pick up or assimilate parents' covert death wishes and aggression in the form of a self-hating thought process. A number of theorists have noted the presence of unconscious death wishes in parents and their effects on children (Rosenbaum & Richman, 1970). For example, Bettelheim (1956/1979) observed that the schizophrenic child's reactions are "strangely similar" to those of prisoners in the concentration camps, and went on to state that "specific events, different for each child, had convinced these children that they were threatened by total destruction all of the time, and that no personal relations offered any protection or emotional relief" (p. 117).

In a similar vein, Dorothy Bloch (1978), child psychoanalyst, has written about children's fears of infanticide and their defense against such fears: "Once I began to probe the function of children's fantasies, it became apparent that they were a means of survival and defended the children against their fear of infanticide" (p. 13).

Bloch cited cases in which preschool youngsters (both boys and girls) assumed the opposite sexual identity in a desperate attempt to escape the perceived danger of infanticide:

> In the cases of the four children who acted out the fantasy of a homosexual identity, each felt his [her] life was threatened by the parent of the same sex. . . . [Each felt] that the parent of the opposite sex preferred him [her] to the other parent . . . [leading them] to conclude that only a change of sex could secure the threatening parent's love and thus save his [her] life. (pp. 69-70)

As noted previously, children identify with the punitive, rivalrous parent, taking on as their own the parent's aggression and adopting the parent's hostile point of view toward themselves. Later, as adults, they often feel the most self-hating and self-destructive in competitive or rivalrous situations.

The Role of Competition and Parental Aggression

When adult individuals are involved in competitive situations in relation to the pursuit of their goals, often negative or self-destructive thoughts become more pervasive. Because of this, many people pull back from competing; on some level, they anticipate the arousal of suicidal voices and the associated rage toward self. In general, they retreat before they are consciously aware of their self-attacks or suicidal voices. Often they suppress these destructive urges and attempt to objectify their aggression toward themselves by projecting the attack as though coming from outside, leading to an essentially paranoid orientation.

In a 12-year study involving over 2,500 women, Rheingold (1964) found that many recalled childhood fears of being killed or mutilated by a hostile, vindictive mother: "The threat of retaliation . . . forces her to abandon her aspirations [to be a better wife and mother] and surrounds all woman-roles with danger" (p. 267).

Rheingold stressed the fact that marriage once again arouses a woman's fear of her mother, a familiar sense of dread that she has lived with since infancy:

> Marriage is a crisis for the woman. . . . Next to pregnancy and becoming a mother, marriage poses the greatest threat because it represents two bold acts of self-

assertion: assuming the status of the married woman and entering into a publicly announced heterosexual relationship. (p. 437)

Similar psychodynamics are operant in families where the male child feels threatened by retribution from an insecure father and later retreats from adult expressions of masculinity. The dynamics discussed here contribute to an understanding of unresolved Oedipal issues. When people feel threatened, they identify with parental aggression toward them as a rival, and they react as if they were the incorporated other.

Later, when the individual finds him- or herself in a competitive situation, the incorporated hateful feelings toward self are aroused. In this manner, Oedipal issues play an important part in self-destructive thought and action, and in very serious cases involve a suicidal outcome. In their work, J. Kestenberg and M. Kestenberg (1987) suggested that "having discovered murderous wishes toward parents, psychoanalysis neglected to deal systematically with the murderous wishes of parents toward their children" (p. 149). In other words, psychoanalysts have focused primarily on the child's rage instead of the parent's, and this has obscured their understanding (Endnote 3).

Case Study

The case of Roger demonstrates a retreat from Oedipal rivalry and provides an example of an individual whose angry competitive feelings were turned inward against the self, giving strong support to the antiself system.

Roger, 38, first entered therapy when he was 19 and suffering from a major depressive episode and persistent thoughts of suicide precipitated by the loss of the relationship with his high school girlfriend. After 2 years of therapy during which there was noticeable improvement in his affective state, Roger developed a stronger sense of self, embarked on a career in computer programming, and eventually started his own business. Several years later, his business expanded and sales increased significantly, bringing him financial success and a sense of accomplishment. He was aware that he had surpassed his father, who was on the brink of financial disaster because of poor business decisions and mismanagement of investments. This significant accomplishment triggered a severe state of anxiety in Roger, which gradually took the form of paranoid thoughts toward other men. At this point, he requested a session to deal with his depression and increased agitation.

In the Voice Therapy session that follows, Roger first describes his adverse reactions to his recent achievements. Later, in recounting his life history, he develops insight into the restrictions he still places on himself in relation to competing with other men for positions of power. He connects his limitations to the fear he felt as a child in the face of his father's explosive anger and rage.

Before I went to Mexico this winter, I felt better than I'd felt in a long time. There were a lot of things that were really going well in my life. I felt good in business. I had a confidence in myself that I had never had before.

The contrast to that is that when I came home, I felt like I didn't care about anything. I had no excitement, no energy. I dreaded getting up in the morning again. I felt depressed. I just wanted to blend away. I wanted to sort of fade into the carpet.

The thing that really shakes me up is that I began to have not really suicidal thoughts, but thoughts in a loud voice, just wanting to rip myself to pieces. In relation to my male friends, instead of feeling really comfortable with them, I started feeling very paranoid with them. At different times, I'd start to feel like men were really angry at me.

During the period of time to which Roger refers, his sister had talked about a traumatic family incident that happened when he was 8 years old, an incident that he had almost forgotten.

Sue started talking about how things were in the family and how my father really was. She went over an event that happened where he wanted to throw me out of the house and made me pack my clothes and was calling a taxicab and they were going to truck me away. I had put it away in my mind that the whole thing was my fault, and I had explained it, like I deserved it on some level, even though I knew it was a horrible event.

But to hear it from *her* point of view made me feel like "God, this thing really did happen to me," and it shook me up, and I was almost angry at her for bringing that whole subject up. Anyway, I realized how much I really wasn't wanted in my family by my father.

Other incidents came to mind as Roger further explored events from his childhood. Two important themes began to emerge: (a) the unremitting threat Roger felt in relation to his father's uncontrollable rage, and (b) his mother's seductive interest in him and her rejection of his father. This intensified his father's jealous hatred and increased Roger's sense of living in constant danger.

I also remember that when I was about 4 or 5 years old, we had this dog. It was a collie and it would always come up and take crackers out of my hand. Once my father came home, and he was angry at the dog for taking the crackers, but I was feeding the dog, so he kicked the dog. He kicked him really hard, and the dog died.

I knew that kick wasn't meant for the dog. It had nothing to do with the dog. It had to do with me. And it was a blind rage. He was furious. He needed an excuse, and he kicked the dog. That scared me.

I remember that I had what I would call a strange relationship with my mother at that time. This is before I went to school. She would take these long naps and

I would lay down with her, during that time, and just sleep with her. And I felt embarrassed—not exactly embarrassed, but I know that contrasted with this thing with my father who was furious with me all the time. It seemed like that just aggravated it.

Roger moved out of the family home when he was 18 and lived with a girlfriend for a year at a ski resort. When his relationship with his girlfriend ended, his world seemed to crumble. Soon after, he lost his job and started taking drugs.

I'd spend all day, because I didn't have a job, sitting in this trailer on the outskirts of town in this terrible place. It was snowing all the time and I hated waking up. One morning I woke up and I decided to kill myself. That had been building for a long time. I was thinking: "Why don't you just end this? Why don't you just be done with this? You feel so bad. Let's just go ahead and just get done with it."

I tried to slit my wrists that night, but my friend came home. I had stopped it beforehand. I said, "I don't want this to happen." But I was feeling really terrible. And that's what made me start therapy.

Therapy helped Roger identify the sources of his self-destructive thoughts, which led to a marked improvement in his self-esteem and life circumstances.

I had my business, which was beginning to work out really well. I felt free and active and I had a sense of myself again. Then things began to change.

Roger goes on to describe the current situation and examines his fear of men in more depth:

I have a feeling that something else is affecting me right now. I'm afraid of standing out. I'm afraid of being taken seriously. I'm afraid of other men looking me in the eye and being acknowledged as an equal.

I feel like I do things in my everyday actions with all men and people in general where I basically check in with them saying, "You don't have to worry about me. I'm fine. I'm not a competitor. I don't have any opinions about anything."

But I feel that I'm at a point where that's visibly not true about me any more. I'm running a business. I have issues with employees to address every day. I have to be strong in those situations, and it's a contrast. It's stupid for me to walk around acting that way.

So if I'm in a conversation with a man and I'm beginning to check in by acting that way, it stands out. I feel like gagging. I feel like throwing up. It makes me sick to my stomach. But I feel like there's a need for me to do that, and I don't like that need.

I actually feel paranoid toward other men in my life like I'm going to get in trouble by continuing to be successful, which is insane, if I really just say it out loud. But it's a gut level fear and it stands out to me.

Roger's case history as recounted thus far in the session demonstrates a pattern that fits the interpretation of the Oedipal complex described earlier. As a child, he was close to his mother, and his father was angry, intensely jealous, and explosive. According to Roger, his father saw him as a rival and wished to dispose of him. This unconscious wish was demonstrated in the incident where he actually put the 8-year-old youngster out of the house. In identifying with his father, Roger took on his father's rage in the form of voices telling him to do away with himself. In psychoanalytic terms, Roger experienced considerable castration anxiety whenever he began to compete for a woman or achieve success in business. At these times, he would turn on himself to the point of having self-destructive thoughts.

The treatment focus in this session was one of exposing the hostile voices as they came to the surface and helping Roger develop an integrated point of view that would allow him to move toward his basic goals without surrendering to the self-destructive process. At this point in the session, Roger discusses in more detail the traumatic incident he described earlier.

That one incident where I got thrown out of the house stands out to me. What really happened that night before I got thrown out was that I was at the dinner table and I was feeling really good and joking around with my mother and my two sisters. We were having the time of our lives. It was a happy time in our family right then.

And my father was sitting there, just looking at the ceiling, just beginning to boil—and then he just blew up.

He just wanted me out. It was like an insane act, and I thought at the time, "He's really jealous. He's absolutely jealous. He wants me out. He hates not being number one in this family."

After that, for years, there was all this talk of military school. "Let's get you out of the house for the summer, let's ship you back East. Let's try to find a nice military school. I can't do anything with this kid."

In my family I was faced with two options. One, I could be the perpetual fuck-up and be looked at as being like a fuck-up and no good and everybody would hate me, or at least my father would hate me. Or I could really try to do something with my life and get killed, basically get killed.

Here Roger verbalizes the self-punishing thoughts and voices underlying his depression.

In terms of these voices I could get into, I wanted to say the specifics of what I felt like since I got back from Mexico. It's a weird image. I don't understand it. The voices are the feelings a rival would have toward someone else. *This* voice is furious, different from the ones I had when I attempted suicide. This one is:

"What are you doing here? You're not supposed to be here. [*Loud voice*] Get out of here. Go find a gun. Find a gun! What would it feel like to suck on a gun? Suck on a gun. Just suck on a gun and then pull the trigger. Pull the trigger. Blow your head off! Just blow your head off!" [*Intense rage, yelling loudly*]

"Blow your brains all over the wall! What would it feel like to have your skull just lift off the back of your head? Smash your head. Smash it! Blast your brains. Put that gun in your mouth and suck on it. Smash it! I don't want a piece left of you. I want you to die horribly. I want you to die in pain, pain, pain! Blow your head off." [*Cries deeply*]

Roger then answers back to the voice from his own point of view and expresses his outrage and pain. His spontaneous insights into the meaning of the sexual symbolism implied in the suicidal image point to an important dynamic in this Oedipal conflict, that is, placating the father while turning his father's sadistic attitudes on himself.

God, God, God! I didn't think about it, but that image of sucking on a gun—he wants me to suck on his dick. What is this? "Fuck you, you fucking asshole. Fuck you!"

It's so weird. It's like he had a sadistic wanting to take a person apart in pieces, just like someone, a Nazi doctor in a concentration camp, wanting to do experiments on people just for the heck of it, to see what happens.

Roger identifies the contents of the sadistic voice he incorporated from his father associated with painful incidents in his childhood:

"If you put a human body in these conditions, what would it look like? What would it feel like?" [*Snide, sarcastic tone*]

"What would it feel like to feel your skull slowly lift off the back of your head and for your brains to come out and for you to still be alive when that's happening? What would that feel like? Wouldn't that be interesting to see that happen?"

What is that? What a stupid thing! He's crazy. He's so crazy. Fucking son of a bitch!

When I was growing up, I always wondered what my fascination was with doctors in the concentration camps wanting to do weird human experiments. It's really the way that I felt like he was. He just has a cold, nonfeeling attitude of wanting to take a person apart, experiment, dissect them, look at them, take them apart, look at the guts. What does this do? How does that connect? The sadistic wanting to do something to humans.

In identifying the sources of his sadistic attack on himself, Roger understands the meaning of the defensive maneuvers he adopted to try to ensure his survival as a child. He makes an important distinction between the voices that drove him to attempt suicide when he was a teenager and the self-attacks he experiences in relation to his current success in the business world.

Roger: I feel like the only way I could have survived there is just to stay out of his way. I had to blend into the carpet. I couldn't stand out. I couldn't keep things organized. I couldn't make even a hint that I was there. I had to be invisible in the family.

Dr. F.: You expressed a lot of intense feelings. How do you feel now after expressing that?

Roger: I feel relaxed and clear. I don't have a lot of noise going on in my brain. My feeling about my own voice is that when it's going full bore, it's like a yell in my brain.

   I also feel like I understand some things. I understand that when I was working at the ski resort, I never heard a voice yelling like that, because I feel like I gave into it before it ever got to a voice. I feel like falling in love with a girl symbolizes going back to a relationship with my mother and giving up on my life, and then when that went away, I had nothing.

   Then it was a quiet soothing kind of voice saying, "You were born a misfit. You never should have lived past birth. You should have died in an incubator." It was a different kind of suicidal voice, but which coincidentally matches my mother's idea about me, when I think about it.

   This other voice has to do with trying to be different in my life in a way that I've never been before in terms of being okay in business, and I would really describe this as just being myself. I'm not holding myself back and it's easy, and my voice is very upset about that, furious. It wants to rip me to shreds.

Dr. F.: You are competing now.

Roger: I'm competing in the real world.

Dr. F.: You are out there in the open, and the voices are more savage and sadistic.

Roger: There are two ways of dealing with the voices. One is to try to do what I'm doing here and to just address it and know what it has to do with. But the other way would be to subtly undo my business over a course of time and to become unsuccessful and to blend away symbolically like I did in my family.

Dr. F.: Placate, as in sucking on the gun.

Roger: Right, basically. To give in, to cave in and kiss up to men again. I understand now why I feel like gagging.

Dr. F.: You either withdraw from competing or face up to these voices and try
to work them through.

Roger: Right.

Several weeks after the session, Roger reported feeling a sense of relaxation
and renewed energy in relation to his business. He spoke of additional insights
he had gained since the session.

In my session, I realized that my father was a crazy man. I never realized it to
the degree that I did in that session. There were reasons why I didn't compete in
my everyday life, because that was the way that I survived in my family, the only
way I could possibly do it.

And those fears followed me. Instead of seeing that my father was really like
that, to the degree that I did the other day, those fears were somehow transmitted
onto every other man in my adult life and on every situation, so I'd have a gut
level feeling of not being able to compete. I'd feel like men were going to kill
me.

I don't have that any more. But instead I feel like it has to do with the past.
It has nothing to do with my real life now.

Discussion of the Session

In the session, Roger developed considerable insight into the origins of his
suicidal impulses and irrational fears of men. He was able to recall important
events from his childhood that had shaped his life as well as his emotional
reactions to these events. Most important, he connected his present-day behavior
to the defenses he was forced to adopt in relation to his father's rage, and he was
able to take back the projections he had made onto other men. He understood
his irrational paranoid reactions to male competitors as a repetition of his
response to the *real* dangers he faced in relation to his father's jealous rage.

The image of sucking on the gun represented a symbolic homosexual impulse
to placate the father, thereby minimizing the ever-present threat from an aggressive, dangerous individual who lived in close proximity to the youngster.
Roger's description of "kissing up" to men was an extension of that same desire
to be safe from aggressive retaliation from symbolic paternal substitutes in his
current life. To protect himself, he felt that he should not be conspicuous, he
should not achieve, he should not conquer in the sense of being successful with
women. Consequently, Roger was unable to be successful in business or with
women without generating the voice process to do away with himself, to destroy
himself.

It is important to note that Roger's father had been treated similarly as a child
and had been subjected to the same kind of sadistic mistreatment by his own

father. During Roger's childhood, his father had made an effort to suppress his rage and control the impulse to act it out, but his aggression would burst out at times in an uncontrollable explosion of sadistic fury toward his son.

In considering this case, one can understand Freud's compelling interest in the Oedipal conflict. Powerful destructive forces exist within many family constellations that arise because of the sexual rivalry between family members. When individuals begin to achieve success in direct competition with a rival or rivals, considerable anxiety and guilt are often aroused, along with tendencies toward self-annihilation. I have found that unusual achievement, both personal and vocational, or attainment of a leadership position often precede periods of self-limiting and self-destructive behavior. This is particularly evident when a person's accomplishments surpass those of his or her parent of the same sex. At this point, a significant increase in self-destructive voices and suicidal ideation is reported.

CONCLUSION

To summarize, in the process of defending him- or herself, the child fragments into the self and antiself. Rather than suffer this fracture, many people side with the enemy within. Later, as adults, they externalize this defensive process in their closest personal ties. Many people retreat to the seeming safety and security of their inner world, which represents, in effect, a form of controlled destruction of the self and the progressive ascendancy of the antiself.

The self is thus a divided and conflicted dynamic relation between itself as self and its antiself. The antiself is induced by ineffective or malignant styles of parenting and socialization that are fundamentally authoritarian and moralistic. This creates within the child a self-hating inner voice that seeks to destroy the very project of becoming a self that gives human existence its most significant meaning. The self is divided against itself, in Kierkegaard's sense, both fearing life and desiring death and desiring life and fearing death. Existentially, this form of despair toward becoming a self in the face of death is not a mere mood or a passing emotion; it belongs to the very structure of the self and, as such, is universal.

ENDNOTES

1. Empirical studies related to the internalization of childhood trauma have been conducted and results reported in "Studies in Self-Representation Beyond Childhood" (Bocknek & Perna, 1994). Results from one study demonstrated a significant correlation between psychopathology

(bulimia) and developmental delay that was uncovered through identification of subjects' self-representations.

In "Parental Representations and Psychopathology: A Critical Review of the Empirical Literature," Bornstein (1993) reviewed studies confirming the hypothesis that dysfunctional parental introjects predict an individual's risk for psychopathology. This researcher also noted that correlations between level of psychopathology and the *content* of an individual's parental introjects were comparable to correlations between level of psychopathology and the *structure* of an individual's parental introjects.

2. Studies regarding individuals' reactions to trauma in general are instructive and point out the adaptive nature of such responses. In summarizing their clinical findings, Noyes et al. (1977) note that hyperalertness and mental clouding (a "dreamlike alteration in consciousness accompanied by dulling of thought and mental imagery") are part of the syndrome of depersonalization that "may well appear in response to anxiety that is severe and potentially disorganizing" (p. 406). They conclude that "depersonalization may . . . represent an adaptive mechanism that combines opposing reaction tendencies, the one serving to intensify alertness and the other to dampen potentially disorganizing emotion" (p. 406).

3. It should be noted that in Sophocles' tragedy *Oedipus, the King* (the myth to which Freud alluded in constructing his theory of the Oedipal complex), Oedipus's father, King Laius, and his mother, Jocasta, colluded in committing the original crime of attempted infanticide against their son.

> And the child's [Oedipus] birth was not three days past when Laius pinned its ankles together and had it thrown, by others' hands, on a trackless mountain. (Hadas, 1967, *The Complete Plays of Sophocles,* p. 94)

Laius and Jocasta's murderous aggression represented a desperate attempt to avoid the fulfillment of an "evil" prophecy foretelling Laius's own murder at the hands of his son. The prophecy may be interpreted as a projection of Laius's fears and rivalrous jealousy onto his infant son.

PART II

Defense Formation

6

The Fantasy Bond and Self-Parenting Process

Those of us who enslave ourselves in the bondage of the mirage of love
are parched for lack of love, and so fearful of giving and getting the love
we lack, so terrified of the real thing, that we create our own hell and
whine and complain that it keeps on not being the heaven we say we
want and want to believe we are in.

R. D. Laing (1985, p. 18)

Psychological defenses that protected people from suffering emotional pain
and anxiety when they were children later play destructive limiting roles in
their adult lives. An individual's defense system functions to keep him or her
insulated from primal pain at the cost of being removed from the deepest
personal experiences.

Psychological defenses are subject to malfunction in a manner that is analogous to the body's physical reaction in the case of pneumonia. The presence of
organisms in the lungs evokes cellular and humoral responses that meet the
invasion, yet the magnitude of the defensive reaction leads to congestion that is

AUTHOR'S NOTE: The substance of this chapter is taken primarily from an article titled, "A
Concept of the Primary Fantasy Bond: A Developmental Perspective," *Psychotherapy, 21* (1984),
pp. 218-225. Used with permission.

potentially dangerous to the person. In this disease, the body's defensive reaction is more destructive than the original assault.

Similarly, defenses that were erected by the vulnerable child to protect him- or herself against a toxic environment eventually become more detrimental than the original trauma. In this sense, people's psychological defenses formed under conditions of stress become the core of their neurosis or psychosis.

I conceptualize neurosis as an inward, self-protective style of living that leads the individual to seek satisfaction more in fantasy than in the real world. It represents an adaptation to the frustration of infantile urges and primal hunger. It is the process of reliving rather than living, choosing bondage over freedom, the old over the new, the past over the now. It is the attempt to re-create a parent or parents in other persons or institutions, or even, if all else fails, in oneself. It is the abrogation of real power in exchange for childish manipulations. It is the avoidance of genuine friendship, free choice, and love in favor of familiarity and false safety. One clings to the emotional deadness of the family and to illusions of security by repeating early patterns with new objects.

In one sense, neurosis is a response to a realistic fear—the terror and anxiety that surround our awareness of death. However, it is a maladaptive reaction when it involves a progressive giving up of one's life in an attempt to alleviate death anxiety. Indeed, most people prefer to exist in a nonfeeling, defended state because to feel for themselves or for another person would make them more aware of their vulnerability and limitation in time.

THE FANTASY BOND

The basic tenet of my theoretical approach is the concept of the fantasy bond, which represents the primary defense against psychological pain. The fantasy bond is an illusion of connection, originally an imaginary fusion or joining with the mother's body, most particularly the breast. The term is used here to describe both the original imaginary connection formed during childhood and the repetitive efforts of the adult to continue to make fantasized connections in intimate associations. This defensive process leads to a subsequent deterioration in later personal relationships. The function of resistance is to protect the individual from anxiety that arises whenever the fantasy bond is threatened.[1]

---

1 Resistant behavior in or out of therapy represents an attempt to maintain psychological equilibrium by minimizing or avoiding both *negative and positive anxiety states.* The latter refers to anxiety derived from positive events and improvement in a person's life circumstances. See Whitaker and Malone's (1981) discussion of positive and negative anxiety in *The Roots of Psychotherapy.*

It is important to differentiate this specific use of the word *bond* from its other uses in psychological and popular literature. It does not refer to "bond" as in "bonding" (maternal-infant attachment) in a positive sense, nor does it refer to a relationship that implies loyalty, devotion, and genuine love (Klaus & Kennell, 1976). The term *bond* is used here to connote a sense of bondage or limitation of freedom.

For the infant, this fantasized connection alleviates emotional pain and distress by providing partial gratification of its emotional or physical hunger. In other words, the fantasy bond is a substitute for love when there is a deficiency in real love and sensitive care in the infant's environment. The more deprivation in the child's early life, the more he or she compensates and depends on the fantasy of fusion.

The fantasy bond arises because of the overwhelming pain and separation anxiety that occurs when the infant is faced with excessive frustration. Winnicott (1958) characterized this type of anxiety as being an emotion far more devastating than frustration:

> Maternal failures produce phases of reaction to impingement and these reactions interrupt the "going on being" of the infant. An excess of this reacting produces not frustration but a *threat of annihilation*. This . . . is a very real primitive anxiety. (p. 303) (Endnote 1)

The Concept of Love-Food

At the preverbal stage, anxiety is intolerable to the infant and creates a dread not only of separation and starvation but perhaps even of death (Bowlby, 1960). Observing these phenomena led to the conclusion that a good mother would possess the emotional resources and affection necessary to provide her infant with ingredients that would enable him or her to develop into a comfortable social being (Winnicott, 1960/1965b) (Endnote 2). Ideally, she would nurture him or her without debilitating anxiety and there would be a true empathy toward the child. I have called the product of this ability on the part of the mother "love-food," which implies both the strength of character and the desire to provide for the need gratification of the infant. If mothers, that is, parents, are immature, weak, and ineffectual, they will fail to provide security for the child. In terms of theory, love-food is necessary for *survival* in both the physical and the psychological sense of the word (R. Firestone, 1957).

When deprived of love-food, the infant experiences intense anxiety and pain and attempts to compensate by providing various forms of self-nourishment, such as sucking its thumb. At this point in its development, the infant is able to create the illusion of the breast. Winnicott (1958) has portrayed this ability of the infant to fantasize the image of the breast. He states, "A subjective phenome-

non develops in the baby which we call the mother's breast" (pp. 238-239)
(Endnote 3).

The infant who feels empty and starved emotionally relies increasingly on
this fantasy for gratification. And, indeed, this process of "self-parenting"
provides partial relief and thus is immediately rewarding. In explaining the
survival function of fantasy in schizophrenia, J. N. Rosen (1953) stated,

> When a wish for something is so important that it involves a matter of life and
> death, then, and only then, does the unconscious part of the psychic apparatus
> spring into action and provide the necessary gratification with an *imagination.*
> (pp. 107-108)

Rosen went on to report the story of a soldier, lost in the African desert, who
imagined that the sand was water and scooped up handfuls of it, which he said
were "wet and cool to his touch and refreshing to taste." Such is the power of
imagination when one is faced with a situation conceived to be one of life-threatening deprivation.

Determinants of the Fantasy Bond

In the early stages of an infant's development, intolerable feelings of dread,
anxiety, and isolation are at times conveyed through the physical interaction
between the mother and child. It is impossible for an anxious mother (or
caretaker) to hide her fears and anxieties from her infant (D. N. Stern, 1985;
Mahler & McDevitt, 1968). In observing rejected infants, my associates and I
have noted an important negative characteristic in their mothers that appeared
very damaging to their offspring. This was the mother's refusal to let herself be
affected or moved by the emotional experience of feeding or caring for the child
(Endnote 4). Other observers have remarked that this type of mother seems to
avoid her baby's loving look or smile at the point when the baby first begins to
recognize her. This avoidance is detrimental to the baby's subsequent emotional
development. The child grows up feeling "not seen," unimportant, and neglected.

The symptoms in this type of infant are a general dissatisfaction indicated by
excessive whining and screaming, an inability to relax against the mother's body,
a desperate clinging to the mother, and a "spaced-out" or pitiful, pinched look
on his or her face. Toddlers categorized with anxious/avoidant or anxious/
resistant patterns of attachment (Ainsworth et al., 1978; Bowlby, 1969, 1973;
Main et al., 1985) exhibit many of the same signs or symptoms.

In terms of the mother-child interaction, it is my contention that the single
most damaging factor is habitual physical contact in the absence of genuine
emotionality; that is, the mother has withdrawn her affect and desire for contact

with the child, but still offers adequate, or even excessive, physical care or affection. In this respect, she is like an automaton (Bolton, 1983) (Endnote 5). Parental role-playing never succeeds in allaying the child's agonizing feeling of being unlovable. In actuality, it confuses the issue and intensifies the fantasy bond.

The emotionally mature or adequate mother, in contrast, has the capacity to tolerate genuine closeness and can move in and out of separation experiences. She offers sensitive care and relieves her child's anxiety without being overprotective. This mother does not routinely try to put her infant to sleep after a feeding, but is interested in maintaining the contact through play and communication. As the child grows older, she offers appropriately varied responses, alternating spontaneous contact with letting go of her offspring. This mother (or father) also copes with acting-out behaviors—whining, excessive crying, tantrums—before these negative patterns become integrated into the child's personality.

THE SELF-PARENTING PROCESS

The fantasy bond represents the child's attempt to parent him- or herself and involves both self-nourishing thoughts and habits as well as self-punishing ideation and behavior. It is a process of parenting oneself both internally in fantasy and externally by using objects and persons in one's environment. The result is a pseudoindependent posture of complete self-sufficiency—a fantasy that one can take care of oneself without needing others. The child experiences this false sense of self-sufficiency because he or she has introjected an image of the "good and powerful" mother or caretaker into the self. Unfortunately, at the same time, he or she must necessarily incorporate the mother's covert rejecting attitudes. These incorporated parental attitudes form the basis of the child's negative self-concept. The process of gratifying oneself internally through the self-parenting process can relieve fear and allay the anxiety of feeling separate and alone. It acts to banish painful feelings of emotional starvation and emptiness to the realm of the unconscious.

The self-parenting process is made up of a *self-feeding* component (Endnote 6) as well as a component of *self-condemnation and self-attack*. Both aspects of self-parenting take on their special character from the internalization of parental attitudes and responses in the process of growing up in a specific interpersonal environment.

The self-feeding aspect of this process is expressed in a wide range of behaviors including fantasy preoccupation, eating disorders, alcoholism, drug abuse, masturbation, and many other self-aggrandizing, self-satisfying, and self-protective maneuvers. Addictive patterns are also manifested in a type of sexuality characterized by a lack of real feeling, an impersonal connection that is used to relieve primitive feelings of emotional hunger.

Self-critical thoughts, guilt reactions, and attacks on self are examples of the disciplinary or punitive aspect of parental introjects. They represent the self-punishing element of the core defense. These parental introjects, both ideational and affective, contribute to feelings of inferiority and omnipotence. They alternatively build up and tear down the self.

Fantasies of fusion and self-parenting systems act as painkillers to cut off feeling responses, which, in turn, interferes with the development of a true sense of self. The end product of this progressive dependence on self-nourishing patterns is a form of psychological equilibrium achieved at the expense of genuine object relationships. Defended individuals seek equilibrium over actualization, that is, they are willing to give up positive, goal-directed activity to maintain internal sources of gratification.

The extent to which children eventually come to depend on this imaginary fusion is proportional to the degree of frustration, pain, and emotional deprivation experienced early in life, prior to the awareness of death. In defending themselves against an overload of pain, children depersonalize, fragment, lose feeling for themselves, and become hostile and untrusting of others. To maintain some sense of ego intactness, they merge with the parent in fantasy, incorporate hostile parental attitudes, and at the same time retain the painful, "primal" feelings of being the helpless, "bad" child. As noted, they develop an illusion of being at once the good, strong parent and the weak, dirty child, and thereby conceive of themselves as a complete, self-sufficient system. There is a feeling of pseudoindependence that detracts from object relations.

For the deprived child, the self-parenting process eventually becomes addictive in itself. Children (and adults) have at their disposal an immediately rewarding means of escaping circumstances that are anxiety-provoking and that lack the ingredients to sustain them.

The formation of the self-parenting process and its long-lasting effect on children's development are illustrated in a case of an agitated baby, E. Although the parents were knowledgeable about children (the mother was a teacher and the father a psychologist), rather than address the issue that their child was exhibiting signs of distress, they simply labeled him "temperamentally hyperactive." Their approach was to attempt to ameliorate the symptoms by offering whatever would immediately placate the baby. The mother described the child as "addicted" from birth. She gave as evidence the fact that "from the very first day, E. was extremely tense, hyperactive, and agitated, but his body would relax completely and he would actually breathe a loud sigh of relief when I put a pacifier in his mouth." His parents continued to offer him painkilling solutions, and over the years he became apathetic and resigned.

The youngster grew up preferring isolation over personal interactions. His sole interest was music, and he spent hours alone in his room, with his stereo or electric guitar. He went on to take drugs, progressing from marijuana to heroin use, and stole money to support his habit. He basically lived at home in a basement room until he was 29 years old, yet his parents were suspiciously unaware of his drug habit. Later he was fired from his first job because of incompetency and tardiness brought about by excessive drug use. He is currently involved in a long-term rehabilitation program.

In this brief example, it is important to note that faulty environmental conditions operant early in E.'s life contributed to his adopting a life of addiction. My conjecture is that E. first became addicted to the pacifier his mother used to "quiet" him. His mother was somewhat withdrawn and preoccupied and she refused to allow him to disturb her inward state. Later, his parents' indulgence and their indifference to his emotional suffering crystallized his tendency to cut off pain by increasingly sophisticated means. In a sense, they trained him to be an addict.

To summarize, the fantasy bond is formed as a reaction to both interpersonal pain and separation anxiety and precedes the child's awareness of death. Regarding the inevitable separations of childhood, I have noted that children progress through several stages. These stages correspond to the successive steps they take in differentiating themselves from the mother and later the father and the extended family. In early infancy (birth to approximately 6 months), children feel utterly dependent on the mother and experience themselves as merged. Later (4 or 5 months to 2 years), there is a gradual accommodation to the reality of being separate from the mother.

Separation anxiety is experienced at every phase of individuation, precipitating a fear of loss of self and a dread of annihilation (Rheingold, 1967; Winnicott, 1960/1965b) (Endnote 7). To compensate, there is an imagined fusion with the mother or primary caretaker. This fantasy connection represents a desperate attempt on the child's part to deny his or her true state of aloneness, helplessness, and vulnerability. By the time children develop a structured concept of their own personal death, they have already established a complex system of defenses against separation anxiety. Indeed, death symbolizes the ultimate separation.

THE IMPACT OF DEATH ANXIETY
ON THE DEFENSE SYSTEM

Sometime between the ages of 3 and 6, children become aware that people die, that their parents are vulnerable to death, and that they themselves cannot maintain their own lives. Their world, which they had experienced as permanent, is literally turned upside down by the dawning awareness of mortality.

In learning about death, most children feel, on some level, that a terrible trick has been played on them. Many become angry or distant from their parents, while others exhibit an intensified clinging or dependency. In general, children try to ameliorate this final blow to their security by regressing to an earlier stage of development where they were unaware of death. Remaining infantile or suspended in a childish state is a primary defense against death anxiety, as aging is associated with movement toward finality. Faced with death anxiety, children attempt to reinstate and reinforce the imagined connection with parents and parental introjects. On a behavioral level, increased preoccupation with fantasy, acting-out, nightmares, signs of depersonalization, and other regressive trends are common during this crucial phase.

Many children have nightmares filled with themes about death and indicating feelings of vulnerability about their bodies. These terrifying dreams seem to occur more frequently in those children who have not yet successfully repressed their emotional reactions to the knowledge of death. For example, Randy, age 3¼ years, woke up crying from a bad dream in the middle of the night. Talking through his tears, he told his mother:

Randy: I am Randy and I am going to be Randy when I get big and till I die. Isn't that sad?

Mother: What?

Randy: That I am going to die. Everyone knows that they are going to die, even Roy [a self-assured 5-year-old acquaintance], even strangers. But they pretend they won't. You know why?

Mother: Why?

Randy: Because when you die all your skin peels off and then you're not Randy any more.

One apparently universal response to the knowledge of death is manifested in a basic paranoid orientation toward life, that is, the fact that death gives rise to a core paranoia that is then projected onto other situations. In some sense, paranoia is an appropriate reaction to existential realities, as powerful forces are operating on humans that are beyond their control and that eliminate all chance of survival. Life as they know it must terminate. Children generalize death anxiety and often develop fears of monsters, ghosts, and other imaginary dangers.

In summary, the point in the developmental sequence when the child first discovers death is the critical juncture where his or her defense system crystallizes and shapes the future. Dating from this time, most people to varying degrees accommodate to the fear of death by withdrawing energy and emotional investment in life-affirming activity and close, personal relationships. The thought of losing one's life, losing all consciousness, losing all ego through death is so intolerable that the process of giving up offers relief from the anguish. To whatever extent they renounce real satisfaction, they rely increasingly on internal gratification, fantasies of fusion, and painkillers. The most powerful and effective denial of death lies in the fantasy bond that the child developed originally as a compensation for environmental deficiencies.

RECAPITULATING THE PAST

The child achieves psychological equilibrium when he or she arrives at a particular solution to the basic conflict between reliance on an internal fantasy process for gratification and seeking satisfaction in the external world. When this equilibrium is threatened by events that contradict the earliest childhood experiences, anxiety is aroused and the individual retreats to a more inward state of parenting the self. One's identity as the "bad" child is disrupted if one is valued or loved by a person who has significance in adult life. To defend against intrusions into this inward state of imagined safety and security, the person uses three major modes of defense: (a) selection, (b) distortion, and (c) provocation. These defense mechanisms are behavioral operations that function to protect the fantasy bond.

Selection

Selection is a method whereby individuals choose present-day "love-objects" to replicate the early family situation. People are resistant to forming associations with significant others who behave toward them in a way that differs qualitatively from the treatment they received as children. They tend to select mates who are similar to one or another parent because they feel comfortable with them. They feel relaxed when their defenses are appropriate. A damaged person externalizes the introjected parental image by using the new partner to maintain the "good" parent/"bad" child system.

F., a somewhat passive man, fell in love with M., a woman who appeared to be affectionate, enthusiastic, and energetic. But he soon came to realize that he was involved in a relationship that was very controlling and critical in a manner similar to his childhood relationship with his parents. Over the course of time, M. became completely dominating and found fault with everything about F. M. provided the definition and rejection so familiar to F. and served to remind him once again that he was "bad." Eventually the relationship became so intolerable that F. left M. There was an immediate improvement in his sense of well-being and feelings about himself, but he was left with a deep sense of nostalgia.

J. grew up in Russia with a hypercritical, punitive mother. To escape her home situation, J. married at a young age. However, her Russian husband continued the tradition of her mother by dominating and patronizing her. J. divorced him and later met T., an American businessman, in Moscow. In spite of a strong language barrier, she fell in love with this new and different "foreign" man and she joined him in America. Even though they came from different cultures and spoke different languages, as they got to know each other better, it became obvious to J. that she had again chosen a man who exhibited the same judgmental and punishing characteristics as her Russian husband and her mother before him. J.'s response to T.'s demands and disapproval was to feel angry and victimized, but nevertheless she accepted his criticisms and maintained her stubborn sense of worthlessness.

Distortion

The individual who uses distortion as a defense alters perceptions of new objects in a direction that corresponds more closely to the members of the original family. Not all distortions are negative. Both positive and negative qualities may be attributed to significant people in the damaged individual's life. Admirable characteristics are exaggerated as well as undesirable traits, but the distortion generally functions to make new figures more closely approximate the important people in the individual's childhood.

The child maintains an *idealized* image of the parent and projects his or her *real* qualities onto others. People who make positive changes in their relationships or in their lifestyle often need to distort the new situation. Numerous case histories have been documented about children previously neglected or abused by their parents, who, when placed with loving foster parents, have distorted their new surroundings and reacted adversely. It is characteristic of the damaged child to attempt to reproduce the circumstances of the earlier environment, no matter how miserable they were. In the following case study, the mechanism of distortion is clear.

Case Study[2]

Kathy was approximately 18 months old when her mother, responding to pressures from relatives, suddenly decided it was time to take her off the bottle and feed her from a cup. The first night she was denied the bottle, Kathy screamed all night. After listening to her daughter's cries through the night, the

---

2 The material in this case study is taken from *Compassionate Child-Rearing: An In-Depth Approach to Optimal Parenting,* Plenum Press (1990). Used with permission.

mother returned to the crib and offered her the bottle. Kathy threw it on the floor and began to suck her thumb. She never took to the bottle again.

In refusing gratification from outside, the toddler had substituted thumb-sucking and subsequently developed other patterns of self-nourishing behavior. This incident—what seemed like a normal step in the weaning process—was a key event in Kathy's deprived existence and acted to solidify well-formed defenses.

Family history. Kathy had been born to an emotionally immature couple in which neither partner was capable of providing nurturance or guidance to their child. Kathy's parents were narcissistic and emotionally deprived individuals. Each had experienced much trauma during their own early years.

The most glaring and puzzling characteristic of this couple's relationship, however, was the fairy-tale quality of their family life that had persisted uninterrupted until the mother, no longer able to ignore the alarming symptoms Kathy was beginning to exhibit, sought professional help. Against the wishes of her husband, she finally took the youngster for evaluation at a child guidance clinic.

Symptoms and analysis. In the initial interview, Kathy, now 4 years old, appeared pale and listless. She had dark circles under her eyes and displayed signs of impoverished affect and symptoms of depression. Her mother reported that Kathy spent long hours in front of the television set and when diverted to other activities would show very little interest. If left alone in a room for a short while, she would often simply fall asleep on the floor, in the midst of play.

Kathy's mother had extreme dependency needs, which had their source in her own childhood and now were focused on Kathy. The combination of abject rejection and intrusive proprietary interest shown by this mother had a draining effect on the youngster, causing her to give up basic wants and needs at an early age, perhaps even prior to the incident with the bottle. That incident served to crystallize in Kathy's mind her parents' long-term neglect and hostility as well as their disregard of her needs as an infant.

Development and presenting symptoms. Kathy's parents were divorced when she was 5, and her parents asked some close friends of theirs to take care of Kathy. They were mature, warm, and loving individuals who had befriended Kathy from the time she was a toddler, and they were moved by her parents' request to try to help her.

During the years she spent with these foster parents, Kathy improved in many areas. With her new family and later with her therapist, however, Kathy acted out the child aspect of the self-parenting process. She pulled excessive caretaking responses from her new parents and indulged in negative, attention-getting behavior that nevertheless gave her a sense of security. When she reached adolescence and tried to develop an adult orientation, she began to regress to a more oral level.

At 15, Kathy developed a serious eating disorder, consisting of compulsive overeating and purging, and at times gained up to 10 pounds within a 2-day period. Whenever she began to function maturely and form more consistent relationships, she would defend herself against her feelings and sense of vulnerability by engaging in compulsive eating. This was a central theme in her life. She found it difficult to sustain long-term friendships and maintained a peculiar indifference or blankness in relation to planning her future or even toward activities typically enjoyed by adolescents.

In Kathy's mind, no new set of parents, no amount of warmth or affection, could induce her to "accept the bottle" again. For many years, she distorted her new circumstances, stubbornly refusing to take a chance again after her early experiences with oral deprivation, rejection, and the dreadful feelings of annihilation and disintegration. She felt compelled to protect herself from potential rejection by engaging in the behaviors she originally used to preserve her integrity and some sense of self. In this way, she molded her new environment to correspond more closely to her traumatic childhood experiences.

Provocation

Provocation was another defense used by Kathy with her foster parents. Beginning with a refusal to keep her room neat, a habit that brought out nagging, angry parental reactions from her foster mother, Kathy progressed to acts of delinquency (shoplifting) and overeating in her bid for negative attention, rejection, and punishment. She needed to prove that she was bad and that others would reject her as her parents had. In a therapy group that she attended when she was 17, she revealed aspects of the underlying pain that drove her to engage in addictive habit patterns symptomatic of her need to "feed" herself.

Kathy: Over the past months I've started to think about myself more and more that I'm bad and that I make people feel bad. I feel like I don't deserve anything myself and I hurt other people, so I should just leave.

I know that I feel happy when I'm losing weight. It gives me a sense of myself in a way, but when I'm overeating, I feel bad. There are things that I do that I know are bad for me, but instead of just thinking that they make me feel bad or they make me feel unhappy, I think I'm bad for doing them and then I don't talk about them. I'm very secretive.

Therapist: It seems that first you do something to isolate yourself, something negative or self-destructive like overeating, then you hate yourself for it and go further into more destructive behavior. It's a cycle.

Kathy: It doesn't happen overnight. It's been happening my whole life. I've felt bad my whole life. I've always felt bad. I just know people hate me.

Therapist: But where did it come from? How did you get a feeling that you're bad?

Kathy: I don't remember specific things, but I do remember feeling hated, or feeling just a coldness or like it didn't matter that I was there, like I was a doll or something, like I wasn't a person.

My mother just wanted a doll, and anything that I needed she hated me for. I feel like she hated me because I had needs. She would have rather had a doll that she could just dress up and carry around with her and show off to people, that would make her proud and that wouldn't need anything.

Therapist: Did you start to feel bad for wanting things?

Kathy: Yeah, I didn't want anything and whenever I did want something, I felt like I was mean, and I still feel that way.

During this crucial period, Kathy slowly and painstakingly shifted her reliance from the addictive pattern of feeding herself, manifested in her eating disorder, to accepting help and support from others. Signs of progress were seen when she broke her habit of first cheating on her diet and then lying about it. During this transition, Kathy reported feelings of resentment and guilt about letting people into her life.

Subsequent follow-up showed that as Kathy gradually became more successful in controlling her destructive eating patterns, her interest in other people and her curiosity about the world, qualities previously submerged in her personality, began to surface. As of this writing, she has regained some feeling for herself and achieved considerable insight into the ways in which she was damaged early in life.

In general, provocation is used by the neurotic person to manipulate others to respond to him or her as the parent did. To a large extent, the individual will behave in ways that provoke angry, punishing parental reactions in others: employees provoke anger and cynicism in their bosses by unnecessary incompetence and inefficiency; husbands and wives provoke each other to helpless feelings of rage by their forgetfulness, by being late for important engagements, and so on. Bach and Deutsch (1979) described this well in their book, *Stop! You're Driving Me Crazy.* Most people are largely unaware of the fact that their behavior may have the specific purpose of provoking aggression or withdrawal in others. Many marriages fail because each partner distorts his or her perception of the other and provokes angry responses to maintain a "safe" distance.

All three maneuvers—selection, distortion, and provocation—work to preserve the introjected parent that the individual later projects onto new associations. The wounded adult anticipates that the loss of the fantasy bond with the loved one would expose him or her once again to the anxiety, fear, and pain endured at a time in childhood when he or she was helpless and dependent. Therefore, at the point where the individual begins to experience more closeness and feels more loving, he or she becomes anxious and retreats to a more familiar, less personal style of relating.

DIMENSIONS OF THE
PRIMARY DEFENSE SYSTEM[3]

There are several major aspects of the primary defensive process, each of which represents an adaptation to the home environment with all its deficiencies and pressures. These defense mechanisms become abnormal because of their intensity or degree, and misapplication to new persons or situations.

The following aspects of the defensive process are not discrete entities or specific defenses but consist of readily observable patterns that tend to overlap to a considerable extent. Therapeutic intervention directed toward correcting one component challenges the entire defensive process.

1. The *idealization of parents* or family is a necessary part of the self-parenting system. Because of the extreme dependency during the early years, the child *must* see the parent as "good" or powerful rather than recognize parental weakness or rejection (Arieti, 1974; Kempe & Kempe, 1978; Oaklander, 1978). The child feels that he or she could not survive with inadequate, weak, or hostile parents, and therefore denies their negative qualities and sees him- or herself as bad. To parent oneself successfully in fantasy, one must maintain the idealized image of one's parent.

2. The *negative self-image,* the "bad" child, exists concomitantly with the idealized image of the parents. In perceiving the parent as good, the child must think of him- or herself as bad, unlovable, and undeserving. The child must interpret parental rejection as being his or her fault because the child needs to see the parents as being loving, competent people. The self-hatred inherent in the negative view of the self originates when the child incorporates the parent's negative attitudes toward him or her. These negative attitudes toward self become a prominent part of the self-concept and are at the center of the individual's self-hatred.

3. The *displacement of negative parental traits onto the interpersonal environment* is a result of the child's blocking from awareness the parents' weaknesses and their negative qualities. To preserve the self-nourishing system by

---

3 The material in the following section is taken primarily from *The Fantasy Bond: Structure of Psychological Defenses,* Human Sciences Press (1985). Used with permission.

maintaining the idealized parental image, the damaged individual projects the parents' weaknesses and undesirable traits onto others.

4. The defended individual experiences a *progressive loss of feeling for self* as he or she increasingly relies on fantasy gratification. Existing in a deperson-alized, inward state, experiencing minimal compassion or self-love, the person feels considerable hatred for self and others. In this withdrawn state, he or she may actually experience little emotional pain or anxiety and feel somewhat content or comfortable. This individual has succeeded in repressing much of his or her emotional distress and generally only seeks help after some sort of environmental stress breaks through defenses.

5. *Withholding* is a holding back or withdrawal of emotional and behav-ioral responses from others. When the child is hurt or frustrated, he or she withdraws the affection or psychic energy invested in the parents or other objects; a kind of decathexis takes place. Extreme withholding reflects a basic fear of being drained and represents a pulling back from an exchange of psychonutritional products, giving to or receiving from objects in the real world. Theoretically, the self-parenting process can be understood as a psychonutri-tional system wherein the individual imagines that there are limited quantities of nourishment available.

6. *Self-nourishing habits and routines* support the core defense. The methods and means of an inward style of self-nourishment begin early in life. As they mature, people substitute more refined techniques of satisfying themselves and alleviating pain. A person's degree of dependency on painkilling substances, habits, and routines clearly indicates neurotic dependence on the primary fantasy process. Emotional deprivation is at the core of addiction and abnormal depend-ency in relationships.

Over the past decade, my concept of the fantasy bond has become integrated into the mainstream of psychological thought and, to some extent, has become familiar to the general public in the form of codependency. Murray Bowen (personal communication, 1987) noted that the concept of the fantasy bond, by providing an in-depth analysis of intrapsychic dynamics operating within the family system, clarified the relationship between individual psychodynamics and family systems theory. Other theorists, beginning with Hellmuth Kaiser (Fierman, 1965) (Endnote 8), have also dealt with the subject of this mode of relating (Karpel, 1976; Wexler & Steidl, 1978; Willi, 1975/1982).

In summary, the fantasy bond originates in early childhood or infancy to fill a gap when there is environmental deprivation; it "nourishes" the self; and it becomes the motivating force behind self-destructive, neurotic behavior. It is a maladaptive solution that occurs not only in the seriously disturbed or psychotic patient but also, to a lesser degree, in the neurotic or "normal" person. No child has an ideal environment; thus all people depend to varying degrees on internal gratification from the primary fantasy bond or self-parenting process.

CONCLUSION

Human beings desire freedom and individuality, but paradoxically they fight stubbornly against change and progress. Ernest Becker (1964) attempted an explanation for the problem of resistance. He asserted,

> The patient is not struggling against himself, against forces . . . within his animal nature. He is struggling rather against the loss of his world, of the whole range of action and objects that he so laboriously and painfully fashioned during his early training. (p. 170)

I suggest that the concept of the fantasy bond—the illusion of connection to the mother—and all the subsequent actions and thought processes are a dynamic formulation of the primitive defensive inner world of which Becker wrote. I see resistance as the holding on to an imaginary connection to others, due to the dread of reexperiencing one's sense of aloneness and helplessness.

Ultimately, resistance functions to protect the individual from experiencing anxiety states that arise from threats to the solution of the basic conflict—the conflict between dependency on inner fantasy for gratification versus a desire for real gratification in the interpersonal world. How one resolves this core conflict determines whether one has a free-flowing, changing existence or a static, rigid, inward posture. The concept of the fantasy bond provides an explanation for the underlying dynamics of the resistance to change. It is the major barrier to a richer, fuller existence.

ENDNOTES

1. Winnicott (1960/1965b) distinguished annihilation anxiety from castration and separation anxiety. He observed that "at this stage the word death has no possible application" (p. 47).

> The result of each failure in maternal care is that the continuity of being is interrupted by reactions to the consequences of that failure, with resultant ego-weakening. Such interruptions constitute annihilation, and are evidently associated with pain of psychotic quality and intensity. (p. 52)

See also Khan's (1963) concept of cumulative trauma. In his synthesis of these concepts, Khan cited a study by Searles (1962/1965b) and commented,

> Impingements which he [the infant] has no means of eliminating . . . set up a nucleus of pathogenic reaction. These in turn start a process of interplay with the mother which is

distinct from her adaptation to the infant's needs. . . . This in turn leads to a dissociation through which an archaic *dependency bond* is exploited on the one hand and a precipitate independence [pseudoindependent posture] is asserted on the other. [italics added] (Khan, 1963, p. 298)

2. Theorists have referred to the "good" mother in a variety of terms: Hartmann (1964) referred to the role of the mother in providing a "protective shield" against overwhelming stimuli as "the average expectable environment," and Winnicott (1960/1965a) used the term "good-enough maternal care" to describe the "holding environment" needed by the infant for ego development. According to Winnicott,

> The mother who is not good enough is not able to implement the infant's omnipotence, and so she repeatedly fails to meet the infant gesture; instead she substitutes her own gesture which is to be given sense by the compliance of the infant. (p. 145)

Wolman (1991) interpreted Winnicott's term "substitutes her own gesture" as referring "to a pattern of intrusive action" (p. 43).

3. Findings from empirical studies supporting the hypothesis that "oneness" fantasies reduce tension have been reported by Silverman, Lachmann, and Milich (1982). Results showed that the message *"MOMMY AND I ARE ONE"* presented subliminally (on the tachistoscope) ameliorated symptoms in schizophrenic patients and in some groups of nonpsychotic individuals.

Mahler's (1974) clinical observations of toddlers are also noteworthy with respect to the inferences she made about the subjective experience of the fantasized maternal image. In noting the mother's absence from the room,

> the toddler's gestural and performance motility slowed down, his interest in his surroundings diminished, and he appeared to be preoccupied with an inwardly concentrated attention. It was as if he wished to "image" another state of self—the state that he had felt at the time when the symbiotically experienced partner had been "one" with him. (p. 100)

The reader is also referred to three essays in the volume *Beyond the Symbiotic Orbit: Advances in Separation-Individuation Theory* (Akhtar & Parens, 1991): "Separation-Individuation Theory and Psychosexual Theory" by Henri Parens, "The Stages of Ego Development" by Stanley Greenspan, (1991), and "Contemporary Infant Research and the Separation-Individuation Theory of Margaret Mahler" by Patricia Nachman. Of particular interest is Nachman's report of clinical studies demonstrating "evidence for some basic form of representational capacity for infants under 7 months" (p. 128). According to Nachman (1991), "Many developmental psychologists see this as the key to further understanding of the internalization process" (p. 128).

4. A number of clinicians have described this form of withdrawal in mothers. Estela Welldon (1988) in *Mother, Madonna, Whore,* drawing on her own clinical experience and the observations of others (Blum, 1980; Glasser, 1979; Greenson, 1968; Mahler, Pine, & Bergman, 1975; Masterson & Rinsley, 1975; J. Rosen, 1953; Steele, 1970), concluded,

> My argument is that motherhood as a perversion occurs as a breakdown of inner mental structures, whereby the mother feels not only emotionally crippled in dealing with the huge psychological and physical demands from her baby, but also impotent and unable to obtain gratification from other sources. (p. 83)

5. Frank Bolton (1983) in *When Bonding Fails: Clinical Assessment of High-Risk Families* described this type of emotionally inadequate parent as one for whom child rearing

> *becomes an idealized image rather than an activity.* . . . Consequently, most interactions in private are shallow and unrewarding. Interactions that take place in public, on the other hand,

are elaborately choreographed to create the image that this parent is being "what a parent should be." (p. 163)

The constant surveillance and demand of the adults around them [the children] resulted in a slowing or retardation of normal personality and emotional development. (p. 162)

6. Kohut's (1977) concept of the "selfobject" is similar in some respects to my concept of the fantasy bond or self-parenting process, in particular the self-nurturing component. Kohut proposed that during the early months of life, "the child's rudimentary self merges with the selfobject, participates in its well-organized experience, and has its needs satisfied by the actions of the selfobject" (St. Clair, 1986, p. 149). Kohut also described the effects of inadequate parenting:

With every denial from the parents, with every delay, which is a kind of denial, something is set up internally. The ego performs internally something that formerly was performed externally by the mother or father. . . . If the loss is traumatic, beyond what the psyche at a specific developmental moment can actually perform, or if it is done in too great a measure, then there will be a gross identification with the lost parent. (Elson, 1987, p. 103)

7. Joseph C. Rheingold (1967), in *The Mother, Anxiety, and Death,* summarized the views of separation, annihilation, and death anxiety prevalent at that time in psychoanalytic literature. Findings from his 12-year clinical study led him to conclude:

I believe that it is not fear of natural death, whether existential or acquired, that determines anxiety, but fear of catastrophic death. One must remember that anxiety manifests itself long before there is any realistic knowledge of death. (p. 188)

8. Kaiser (Fierman, 1965) described the universal psychopathology as "the attempt to create in real life by behavior and communication the illusion of fusion" (pp. 208-209). According to Kaiser, this "delusion of fusion" can be observed in the therapy setting: Transference is another attempt on the part of the patient to fuse with a parental figure to avoid being a separate individual.

7

The Fantasy Bond in Couple Relationships

ⓔⓧⓔ

After living together and being in love for awhile, they begin to feel tied
to each other, bound to each other, connected to each other. They are not,
except in fantasy. Moreover, they may even go on to feel that they are
not separate individual human beings, each with their own centers,
points of view, destiny, each with their own deaths awaiting each,
separately, but they, we, two, have become one. Who could ask for
anything more? Alas, this also is fantasy. However intimately at one we
are, *we* could not feel *at* one, *as* one, unless we are not one.

R. D. Laing (1985, p. 17)

It is commonly thought that marital relationships deteriorate because of the
routines and familiarity that characterize married life. The mistaken notion
that "familiarity breeds contempt" confuses causes. The real source of marital
strife is the neurotic predisposition of each member of the couple. Their
individual defenses lead to the substitution of a fantasy bond or addictive
attachment in place of genuine loving and respectful relating. This sacrifice of

AUTHOR'S NOTE: The substance of this chapter is taken primarily from an article titled,
"Destructive Effects of the Fantasy Bond in Couple and Family Relationships," *Psychotherapy,*
24 (1987), pp. 233-239. Used with permission.

independence for the illusion of enduring love and connectedness destroys the excitement and vitality manifested in the early phases of the relationship.

The key issues in conflicted couples are not the "wrong choice of partner," economic hardship, sexual incompatibility, or an imbalance of power. Each individual's lack of tolerance for feeling the closeness of another human being, man's essential aloneness, and men and women's fear of rejection and potential loss are at the core of marital and family distress. Indeed, most people have a fear of intimacy and at the same time are terrified of being alone. Their solution is to form a fantasy bond—the illusion of connection and closeness that allows them to maintain emotional distance while meeting the social obligations of marriage and family.

Satisfactions achieved in fantasy by the child and later the adult gradually come to be preferred over real gratification because they are under the individual's control. Once an illusion of connectedness with another person has been formed, experiences of real love and intimacy interfere with its defensive function, whereas symbols of togetherness and images of love strengthen the illusion. Anything that arouses an awareness of separateness or a nonbonded existence can be anxiety-provoking, will give rise to hostile feelings, and will therefore be resisted.

Wexler and Steidl (1978) concluded that most couples avoid experiences that disrupt their illusions of oneness. They described a state of "merged identity," where couples regress to an earlier symbiotic state "in the face of separation anxiety." In their analysis, they wrote, "Adults who seek to fuse with their mates are in many respects like the toddler who seeks to fuse with his mothering person" (p. 72). Mark Karpel (1976), in discussing manifestations of mature versus immature relationships, cautioned: "Features that characterize *less* mature forms of relationship [pure fusion and ambivalent fusion, among others] will always be present to varying degrees at varying moments" (p. 81).

Fantasy bonds exist as implicit defensive pacts between individuals. Members of the couple or family conspire both to live with and protect each other's defended lifestyles. They collaborate to preserve a fantasy of love. R. D. Laing (1961) demonstrated how "collusion" is an important relationship dynamic:

> Two people in relation may confirm each other or genuinely complement each other. Still, to disclose oneself to the other is hard without confidence in oneself and trust in the other. Desire for confirmation from each is present in both, but each is caught between trust and mistrust, confidence and despair, and both settle for counterfeit acts of confirmation on the basis of pretense. To do so *both* must play the game of collusion. (pp. 108-109)

Laing's analysis of the development of collusion is similar to my conceptualization of the process of bond formation by the couple. Individuals who have been damaged in their earliest experiences are reluctant to reveal themselves in new relationships. They are resistant to taking a chance on being hurt again. The tragedy of their retreat from their original positive investment and involvement with each other is compounded by mutual self-deception.

DESTRUCTIVE EFFECTS OF THE FANTASY BOND IN COUPLE RELATIONSHIPS

The process of forming a fantasy bond greatly reduces the chance of achieving a successful union. Conversely, to the degree that a bond is *not* formed and the couple remains free, realistic, and independent, the relationship can still develop and flourish. However, most men and women are unaware of their strong propensity for giving up their individuality to become one half of a couple or to merge themselves with another person for purposes of security. Indeed, early manifestations of this damaging connection in mother-child interaction are often mistaken for positive attributes of mothering. Couples that appear to be merged or uniform manifest the same deceptive appearance of closeness.

Using the maneuvers of selection, distortion, and provocation, people are able to externalize the fantasy bond, thereby re-creating negative aspects of the family with new attachments (Endnote 1). They preserve the internal parent by projecting his or her image onto a new object. These projections foster alienation.

The Development of a Couple Bond

Men and women are most likely to form romantic attachments at a time when they are on the upgrade psychologically, often at the stage where they are breaking dependent emotional ties with their families. They are experiencing a stronger sense of self as they feel separate from the family bond. In this phase of development, the newly independent person actively seeks friendship and new relationships. As the person reaches out and risks more of him- or herself emotionally, he or she attracts others with the resulting vitality and enthusiasm. In a new love relationship, one exists, for a while, in a relatively undefended and vulnerable state, typically referred to as the "honeymoon stage."

In their coupling, conflict develops because people strive to maintain their defenses while, at the same time, they wish to hold on to their initial feelings of closeness and affection. The two conditions tend to be mutually exclusive. In a relatively short time, either one or both members of the couple choose to sacrifice friendship and love to preserve their respective defended states.

Early Symptoms

The condition of feeling or being in love is fragile and unstable at the inception of a love relationship. Fear of loss or abandonment, a dread of being rejected, together with the poignancy and sadness evoked by positive emotions, sooner or later become intolerable, particularly for those individuals who have suffered from a lack of love and affectionate contact in their early lives. Because they are afraid of feeling vulnerable, most men and women retreat from being close and gradually, albeit imperceptibly, give up the most valued aspects of their relationships.

As a couple's relationship unfolds, symptoms of the fantasy bond become more apparent. People who in the beginning spent hours in conversation start to lose interest in both talking and listening. Spontaneity and playfulness gradually disappear; feelings of sexual attraction generally wane; and the couple's sex life frequently becomes routine or mechanical.

As the partners begin to withhold the desirable qualities in themselves that attracted the other, they tend to experience feelings of guilt and remorse. Consequently, both begin to act out of a sense of obligation and responsibility instead of a genuine desire to be together.

Another symptom of deterioration is a lack of direct eye contact between the partners. People who once gazed lovingly at each other now avert their glance. This symptom of diminished relating is indicative of an increasingly impersonal mode of interaction. The style of communication becomes dishonest and mis-leading, for example, making idle conversation, speaking for the other, inter-rupting, talking as a unit or in the stylized "we" instead of "I," and bickering. Later on, they manipulate by making each other feel guilty and often provoke angry or parental behavioral responses. Self-doubts and criticism are often projected onto the mate, leading each person to complain about the other. They are critical as their spouses fail to live up to their prior expectations (Lederer & Jackson, 1968; M. Solomon, 1989) (Endnote 2).

One couple, married for 3 years, had settled into a routine of blaming each other for the slow erosion of the genuine love and affectionate feelings that had existed between them at the inception of their relationship. A., the wife, com-plained that she felt guilty about being free and felt increasingly obligated to spend all of her time with her husband; B. revealed that he felt resentful and puzzled that A. no longer wanted to share the activities with him that she had originally enjoyed.

In an in-depth interview, each partner attempted to objectively trace the causes of this deterioration, examining various aspects of a crucial turning point in their relationship. Following are excerpts from the interview:

Husband (B.): [*To wife*] When I realized that I had fallen in love with you, when I really knew that you meant a lot to me and I told you, I became self-conscious. I began to feel strange around you and around our friends. Now that everybody knew that we were in love, I got scared of being rejected. I thought to myself: "What if she rejects you now? You're a fool! A real sucker!"

Wife (A.): I know that when you told me, it was a turning point for me, too. After that, I didn't feel like doing the same things together that we had always enjoyed doing. I had a feeling that things were being demanded of me. I began to think of you as being a really demanding, bossy person. I thought that I didn't have any time left for myself, that I always had to be doing things with you, or for you.

B.: But it appeared that I was demanding because I felt hurt and angry. When we first lived together, you were so sweet. When I came home from work you were always so happy to see me. But later, you were different and I was angry and pained by your lack of interest. I tried hard not to act on my anger, but sometimes I pulled away when I became really discouraged about the relationship.

A.: I remember at the time, I started thinking things that would stop my actions, like: "Don't show him you're enthusiastic to see him. Just sit there, besides, what's the big deal? He's not that great. He's kind of an awkward person, lazy, passive . . ."

I really started picking you apart in my mind. I realize now that I really *did* believe those critical things I was thinking about you. What I understand today is that you haven't changed that much in the years we've been together. But I have.

Looking back, I can see how I've twisted you in my mind, to protect against seeing myself differently than I was raised to believe I was. I had never thought of myself as a soft, loving woman. But your feelings for me made me feel differently about myself—made me feel like I was really lovable. I couldn't live with that different identity, so I twisted everything, to do away with that new feeling about myself, and I hurt you in the process. [*Sad*]

In this case, it appeared that A. had reacted adversely to being chosen and loved by B., and implicitly believed her critical thoughts about him. She tended to act on the directives of her voice and played out the role of a petulant child, responding inappropriately to imagined obligations and demands. In the interview, she again began to see her husband from her own point of view and felt deeply about the damage that had occurred in the relationship. During the course of therapy, both individuals were able to recapture some of their original feelings of tenderness and love.

In general, when I have seen couples together for conjoint therapy sessions, they are hypercritical of each other's traits, assign blame to their mates for deficiencies in the relationship, and generally manifest considerable hostility. Yet, in spite of their stated attacks, on another level, individuals in a bond strive desperately to maintain an idealized image of the partner.

In a typical interaction, the husband may complain about his wife's withholding, dependency, and childishness, while the wife in turn may enumerate her husband's coldness, noncommunicative style, and other shortcomings. It becomes apparent that they are accurate in their description of the other's behavior. When asked why they stay together, the usual response is "because we really love each other." It is difficult to believe in this pronouncement of love when habitually destructive patterns are established.

Although there is a diminution of real affect or feeling in a fantasy bond, nevertheless, dramatic emotional reactions to imagined losses or threats to the fantasy bond are common. This emotionality is often mistaken for real caring about the relationship. As the process of deterioration continues, the couple's emotional responses become progressively less appropriate to the real situation and contain elements and distortions based on the frustrations and pains of their respective childhoods (Benjamin, 1988). Now each individual implements the other's neurosis and strives to preserve the fantasized connection.

Complementary Traits, Mate Selection, and Formation of the Fantasy Bond

Part of the fantasy bond is present even during the early stages of the relationship. People often seek compensatory qualities in their partners. A person who is aggressive looks for someone who is somewhat passive. A spontaneous, lively person is attracted to someone who is controlled, quiet, or retiring. Paradoxically, in this attempt to counteract their weaknesses and shortcomings, each partner's inadequacies are in fact strengthened. Both partners tend to feel progressively more self-hating and dependent. Perversely enough, the very qualities that initially attracted them are frequently the ones they come to criticize and resent.

This dynamic was evident in the case of BF and RF, who separated after 7 years of marriage. The couple met in high school, fell in love, and were married 2 years later. At that time, BF was quiet, somewhat passive and introverted, whereas RF was gregarious, outspoken, and energetic. As the years passed, RF's more forceful personality increasingly overshadowed BF's retiring nature, and serious problems developed in the relationship. In an interview that took place several months after the separation, each recounted how the relationship had gradually deteriorated.

RF: I remember that in the beginning we were both independent. But pretty quickly, I began to control the relationship. I controlled what we did, where we went—it was always my idea. I wanted to be in control, to say which movie we went to see, who we went out to dinner with, what we did every night. I wanted everything to be my way. And it always turned out that way, almost always.

I can see now that over the years, the more I took control, the less attractive you became to me, and the more I felt like I was just an extension of you, you were an extension of me. I felt so connected. I felt like you were almost part of my body, I mean, really.

Dr. F.: [*To BF*] What do you think happened in relation to this?

BF: What she is saying is accurate. I really succumbed to that, to that need to be controlled. I gave up something in myself in looking for direction or something.

Dr. F.: You turned to her for direction, more and more, it seems like.

BF: Yeah, I would turn away from my wants and my friends in some sort of a need for that direction.

RF: I remember hating you for letting me control you. I mean, I hated you for it even though I wanted it so bad. I know it was something I worked at all day long. I was aware of doing it all the time. But every time I hated you for it, still.

BF: It's like I lost my point of view about things. If you had asked me, "What do you want to do now?" I didn't know. And it wasn't a conscious thing—it just wasn't there.

As the interview progressed, BF and RF explored the early family dynamics that they felt contributed to the deterioration of the marriage.

Dr. F.: What accounted for this? What do you think made you need to control or want to control?

RF: It felt like if I didn't control you, you wouldn't be there. If I didn't control you, you would never choose me, you would never be there. I wasn't going to be likable enough to be chosen. I had to make sure it happened. I had to make sure that you were going to be there, that you would choose me, that you would go to the movies with me that night. But it became lifelong, you know, that you would always be there.

Dr. F.: If he would be free, he would leave. You would lose him.

RF: I felt so unlovable, all the time, that I was surprised that I was chosen in the first place. I was thrilled that somebody wanted to be with me that much. So I had to hold on to it. I didn't think it would ever happen again. I never thought you would feel that way again. I had to hold on to it because I just didn't think that I was worth it. I just didn't think that I was worth somebody choosing me even two days in a row to be with, to even be friendly with.

Dr. F.: Why were you so insecure that you thought he would leave if you didn't tie him to you in some way?

RF: Because that's exactly how my mother was. The relationship between my parents was like that. That's what I learned about. All my sisters were like that. I didn't know there was any other way.

I saw my mother controlling everyone in the family, including us, in the same way, to make sure we would always be there, to make sure we would always come back and we would always love her or act like we loved her, but I never felt like I was lovable enough to deserve it.

Dr. F.: [*To BF*] What accounted for your surrendering? What were your fears? What was driving that behavior, do you think?

BF: I know that my mother controlled my life—she controlled the whole household. She was very intrusive. It's almost like I didn't have a life then. I was led around and told where to be and what to feel. She wouldn't leave me alone to feel anything. I couldn't feel bad if I wanted. She had to pick at me and figure out what it was, what was bothering me. I couldn't feel prideful or a sense of accomplishment. She would snatch it away or she would take it as her own success.

I really felt like I lost a lot of time during those years, that I don't know what I felt. [*Sad*]

Later:

Dr. F.: So even though you had a strong initial attraction and really nice feelings toward each other and you were nice people and kind and loving to each other, you couldn't survive your defenses. Your early life experiences interfered with your moving ahead in your life, each of you.

RF: I didn't really see you any more as a person, like I had no feeling for you as a person, as a human being. It's like you were just a toy somehow, or a device that was keeping me alive almost.

Dr. F.: Like an addiction?

RF: Yes, like an addiction, not like a human being. I didn't feel like you were alive, almost, like a human being, or that you had any feelings. The reason it makes me sad is because it makes me feel for myself as a person, but also for you as a person, and how we really have struggles. But it's not each other's fault.

Dr. F.:   It's a sad story, really, how people are trapped in the past, so much, and that you keep on repeating it. But it had nothing to do with each of you. That wasn't the problem. You weren't each other's problem at all. But these fears and this lack of self and lack of feeling for yourself really caused the trouble.

This interview had an unusual effect on BF and RF. It enabled them to remain friends after the separation and to maintain positive feelings for each other. What occurred in the actual session is that understanding the source of their difficulties, that is, tracing them back to issues in their own personal lives growing up, gave them a sense of compassion for themselves. Each could see that they weren't to blame for the deterioration of their relationship. In the accepting atmosphere of the interview, they stopped blaming themselves and each other and instead developed insight into early family interactions that had contributed to their insecurity and necessitated the formation of defenses.[1]

Couple Bonds:
Addiction to the Other as an Ultimate Rescuer

> As a rule, we find . . . in modern relationships . . . one person is made the god-like judge over good and bad in the other person. In the long run, such symbiotic relationship becomes demoralizing to both parties, for it is just as unbearable to be God as it is to remain an utter slave.
>
> *Otto Rank (1941, p. 196)*

Most people expect far more security from couple relationships and marriage than it is possible to extract. There is an expectation that all of one's needs will be met in the relationship. In that sense, one's husband or wife becomes the source of all happiness. The burden these anticipations put on the relationship is enormous; obviously, no one person can fulfill such unrealistic expectations or live up to this idealized image. However, people's actions indicate that they believe, on some level, that by submitting their individuality to a more "powerful" person as in a bond, by giving up their independence and points of view, they are somehow achieving safety and immortality.

---

1 The material in this interview is excerpted from a video documentary, *Bobby and Rosie: Anatomy of a Marriage* (Parr, 1989).

This type of demand on a relationship destroys the equality, genuine companionship, and spontaneous affection. The partners generally alternate between submission and dominance, playing the parent and then the child. Indeed, when a person perceives his or her mate as he or she really is, a mortal human being with flaws, weaknesses, and blemishes, the response is often one of anger and disillusionment (Sager & Hunt, 1979).

Ironically, a satisfying sexual experience can be a major disruption to the bond or the fantasy of being connected. The sex act is a real, but temporary, physical connection followed by a sharp separation. Physical intimacy is close, affectionate contact with a subsequent break in contact; real communication involves sharing of thoughts and feelings followed by a distinct awareness of boundaries. There is often resentment inherent in each of the separations that inevitably follow real closeness, although the anger and hostility can be unconscious.

In a fantasy bond, the sense of separateness is avoided. Moving in and out of closeness is intolerable to those people who have become dependent upon repetitive, habitual contact without much feeling. For example, a woman may withhold her full sexual response—real satisfaction—to avoid union and subsequent disconnection and separation. People avoid real communication because expressing their views implies that they are an entity, that they count, that "they have a vote." This stimulates the fear of separateness and aloneness. I have concluded that most people avoid intimate sexuality, physical affection, and honest communication because they refuse to face the fact that each of these transactions has an ending and necessitates letting go. Each small ending can remind them that everything eventually ends—in death. Establishing an imaginary connection with another person can become a major defense against this unbearable anxiety. Genuine love and intimacy challenge the primary fantasy of connection and arouse an acute awareness of mortality (Endnote 3).

The fear of object loss, which is akin to the fear of losing the self through death, can lead to a withdrawal of loving responses. A seemingly insignificant negative event is capable of precipitating this fear that exists at best only on the periphery of one's conscious awareness.

For example, late one evening, a couple watched the story of Lou Gehrig's life on television. The young woman, who was affectionate, outgoing, and very much in love with her husband, identified closely with the wife of the famous baseball player. At the point in the story where Lou Gehrig died, she felt a rush of deep sadness, picturing the emptiness of her life should *her* husband die.

The next morning she was uncharacteristically cool and aloof and pulled away from her husband's embrace. Much later, the woman realized she had reacted adversely to the reminder of death that she had seen exemplified in the film.

As people involve themselves in this fantasy operation to avoid the fear of loss, they find their lives increasingly hollow and empty. Yet the pull to believe that immortality can be achieved if one is loved by another is irresistible for most people.

Form Versus Substance in Marital Bonds

Most individuals who form and maintain destructive ties are unable to accept the reality of their lack of feeling and the alienation from their loved ones. Ashamed and unable to live with this truth, they attempt to cover up their lack of feeling with a fantasy of enduring love. They begin to substitute *form,* that is, routine, role-determined behavior, all the customary conventions that support "togetherness," for the real *substance* of the relationship—the genuine love, respect, and affection.

The conventional form of relating is made up of routine behavior patterns and superficial conversation or chatter that partners depend upon to maintain their fantasy of closeness. More significantly, the habitual style of communication or lack of communication serves the purpose of maintaining distance while preserving the pretense of love (Bodin, 1996) (Endnote 4).

Withdrawal of Desirable Qualities

In a couple bond, each partner attempts to regulate the flow of love and affection, that is, the amount of gratification the mate gives. By holding back qualities that are most admired or valued by one's mate, one can turn a partner's love into anger or even hatred. By provoking a mate with a variety of manipulations, one can diminish the partner's loving feelings and so maintain a more comfortable distance while keeping one's defenses intact. Through withholding and manipulation, each individual is able to control and limit the other's positive feelings. This withholding behavior, often subtle and difficult to identify, damages the relationship, sometimes irrevocably. Both parties become more inward and defended against each other as these patterns become well established. I have found that withholding plays a central role in marital disputes and is a major source of anger and disillusionment in long-standing relationships.

Male Vanity and Female Control in a Bond

Vanity is a fantasized image of the self that originates when parents substitute empty praise and a false buildup as compensation for the absence of real love, appreciation, and acknowledgment. This image becomes a form of self-gratification, and the adult continues to gravitate toward other people who will praise, flatter, and approve of him or her.

Vanity in a man and the corresponding buildup from a woman are relatively common in our society. Stereotypical views of male superiority and strength and female inferiority and weakness support these dynamics in marital relationships. Men are implicitly taught that they should be the ruler of the household, the preferred choice of their mates, the great lover, superior to other males. The man who has an inflated self-image characteristically selects a woman who offers him the same kind of special treatment his mother provided. A man who is trying to compensate for feelings of sexual inadequacy or other weaknesses, real or imagined, can easily find his counterpart. In many marriages, there is a strong commitment to flattering the man and shielding him from comparisons with other men. Typically, the woman praises her husband and caters to him in his presence but talks about him in derogatory terms behind his back. The man senses on some level that the buildup is a lie, but still craves it.

Whenever the man's ego is threatened—by a hint of infidelity, by his wife's attention being diverted to career, school, or child rearing, or by a break in the flow of flattery or catering—he may feel abandoned or devastated. His underlying feelings of self-hatred and self-doubts are exposed.

An unsuccessful artist had been told by his mother as a child that he had artistic talent. She lavished praise on him and raved about the great artist he was to become. Later, when his wife suggested that he try to find a job to supplement his sparse income, the man went into a deep depression.

For years, he had fantasized a bright future, imagining that his next painting would be a masterpiece. He was convinced that he would soon receive wide recognition as well as financial success. His wife's acknowledgment that he wasn't adequately supporting his family demolished his fantasized image of himself as a great artist as well as his dreams of the future. He turned his rage against himself and punished his wife by becoming depressed and even less productive.

Withdrawing unrealistic support and indirectly attacking a man's inflated image can have far-reaching consequences. When a man's sexual relating is dependent on his wife's buildup, her interest or lack of interest in sex exerts a great deal of leverage in the marriage. If the woman holds back her sexual response, her mate is confused, frustrated, and threatened in his basic feelings about himself as a man. If he is vain, his image of himself as a lover is weakened considerably by this manipulation. In this manner, women are able to effectively control the couple's emotional life. Faithfulness on the part of the woman is an essential ingredient for safeguarding male vanity. Any possibility of a comparison sexually or any hint of an attraction on the part of "his woman" to another man can arouse deep feelings of insecurity and self-hatred in a man (Endnote 5).

A woman is able to control the man in her life not only by manipulating his vanity or maintaining his illusions but also by acting weak, childish, or inferior. By pretending that he is more intelligent, by deferring to him in social situations, or by casting him in the role of a "father," a woman gives her partner a false sense of importance that distorts his sense of reality. These manipulations support the man's fantasized image of superiority as effectively as flattery or exaggerated praise.

FRIENDSHIP AND LOVE RELATIONSHIPS

In contrast to bonds, real friendship and loving relationships are characterized by freedom and genuine relating. In a friendship, a person acts out of choice, whereas in a fantasy bond, he or she acts out of obligation. Therefore, friendship has therapeutic value, whereas the types of bonds described here are antitherapeutic in nature. People cannot be coerced into feeling the right or correct emotion, and when they attempt to make their emotions conform to a standard, their affect becomes shallow and inappropriate and they lose vitality.

Men and women can remain close friends if manifestations of the fantasy bond are understood and relinquished. Healthy relationships are characterized by each partner's independent striving for personal development and self-realization. In a loving relationship, open expressions of physical and verbal affection are evident, as illustrated in Figure 7.1, "Couple Relations Chart." Acting out of choice leads to a feeling of joy and happiness while diminishing one's self-hatred. Hostility and anger are not acted out but brought out in the couple's ongoing dialogue. Negative perceptions, disappointments, and hurt feelings can be dealt with, then dismissed, without holding grudges. In the type of relationship that is growth enhancing, partners refrain from exerting proprietary rights over one another. Each is respectful of the other's boundaries, separate points of view, goals, and aspirations (Endnote 6).

The fact that many people prefer to pursue relationships in fantasy and reject genuine friendship and actual love in reality accounts for a great deal of their seemingly perverse or irrational behavior. An individual's fantasy source of gratification is threatened by genuinely satisfying experiences. For this reason, people's actions are often directly contrary to their own best interests. Understanding the dynamics of the fantasy bond helps explain self-limiting and self-destructive behavior that interrupts the flow of goal-directed activity.

THERAPEUTIC APPROACHES

A major problem with many psychotherapies is that both the therapist and the patient refuse to challenge the core defense—the fantasy bond. Intense reactions and strong resistance are inevitable when separating from illusory connections with one's family or mate. For this reason, the therapist is often afraid of retaliation from family members. Furthermore, therapists may conform

Ideal Relationship	Relationship Characterized by a Fantasy Bond
1. Separate identity	1. Merged identity (illusion of fusion)
2. Equality	2. Dominance/submission
3. Independence	3. Insecurity and excessive emotional dependency
4. Eye contact	4. Limited eye contact
5. Respect for each other's boundaries	5. Overstepping boundaries
6. Loving operations	6. Nonloving operations
a. physical affection	a. coldness
b. consideration	b. insensitivity
c. respect	c. criticality
d. companionship	d. inwardness and isolation
e. support	e. hostility
f. spontaneity	f. routines
g. positive sexual relating	g. sexual dysfunction
7. Realistic appraisal of self and other — both good and bad	7. Buildup and tear down of self and other
8. Nondefensive — open to feedback	8. Defensive posture (angry reactions to feedback)
9. Open to give and take with the other	9. Pseudoindependent and self-nurturing
10. Respect for the goals of the other separate from self	10. Other seen only in relation to self
11. Open system — nonexclusive — extended family system— open to friends and outsiders	11. Closed system — exclusive of others

Copyright © 1996 by The Glendon Association

Figure 7.1. Couple Relations Chart: Positive and Negative Modes of Relating

to standard beliefs about the sanctity of the family unit (or preserving the couple) as protection against seeing the destructive processes within their own marriage or family.

Once a fantasy bond is formed, many patients falsely equate breaking the bond with terminating the relationship itself. In actuality, exposing destructive ties opens up the possibility of a renewed and better relationship. In this context, it is important for patients to recognize that, for the most part, divorce or rejection of the other may represent a step backward into an inward, unfeeling, or self-denying life. Despite the many rationalizations offered for breaking up or leaving a long-standing relationship, in the majority of situations, patients are preserving their defensive structure rather than moving toward a positive life choice.

Unless manifestations of the bond are identified and consistently challenged, there will be no sustained therapeutic progress. Therefore, in an effective psychotherapy, destructive bonds are exposed and understood in the context of an individual's fears and anxieties. This approach assists the couple in relating to each other on a more positive basis and frees them to experience genuine loving feelings.

CONCLUSION

The fantasy bond represents a neurotic solution in that human beings depend on inner fantasy for gratification and progressively give up actual gratification in the real world. In their coupling, men and women surrender their individuality and unique points of view for imagined safety and eternal love.

In forming a fantasy bond with our loved one, we deny the inevitability of our personal death and block out the terror of dying. The illusion of being connected to another person gives us a sense of immortality, a feeling of living forever, but robs us of day-to-day life. In contrast, living in an undefended, nonfused state forces us to face our existential aloneness and separateness. Indeed, the addictive and compelling nature of the fantasy bond lies in the fact that it denies death and relieves our anxiety about the future. The drawback is that it creates a powerful resistance to living a free, independent existence in harmony and genuine closeness with our loved ones.

ENDNOTES

1. In his classic study, *Family Therapy in Clinical Practice,* Murray Bowen (1978) described the typical couple:

In the average nuclear family living apart from the parental family . . . the spouses are emotionally "fused" with each other and with the children, and it is difficult to get far beyond the fusion or to do more than react and counterreact emotionally. (p. 545)

Boszormenyi-Nagy and Spark (1984), in *Invisible Loyalties,* also discussed the intergenerational transmission of patterns of reciprocity and obligation within family systems.

2. Descriptive accounts of the myths of marriage that distort people's expectations of the marital state and predispose disappointment can be found in *The Mirages of Marriage* by William J. Lederer and Don D. Jackson (1968). Partners also tend to depend increasingly on each other for

affirmation of their feelings of self-esteem or self-importance. Miriam Solomon (1989), in *Narcissism and Intimacy,* discussed the development of defensive collusion formed by partners with a "history of narcissistic vulnerability": "A collusive contract maintains the consistency of each partner's perceptions. In that way, neither is forced to deal with overwhelming negative feelings about oneself. . . . Any change in the system reactivates defensive rather than adaptive mechanisms" (p. 95).

3. David M. Schnarch (1991) emphasized existential issues in discussing problems in intimacy in his book *Constructing the Sexual Crucible:*

> Love signals our eventual final death. . . . Like love, life itself is something we won't let go of, but which we refuse to accept anyway. . . . Loving is not for the weak. . . . There is an alternative escape route that many people take: to not love the partner too much. (pp. 594-595)

4. Problems in communication were found to be a major factor in divorce in a longitudinal study conducted by B. Parker and S. Drummond-Reeves (1993). Bodin (1996) has described the development of a scale to assess relationship conflict that includes a number of items related to forms of dysfunctional communication.

5. Robert Wright (1994) reported a study by evolutionary psychologist David Buss in which men imagining sexual infidelities on the part of their wives exhibited a significant increase in heart rates, whereas women experienced distress when imagining emotional infidelity. Buss and Schmitt (1993), in their article "Sexual Strategies Theory: An Evolutionary Perspective on Human Mating," conjecture that "sexual jealousy is one adaption for the problem of paternity uncertainty. . . . Male sexual jealousy apparently functions to guard a mate and to dissuade intrasexual competitors, thus lowering the likelihood of alien insemination" (p. 216).

6. Beavers and Hampson (1990) defined "optimal" families along a number of dimensions. They concluded that

> in these families . . . intimacy is sought and usually found, a high level of respect for individuality and the individual perspective is the norm, and capable negotiation and communicational clarity are the results. There is a strong sense of individuation with clear boundaries; hence, conflict and ambivalence (at the individual level) are handled directly, overtly, and (usually) negotiated efficiently. (p. 48)

In *Sexual Animosity Between Men and Women,* Gerald Schoenewolf (1989) described the "Harmonic Couple" in terms of a lack of narcissism in each partner and a complementarity between male assertiveness and female receptivity: "The relationship becomes one of mutual respect and interdependence, in which neither is dominant" (p. 119).

8

Manifestations of the Inward Process

> I consider many adults (including myself) are or have been, more or less
> in a hypnotic trance, induced in early infancy: we remain in this state
> until—when we dead awaken, as Ibsen makes one of his characters
> say—we shall find that we have never lived.
>
> *R. D. Laing (1969/1972, p. 82)*

In this perceptive and compelling quote, Laing refers to a state of mind and a lifestyle that I have observed for many years. The majority of individuals in our culture exist in a dazed state, removed from feeling and unaware that they are deeply involved in a process that diminishes their human qualities. Their emotional deadness precludes an awareness that they are living out a life that is not really their own. I have come to understand that this lack of awareness is a major characteristic of an inward state that affects the lives of most people.

Unfortunately, to comprehend people's narrow focus and loss of experience, it is necessary to take an incisive look at one's defenses. A person must not only overcome powerful resistances that defend against psychological pain but also the social pressures that militate against this development. In this chapter, I will attempt to explain this form of depersonalization, illustrating the psychodynamics involved in alienation and self-limitation. I contrast the potential for men and women to spend the larger portion of their lives in an honest, open, and outward state of self-realization with the majority of people who lead self-defeating, emotionally impoverished lives (Endnote 1).

The process of becoming inward and neutralizing experience cuts people off from feeling for themselves and others. In this self-protective state, they look inward, at themselves, instead of outward toward other people. The inward state is characterized by feelings of self-consciousness rather than feelings of being conscious of self, or centered in oneself. The ability to give and accept love is seriously impaired when one is in an inward state.

There are a thousand ways of eliminating those attributes that make one uniquely human. The compulsive TV viewer or video game player numbs his or her senses; the workaholic loses him- or herself in his or her job; and the cocaine addict drugs him- or herself into a state of oblivion. There are a wide variety of lifestyles and addictive habit patterns, many socially condoned, that function to alienate people from themselves: the self-sacrificing ascetic denies him- or herself sexual experiences and other pleasures of life; the loner avoids personal contact with potential friends; the lover clings to a relationship with the other and gives up his or her individuality; the businessman/woman develops an ulcer; the despondent teenager obsesses about suicide; the schizophrenic retreats into a waking nightmare.

CONDITIONS CONDUCIVE TO
THE RETREAT INTO INWARDNESS

As described earlier, the process of becoming inward and self-protective is a response to negative environmental conditions that are damaging to psychological development. In considering the optimal situation for the newborn infant, an analogy can be made between the developing child and flora and fauna. It is obvious, for example, that plants and animals need certain basic elements to survive and grow; similarly, human beings require specifiable environmental conditions to reach their full potential for physical and emotional development.

The infant needs food, water, warmth, shelter, and an optimal amount of audiovisual and tactile stimulation to survive. It has been well established that insufficient physical contact can cause "failure to thrive" syndrome and death in infancy. Although receiving less critical attention, there are many cases of overstimulation, such as rough or insensitive handling, violation of the boundaries of the child, and excessive touching on the part of emotionally hungry or immature parents that can be equally destructive to the functional integrity of the individual.

Human beings are social animals and each person has a basic need for affiliation with others. The growing child requires contact with an empathic, affectionate adult or adults who are mature enough to be able to provide control and direction. Under ideal conditions, the interpersonal environment would offer close, genuine experiences that would enhance the individual's search for meaning in life.

It is difficult for us as adults, who are distant from and out of contact with the world of our childhood, to identify the events or environmental conditions that acted as roadblocks to our development. The elements that relate to what Winnicott (1958) referred to as the infant's "going on being" are often subtle and therefore not easy to pinpoint. Although the long-lasting effects are more apparent, it is difficult without in-depth analysis to establish the correlation between early environmental failures and their consequences. On the other hand, if we are sensitive to the child's essential humanness, we can observe the personal qualities trod on or tampered with by parents in the course of socializing their children. In many families, children's expressions of love and affection, their reaching out to touch the world, their drive to explore and manipulate their surroundings, their exhilaration in jumping, dancing, and moving about freely, their delight in hearing the sound of their own voice, their enthusiasm and feelings are subtly or not-so-subtly discouraged, controlled, punished, and squelched by well-intentioned, albeit defended, adults. Finally, a child's spirit may be subdued altogether as he or she adapts to a situation from which there is no escape.

OBSERVABLE SIGNS OF FRAGMENTATION AND THE INWARD STATE IN CHILDREN AND ADULTS

Even in very young children, one can observe the early signs of withdrawal or retreat from the self, as shown in Figure 8.1. These characteristics are entrenched by the time the individual reaches adulthood. The inward person (a) is not centered in him- or herself; (b) has a tendency to avoid genuine eye contact; (c) tends to be excessively dependent or anxiously attached; (d) makes connecting responses that arouse guilt, emotional hunger, anger, and a sense of obligation in the other; and (e) is to varying degrees cut off from feeling or is inappropriate in his or her emotional responses. There are often melodramatic reactions to trivial or unimportant incidents, yet little or no response to significant life events.

When faced with pain, children make the best adaptation possible to preserve a form of rationality, sanity, and equilibrium. A balance is formed between self-fulfilling dimensions of the personality and self-limiting dimensions. As a result of developing defenses, all people exist in conflict between an active pursuit of goals in the real world and a defensive reliance on self-gratification. Retreat to an increasingly inward posture represents, in effect, a form of

Observable Signs of the Healthy Individual	Observable Signs of Fragmentation in Children and Adults
The healthy, spontaneous, centered individual seeks external gratification. Aggression is directed at the source of frustration.	The damaged or excessively defended individual seeks gratification internally in fantasy and tends to sabotage successes in reality. Aggression and rage are directed at self and others as an alienation process.
The healthy individual generally manifests:	**The defended individual manifests:**
(1) A self-possessed state, as contrasted with elevated anxiety states and emotional deadness (2) A lively, appealing quality (3) Eye contact—personal relating (4) Independence (5) Feeling responses	(1) A cut-off or agitated state (2) Unlikable characteristics—character defenses are etched into physical appearance, posture, and expressive movement (3) Lack of genuine eye contact—impersonal relating (4) Dependency relationships and connecting responses (5) A lack of or inappropriate affect

Figure 8.1. Manifestations of Mental Health (Self) and Fragmentation (Antiself System)

controlled destruction of the self. Neurotic symptomatology, personality disorders, and repetitive, self-defeating behaviors are closely related to a negative resolution of this basic conflict. A particular style or mode of defense will tend to generate specific symptoms, that is, compulsive-obsessional disorders, psychosomatic illness, delusions, or other forms of psychopathology. These patterns of defense tend to persist and become habitual, leading to progressive problems in broad areas of functioning.

Anything that threatens to disturb an individual's solution to the core conflict arouses fear. Movement in any direction, that is, a retreat further into fantasy and self-parenting or movement toward external goal-directed behavior, is accompanied either by negative or by positive anxiety (Whitaker & Malone, 1981). The rise in anxiety results in both aggressive and regressive reactions. This phenomenon can be observed in a wide range of situations. The dynamics

OPEN/OUTWARD VS.	INWARD/SELF-PARENTING
Goal-directed behavior Self-fulfillment Self-affirmation	Seeking gratification in fantasy Self-denial Self-destructiveness
Lack of self-consciousness Realistic self-appraisal Self-assertion	Exaggerated self-consciousness Hypercritical attitudes toward the self Passivity and victimized stance

Adaptability
Facing up to pain and anxiety
    with appropriate affect
    and response
	Nonadaptability
	Utilizing routinized habits,
	    addictive personal relationships,
	    and substances as painkillers

Relatedness to others Feeling state Social involvement	Impersonal relating Cutting off or withdrawal of affect Isolation

Genitality
 	
Maintaining a separate identity
Search for meaning and
    transcending goals
	Masturbatory and addictive
	    sexuality
	Merged identity and fusion
	Narrow focus

Figure 8.2. Open/Outward Lifestyle Versus Inward/Self-Parenting Lifestyle
SOURCE: This figure is adapted, with permission, from an article titled "The Psychodynamics of Fantasy, Addiction, and Addictive Attachments," *American Journal of Psychoanalysis, 53* (1993), 335-352.

explain perverse reactions to unusual achievement, positive acknowledgment, and satisfaction in a love relationship. Patients' negative responses to progress in psychotherapy can be understood in this context.

OPEN, OUTWARD LIFESTYLE
VERSUS AN INWARD STATE

Psychological functions and addictive propensities can be represented on parallel continuums, ranging from an outward lifestyle of pursuing goals in the real world to an inward lifestyle characterized by fantasy, passivity, and isolation. The functions delineated in Figure 8.2 exist on a continuum of healthy functioning to serious maladjustment.

Essentially, inwardness or desensitization to one's feelings refers to an insidious process of regarding oneself more as an object than as a person. To varying degrees, all individuals block out feelings and emotions in a manner that causes them to deviate from the true course of their lives. Each person develops specific, idiosyncratic methods for dulling, deadening, and disconnecting from his or her experiences. People have strong tendencies to live out their lives largely in the destructive antiself system or defended posture, resisting individuation and unique experiences in life.

As discussed, an important characteristic of the inward state is that of re-creating the original conditions within the family by (a) selection, (b) distortion, and (c) provocation of others. These maneuvers support defenses that prevent the individual from changing his or her self-concept or identity in the family. They maintain a form of control that minimizes risks and avoids challenges in personal relationships. In using these machinations, people are choosing to relive rather than live their lives.

MANIFESTATIONS OF
THE INWARD STATE

A Retreat Into Self-Parenting

As described earlier, when children are deprived of emotional sustenance, they gradually compensate with fantasy gratification. They develop an imaginary self-parenting process or fantasy bond in which they are both the parent and the object of parenting. They tend to both nurture and punish themselves. The damaged child or adult tends to spend a large part of his or her waking life dominated by conscious or unconscious fantasies that lead to distortion of everyday experiences. This preoccupation is far more extensive and inclusive than the person realizes. It must be distinguished from simple daydreaming, creative fantasy, or the mental activity of planning for the future. As described in Chapter 7, aspects of the self-parenting process are later externalized in the form of addictive interpersonal relationships.

Preference for Fantasy Gratification
Over Real Achievement

Reliance on fantasy gratification tends to be progressively incapacitating as it interferes with adaptive responses. In a sense, they are mutually exclusive pursuits. In choosing to defend themselves, people often prefer fantasy, a self-soothing mechanism that is immediately rewarding, over active competition for life's rewards.

The important issue here is that fantasy and addictive habit patterns actually deprive the person of the necessary ingredients for a happy life. The tragedy is that most people never fulfill their destiny as unique individuals because they are not free enough to move toward a warmer, richer, more positive environment than they experienced during their formative years. Their tendency is to retreat from people, relationships, or circumstances that would meet their needs, while maintaining an illusion that they are acting in their best interests.

Passivity

An inclination toward passivity is one outcome of a defensive solution to the core conflict. Images and symbols of success are extremely important to people who prefer fantasy over the pursuit of real goals; they care more about how they appear than they do about actual personal satisfactions. They are reluctant to initiate actions that could lead to progress because real achievement would remove them from their fantasy world and disrupt the self-parenting process that they have depended on since early childhood.

The passive person moves toward a state of nothingness, an unfeeling, dead space. He or she experiences spontaneous activity or productive work as an unwelcome intrusion. Moreover, the activities he or she is willing to engage in are usually habitual and routine, providing minimal stimulation, offering a false sense of certainty and permanence, and acting to dull feeling reactions. Passivity tends to foster a victimized, paranoid posture in which a person perceives forces acting on him or her rather than seeing him- or herself as acting upon the environment.

A Victimized Orientation Toward Life

The self-protective, defended person finds it exceptionally difficult to cope with adversity. He or she generally succumbs to and is overwhelmed by negative events and circumstances. There is a tendency to complain and dwell on frustrating situations instead of experiencing anger and taking appropriate action. The anger that one would ordinarily feel in response to frustration is rationalized and transformed into a feeling of being hurt or victimized. This posture fosters attitudes of blame and righteous indignation that progressively incapacitate the individual. It gives rise to a chronic low-grade, internalized anger that feeds on itself without a real outlet.

Feelings of being wounded and playing the victim cause people to deal with life in judgmental terms and "shoulds." They operate on the basic assumption that the world should be fair: "I should have been loved by my parents." "After all I've done for them!" "That's no way to treat a person," and so on. Their preoccupation with rights and shoulds even when justified are irrelevant to problem solving. Even in the worst of circumstances, such as confinement in a concentration camp, one would be better off planning tactics of survival or escape rather than focusing on injustice and wrongdoing (Endnote 2).

Another important dynamic underlying passivity and a victimized orientation lies in the mistaken notion that many people have about love. Many individuals equate an internal feeling of love with behaviors that are loving. They *imagine* that they love another, yet fail to express this love through action, that is, through affection, tenderness, or consideration of the other's well-being. Because their internal fantasy of love fails to reach the other person and is usually not reciprocated, they are left feeling foolish, righteous, and indignant.

Treating Oneself as an Object

To varying degrees, all people feel self-conscious, view themselves as objects, and see themselves through the eyes of others. Laing (1960/1969) described self-consciousness as *"an awareness of oneself as an object of someone else's observation"* (p. 106). This phenomenon is seen in an exaggerated form in psychotic delusions of reference.

In a sense, people who self-consciously view themselves as objects have turned their eyes in on themselves rather than focusing their gaze outward toward the world and others. This internal scrutiny or self-centeredness (the opposite of self-love or genuine self-interest) leads to distortions of reality.

In relating to themselves in this manner, most individuals become casually remote, give little or no value to their feelings or experiences, and at times are careless about or disregarding of issues involving their physical health and emotional well-being. When a person allows his or her appearance or surroundings to become cluttered, dirty, or unattractive, there is an indication of pathology. People who characteristically hang on to a problem and remain indifferent to solutions, or who are resistant to logic or reason that would improve their situations, are exhibiting manifestations of a self-destructive, inward lifestyle.

The posture of disregarding oneself originates in early relations within the family. Many adults report that they were treated as objects or possessions by parents who believed that their children belonged to them in a proprietary sense. They revealed that they were intruded on with a lack of respect for their boundaries, that their parents lived vicariously through their achievements, and that they were generally unseen or seen through critical, unfriendly eyes.

In trying to avoid the direct experience of emotional pain, defended individuals have less and less tolerance for anxiety and attempt to narcotize themselves with painkilling substances. They are removed from themselves and their everyday experiences and tend to think of themselves as "the poor, misunderstood child," valiantly contending with a hostile world, the "noble child syndrome." Operating from this perspective, they give themselves approval and praise or reward themselves for success, while denigrating and castigating themselves for errors or failures. In a sense, they pat themselves on the head when they are "good" and lash out at themselves when they are "bad."

Unfortunately, a good deal of "inner child" therapy or recovery group work supports this dimension of inwardness. Any manner or means of self-parenting, reparenting oneself, or treating oneself as an object is detrimental, no matter how kindly or upbeat. When people view themselves as forlorn children in the sense of attempting to minister to their "inner child" and offering themselves the loving care that they were deprived of in childhood, it actually fosters painful regressive states. It is of utmost importance for people to be themselves in an ongoing motivational state, experiencing their emotions rather than observing or attending to themselves. Living an outward life, while at times anxiety-provoking, eventually silences internal "voices," freeing up energy for active pursuits.

Isolation

Isolation is a key aspect of an inward self-destructive lifestyle. It can be a significant sign of suicidal intent and a central element in actual suicide. Self-critical attitudes and cynicism toward others lead to an avoidance of meaningful social relationships. The person addicted to inwardness rationalizes his or her retreat with voice statements (experienced in the second person) such as the following: "You need your own space, more quiet time." "You need time alone to think things over," or simply "You're too busy" or "You don't have enough money to go places or do things." However, he or she typically spends this time alone, brooding, feeling victimized, and indulging in cynical revengeful fantasies and other forms of self-defeating thoughts. The inward state is characterized by an involvement in meaningless, ritualistic habit patterns that distract one from important pursuits. Individuals who are self-protective and isolated also tend to be narcissistic, self-comforting, and self-pitying.

A study by Gove and Hughes (1980) indicates that inwardness as exemplified in social isolation is related to self-destructive behavior. They demonstrated that alcoholism and suicide are two forms of social pathology that relate to social isolation, operationally defined as living alone. These self-destructive behaviors were found to be much more prevalent in those living alone than in those who lived with others. This study agrees with the results found in studies of student suicide (Seiden, 1966) and in research relating high suicide rates to areas of low population density with its resultant physical and social isolation (Seiden, 1984).

Withholding and Self-Denial

Withholding patterns and self-denial are important aspects of the inward process. *Withholding* refers to a holding back of positive responses, talents, and capabilities as a form of microsuicide or retreat from life. Whenever an individual withholds behaviors or qualities that were once an important expression of his or her personal motivation, that person is no longer goal-directed and becomes more oriented toward failure.

The withholding person resists involvement in emotional transactions, refusing to take love in from the outside or to offer love and affection to others. There is an absence of give and take that keeps relationships at bay, a generalized reduction of commerce with others characterized by the reluctance or outright refusal to exchange products. Withholding in the broader sense is not only limited to the holding back of affection and sexuality but relates also to limiting one's capabilities, avoiding or retreating from leading a productive life. Patterns of withholding are prevalent in the workplace, where passive-aggressive behaviors of procrastination, fatigue, incompetence, insolence, and other nonproductive work styles are often manifested. Passive-aggression may be directed outward toward others as a disguised form of hostility or against the self as a pathological example of self-denial and self-limitation.

Wherever it manifests itself, withholding is governed by internal voices that modify one's behavior. Free-flowing feeling responses are inhibited by destructive thought patterns such as in the following: "Why should you go out of your way for her?" "This job is stupid, the boss doesn't know what he's doing." "She doesn't love you." "They don't care about how you feel." "Who does he think he is?" or "Hell, who needs him or anyone?" The withholding individual may or may not be conscious of this underlying thought process, but nevertheless it controls his or her destiny.

Children cannot win in any kind of power play or showdown with parents and must therefore resort to indirect means to assert themselves. Withholding is a form of control through weakness that is often effective in manipulating the interpersonal environment. Minority groups, women, and children are more prone to use passive techniques in an attempt to control their surroundings because they have been disenfranchised from positions of power.

Environmental conditions that foster the development of a withholding posture in life have an adverse effect on personality development. The withholding individual is plagued by internal rage and guilt, leading to an unhappy, unsuccessful life. An intrusive parent who disregards the personal boundaries of the child, a sadistic parent who delights in denying the child gratification, an immature parent who attempts to feed off the child's accomplishments, or a family atmosphere characterized by neglect and/or hostility is most conducive to the defense mechanisms of withholding and self-denial.

Finally, people who inhibit their responses, whether in the work arena or in personal relationships, need to make sense out of their seemingly perverse tendency to avoid fulfilling essential goals. They use rationalizations or ostensibly realistic reasons to justify behaviors that support a restrictive, self-limiting lifestyle. They may even pride themselves on behaviors that are essentially against their own interests. In learning about their inwardness and attempting to triumph over debilitating forces within their personality, growing individuals must learn to challenge these defensive rationalizations.

Lack of Direction in Life:
A Diminished Sense of Values

One of the most tragic consequences of the "processing" that children go through in the developmental sequence is that they grow up with a weakened, fragmented, and fragile sense of self. Very early in life, children disconnect from themselves and lose touch with their basic wants and desires. Cut off from real experience, they find it difficult to express or even define their emotions. If one loses touch with one's wants and needs, it is difficult to identify the source of one's angry feelings. Even if a person develops an "I don't care" attitude and inhibits or represses his or her needs, they are still operant, and when frustrated, mobilize aggressive reactions. This leads to a state of agitation and bewilderment with a corresponding depletion of energy and vitality.

Adult individuals who fail to pursue their goals lack a basic integrity and therefore cannot communicate honestly; in denying their goals or priorities, they deceive themselves and others. On the other hand, if they acknowledge wants that they withhold or motives they fail to pursue, their manifest behavior contradicts their expressed desires. In other words, people who have been damaged don't want what they say they want or behave according to their own interests. When their actions fail to echo stated values, people are duplicitous in their communications, and their mixed signals are confusing and harmful to others, particularly their children.

The process of progressive self-denial, self-deception, and rationalized dishonesty described above leads to a demoralized state of emptiness and futility. A clear-cut sense of direction is lost, and the inward person fails to develop a moral code of his or her own. He or she becomes either submissive or defiant in relation to other people and moral precepts; both responses lack independence because they are reactions to external forces. Neither reflects a powerful, self-directed orientation or clear-cut point of view with which to navigate through life.

A Negative Self-Image
and Cynicism Toward Others

Most people cling to negative attitudes toward themselves, hold on to the way they were perceived in their families, and find it extremely difficult to adapt to a more positive or realistic point of view. The process of self-defamation is closely related to the defense mechanism of idealizing parents and family and has been reported in children as young as 2 or 3 years old.

Negative attitudes and assumptions about other people also originate as responses to traumatic events in childhood. Primarily, anticipations about the world are based on early experiences within the family. If the general atmosphere at home is hostile and the parents are inadequate or untrustworthy, the child's feeling reactions to these conditions will later be transferred to new situations and new objects. As an adult, the person will distort people and events, responding to them with negative or fearful expectations. The interview that follows illustrates the manner in which parental behaviors are projected onto others, thereby distorting the social milieu.

Case Study

The case in point illustrates the process in which a woman experiences a temporary regression of serious proportions and describes the dynamics of her retreat from her closest relationships into an isolated, inward behavior pattern. After a seemingly innocuous phone conversation with her parents, S. became depressed, agitated, and cynical toward her friends. Initially she was unaware of the depth of her regression or of the precipitating factors. Finally, troubled by self-destructive, suicidal thoughts that pervaded her thinking, she talked about her distress to a close friend and began to uncover the reasons for the dramatic transformation in her emotional state. At this point, she volunteered to meet with me to further investigate the dynamics underlying the regressive episode.

The interview began with S., a successful psychological assistant, recalling the event that immediately preceded her withdrawal:[1]

> *S.:* What happened originally was that I had a couple of phone calls from my parents, who live back East. I had invited them to come out to visit me, and I wanted to treat them differently than I've treated them almost my whole life as an adult. My usual way of treating them was sort of angry and belligerent and nasty. That was a way of being that didn't make me feel good, to treat anybody like that. So I wanted to try to treat them decently, just in a friendly way.
>
> But in the conversation with my parents, when I invited them to come out to visit me, they said that they didn't want to come out, or they couldn't. Whatever the reason was, the end result was that they weren't going to be coming.

---

1 This interview was videotaped and made into a documentary film titled *Inwardness: A Retreat From Feeling* (Parr, 1995b).

I *thought* that I felt good from the conversation because I had been friendly to them and I sort of forgot about it. I was relieved in a way that they weren't coming because it's usually an uncomfortable situation when they visit.

But then about 6 weeks or so after that, I noticed funny things about myself. I felt that I wasn't living in 1995, in the present. I had come to be distorting almost everything, interactions with friends that I'm really close to and that I really like and love. I was hearing everything wrong, distorting everything.

Dr. F.: After the phone call.

S.: Yes. Everything seemed different to me. I heard people saying critical things to me when they weren't being critical. My whole point of view changed. I started hating people, being critical of them, seeing them in a cynical way. And also being critical toward myself, but that realization came later.

I couldn't understand what it was coming from. I didn't know why, why am I back to this old way of being? And it wasn't appropriate to anything. In fact, I was superimposing an old way of being onto a current situation and current people that absolutely did not fit. I was hearing people being angry when they weren't.

Dr. F.: So how did that connect in your mind (with the phone call)?

S.: Just the contact with my parents, even though it was seemingly benign, sent me back to an old image of myself, an old mood, an old style of living.

Dr. F.: It seems like you were really vulnerable in that phone call.

S.: Yes, because in the conversation, I didn't exhibit a defense that I usually had, which was a nasty way of being. It was a deliberate thing that I tried to do, to be friendly to them, but it did leave me being more vulnerable.

S. then recounted the steps she took to begin to reverse this distorted view and her downward spiral, which allowed her to emerge from the inward state into which she had retreated.

Dr. F.: How did you come out of that state where you were progressively feeling worse and worse after the phone call?

S.: First of all, by mentioning it, by saying, noticing that I felt really bad.

Dr. F.: So you broke the pattern in a way.

S.: Just by saying something, "Look I feel really bad and I don't know why." Just to my friends. That was a break that interrupted the whole pattern.

Then the battle was more than halfway won, just by saying something, by letting somebody in, by looking at people like they were my friends. But I struggled with myself for a long time before I said that.

I knew I was feeling bad for a long time before I said something. I had expected my friends to be angry. In that inward state, I expected that if I said, "Look, I'm feeling bad," they would say, "Look, if you're feeling bad, just get out of here until you feel better and come back when you're feeling better," which is so uncharacteristic of how I know my friends of 20 years to respond to me.

Dr. F.:   So after talking, just mentioning how bad you felt, trusting people that much—

S.:   Then I was back in this world. I knew that people were my friends.

Dr. F.:   How did you come to the insights?

S.:   Just trying to trace back when the last time was that I felt good, what was the last significant event that happened. At the time, I didn't even give that phone call any significance because I thought I came out of it feeling good. But I was really wrong. I felt hurt.

Dr. F.:   Then when you caught on to the fact that it started from the phone call, what happened then?

S.:   Then I saw how I was superimposing the original situation of how I lived as a kid on people and situations in my everyday life, then I started to feel so much better.

Dr. F.:   What happened when you had that realization?

S.:   First I felt huge relief, just so relieved to have a break in it. Like I could just sigh, just relax. It was the opposite of being tense and wound up.

Over the course of the interview, it became clear that after the call to her parents, S. had projected feelings of being rejected by them onto her friends and responded as though *they* were angry and rejecting. This distorted view caused her, in turn, to criticize her friends and to desperately seek isolation and distance, a pattern that was characteristic of her childhood reactions. She mistakenly perceived current social interactions as being hurtful and potentially dangerous rather than acknowledging the truth of her childhood experiences.

S.:   I think that in some way, I was hurt by my parents' rejection, but I didn't see the rejection consciously for a while, for about 6 or 8 weeks.

Dr. F.:   But you saw it everywhere else.

S.:   But I saw it everywhere else. I saw people as rejecting me, even though they weren't. That's what I superimposed on people, that they were rejecting me. So little by little, I cut off relationships that had been very important to me and became more and more isolated. I was desperate for the isolation and scared without it. I was conniving in my mind to arrange situations where I could be alone.

When this process is operating, I feel desperate, like my life depends on maintaining a certain amount of separation between myself and people. Being critical of other people is very much in the service of that because it's a way of justifying my distance from them. Just seeing faults in them that justify my not liking them. I have a reason not to like anybody. I mean, I could find fault with anybody.

S. described the inward state she was in as analogous to an addiction. She revealed that preserving her isolation led to increased alienation from others and contributed to a nonfeeling, depersonalized state.

S.:   In talking about inwardness, I've come to see it as an addiction in a way, like people become addicted to drugs or to food or to TV watching. I see it as my strongest addiction. Or I even think in a general way, it's the strongest addiction a person can have.

Dr. F.:   What are you addicted to? What are the symptoms? What are the things you are drawn to when you say you're addicted to being inward?

S.:   If I'm in a room full of people, isolating myself in my own mind by just thinking those kinds of critical thoughts or cynical thoughts, then automatically, I'm going more in that direction.

Dr. F.:   How is the inwardness hurting you in your life?

S.:   It interferes with the depth of my relationships with people tremendously. Even though it's so much less than it was. With people who I really love, it keeps me separate. It's a way of protecting myself all the time unless I make an effort not to do it.

I've heard that people in Alcoholics Anonymous wake up in the morning and they say, "I'm an alcoholic and today I'm not going to do such and such. I'm not going to have a drink." I feel like that with myself, that I'm an inward person. And today or this hour, I'm going to make an effort not to be this way. I'm not going to see people in a negative way. I'm not going to dwell on negative characteristics about them so that I could just hate them easily.

I know that there are other habits that I do, like driving by myself. I don't have to drive hardly anywhere by myself because there are people who I can drive back and forth to work with. Why not make it that kind of situation? But I choose to drive alone.

Dr. F.:   So you choose to be isolated.

S.:   I choose to be isolated when I can justify it. I look forward to it. But it's a
state of not feeling and not being vulnerable, not being vulnerable to
my own feelings or to seeing someone feeling something towards me or
for me. That's what I try to avoid.

Dr. F.:   Loving or being loved.

S.:   Not feeling my own loving feelings, and not allowing people to feel that
way towards me.

S. reported that before she revealed to her friends that she felt depressed, she
had experienced increasingly angry, hateful thoughts toward everyone. Examining the dynamics of these distorted perceptions at a deeper level, she recognized that her depression and agitation were reminiscent of the way she had felt
as a child.

Dr. F.:   How did you feel when you reached rock bottom?

S.:   Angry and hateful every second of my day. Distracted by hatefulness.
Distracted by hating to the point where I couldn't think about anything
else.
That's a state that I recognize as how I lived as a kid pretty much of
the time, angry and hating. Angry, all the time angry, and hateful. The
word hateful, that reminded me of how I lived as a child. That was
hateful and like this [*Pulls shoulders in*]. Defended, insulated.
I was raised by a woman who I see as extremely intrusive in every
way, physically, emotionally, and the way that I coped with it, the way
that I came to cope with it as a child was just to be extremely inward
and quiet. Almost never talking, especially to my parents.
Then I had nowhere to go with it. I didn't have friends. I didn't have
anybody to talk to about it. I felt wound up like a spring that's going to
explode, but never having a release for it. But that's the state that I was
into recently as an adult. That's how I felt, that wound up and removed.

Several days later, S. recalled a fact she unconsciously neglected to mention
at this point in the interview, that is, that during her regression, she had
experienced suicidal thoughts. She remembered that savage self-attacking
voices intruded on her thinking whenever she was alone, and went on to admit:

S.:   I began to feel angry that I had made a resolution some years ago to not
kill myself. Now I felt hemmed in, trapped by that resolution. I had
self-destructive thoughts at unexpected times, a voice that baited me:
"Why don't you just kill yourself?"

As the interview continued, S. verbalized specific self-destructive thoughts that caused her to avoid close times with her children. These particularly malicious voices tended to occur immediately following an especially positive or happy interaction with her children.

S.:   I have two children. But my relationships with them are very limited. When I've allowed there to be a sweet interaction between me and one of my own children or another child, I have such extreme reactions. Immediately afterward I have a thought that I should kill myself.

A crazy thought that I should just get rid of myself, literally kill myself. That's the thought, even though it's very far removed from action.

Dr. F.:   What does that mean to you?

S.:   Those kind of situations in relation to a child are very different than I remember being treated, in a sweet way. And it's also very different from how I see my own mother, how she was with me.

Dr. F.:   So when you're kind and touched and emotionally close to a child, you feel different from your mother. But why the anger toward yourself? What does that mean to you? Just let yourself feel it.

S.:   [*Sad*] It was like I'm betraying a way that I was brought up to be. I'm betraying her by being different. Also, it makes me see the truth of what happened to me. Somehow, being different makes it more apparent to me how I was really treated. It's a painful situation to recognize.

Dr. F.:   So if you treat your children by being especially kind, it brings out a lot of pain. It makes you turn on yourself.

S.:   And also if I allow that kind of relationship with my boyfriend, if I allow myself to feel loving or just be myself in a way that he would naturally love me back. I'm afraid of having that same kind of reaction like that angry reaction towards myself. And I think that that's part of why I'm stubborn about giving up this way of seeing myself.

Near the conclusion of the interview, S. developed considerable insight concerning the defensive function of inwardness. She realized that as a child, being inward and isolated had protected her from experiencing intense anger and fear reactions to a situation from which there was no escape. She indicated a desire to interrupt ongoing inward patterns in her daily life to minimize the chance of a recurrence of a regressive episode.

Dr. F.:   When you feel the pain of how you were treated, it seems more likely you'd feel angry at the way you were treated. Why are you angry at yourself?

S.: One thing that you just said reminded me that as a young child of around 4 and 5, I actually remember feeling so bad in the situation that I was in, that I would think about the only way that I—that if things got so bad, I could kill myself. Those are actual thoughts that I really remember having a lot of the time.

Dr. F.: Maybe the same thing that was happening then is still happening. You're really not angry at yourself, but it's turned on yourself.

S.: That's the only option that I saw then because I was so angry I didn't know what to do with it. And I either had to direct it outward or inward, but the anger was so great that I was afraid of directing it outward, because I was afraid that I'd really kill somebody. I lived as a kid, feeling like a murderer.

Dr. F.: To murder or to kill yourself.

S.: Or to kill myself. Those were my only two options because of the rage that I felt. And I was really afraid that I would do it. I was afraid that I had so much anger that I would actually kill somebody. So now when I'm in a vulnerable situation, I flip back to the same dilemma, and I'm going to kill them or myself.

Dr. F.: So when you're vulnerable, you feel the pain of how you were treated. It comes back to you, instead of being angry at your mother or father.

S.: I direct it towards myself. But I don't let myself get into that vulnerable a situation. That's why I avoid the whole issue by not letting it happen. By being inward, I don't have to deal with the whole situation.

Dr. F.: Maybe connecting this idea about anger would be helpful and seeing that really you had no alternative then. That you had a murderous rage from the way you were treated, and that the only outlet that you had for it that was acceptable to you—

S.: Was to direct it inward.

Dr. F.: —against yourself. And that's rekindled every time that you're really open and vulnerable.

S.: When these feelings come up, I still get afraid, and then I do whatever I have to, to maintain enough distance so that I'm *not* afraid. So I would have to go through withdrawal. I would have to sweat through the fear that I still feel, even though it's inappropriate now.

It feels so much better to say it to you, than to have it in my mind. I feel totally relaxed now. It's like I gave in to something to make this interview an outward conversation instead of a struggle that I'm trying to have just by myself.

Dr. F.:   Which is part of the inwardness itself. But also there's a solution pointed out in terms of the analogy of the drug addiction, that you have to sweat it out. For example, with your children, instead of withdrawing and holding yourself back, sweating it out would involve being with them. Even though you had these negative thoughts, you wouldn't discontinue the positive actions to get rid of the negative, attacking thoughts on yourself.

Maybe just understanding the connection between that rage being directed outward and then your retreating from that to hurting yourself or wanting to hurt yourself, could be of help, too, in sweating it out.

In the months that followed, S. regained her composure and good feelings about her life and went on to challenge other dimensions of her syndrome of inwardness. The exposure of her inward patterns and insight into their dynamics facilitated an important movement toward a better life, one that would most likely interfere with the possibility of a repetition of this type of serious regression in the future.

CONCLUSION

The inward state is an addictive, painkilling mode of defense adopted by the child when faced with environmental deprivation and external threat. The child's renunciation of the true self and his or her retreat to an emotionally deadened existence is the best adaptation that he or she can make in the struggle to preserve some rudimentary sense of self in the midst of toxic influences. These self-protective measures help an individual to survive an unhappy childhood at the expense of a richer, fuller life as an adult. They serve to restrict or eliminate the possibility of intimacy in close relationships and significantly reduce the person's capacity for relating to his or her offspring.

On an unconscious level, inward people gradually give up goal-directed activity and avoid real gratification to cling to the safety of an internal world over which they have complete control. The process of nurturing themselves in the inward state becomes addictive because it has immediately rewarding properties that dull psychological pain. Becoming aware of this process is essential for understanding and facilitating human beings' growth potential. It is important to emphasize that all people will encounter internal and external pressures as they emerge from a self-protective, inward state and face painful truths about their lives. However, despite our defensive idealization of the family, the overwhelming evidence connecting personal limitations with disturbances in family interactions must be assimilated. We must overcome our prejudices and are duty-bound to scrutinize and expose the causative factors that predispose inward patterns and the resultant misery caused by a defended approach to life. Understanding these dynamics is all the more important because the damage, whether clinical or subclinical, is far more extensive than we would like to believe.

ENDNOTES

1. Christopher Lasch (1984), in *The Minimal Self: Psychic Survival in Troubled Times,* delineates a number of dimensions of what he terms the "survival mentality," that is, tendencies he has observed in a large majority of individuals in our modern "narcissistic culture." These "everyday survival strategies" include a "restriction of perspective to the immediate demands of survival; ironic self-observation; protean selfhood; emotional anesthesia" (p. 94). Lasch's descriptive accounts bear a strong resemblance to the "inward" tendencies depicted in this chapter. Lasch writes,

> We arm ourselves emotionally against the onslaught of everyday life . . . by concentrating our attention on the small, immediate obstacles that confront us each day. . . . Survivors have to learn the trick of observing themselves as if the events of their lives were happening to someone else . . . a withdrawal from the beleaguered self into the person of a detached, bemused, ironic observer. . . . Role-playing, another strategy repeatedly recommended by survival manuals, serves not only to project an appropriate image of energy and confidence but to protect the self against unseen enemies, to keep feelings in check, and to control threatening situations. . . . Emotional disengagement serves as still another survival mechanism. (pp. 95-98)

2. Viktor Frankl (1954/1967), in his chapter "Group Psychotherapeutic Experiences in a Concentration Camp," asserts that in the German concentration camps,

> it seemed that the physical-psychic collapse was dependent upon the spiritual-moral attitude; and this attitude was a free one! And though on entering the camp everything might be taken away from the prisoner, even his glasses and his belt, this freedom remained to him; and it remained to him literally to the last moment, to the last breath. It was the freedom to bear oneself "this way or that way," and there *was* a "this or that." (p. 98)

PART III

Methodology

9

The Concept of the
Voice and Voice Therapy

Unconsciously . . . people inflict punishments on themselves to which an inner court has sentenced them. A hidden authority within the ego takes over the judgment originally expected of the parents.

Theodore Reik (1941, p. 10)

HISTORICAL DEVELOPMENT OF
THE CONCEPT OF THE VOICE

Background and Evolution
of Voice Therapy Theory

My life's work as a psychotherapist has focused on the problem of resistance. In my study of people's resistance to change, I had always been deeply perplexed by a seemingly paradoxical phenomenon: the fact that most people consistently avoid or minimize experiences that are warm, successful, or constructive. I was

AUTHOR'S NOTE: Portions of the material in this chapter are taken from *Voice Therapy: A Psychotherapeutic Approach to Self-Destructive Behavior,* Human Sciences Press (1988). Used with permission.

searching for an answer to the question of why most individuals, in spite of emotional catharsis, understanding, and intellectual insight, still held on to familiar, destructive patterns of the past and refused to change on a deep character level.

In our years of study, my colleagues and I observed clinical material that expanded our understanding of human self-destructiveness. As we addressed the problem of microsuicidal and suicidal ideology in our patients, we became increasingly involved in the cognitive processes associated with self-destructive behavior.

All along, we were concerned with the stubborn resistance to changing a conception of self that was self-critical or self-accusatory. In our work with schizophrenic patients, it became increasingly clear that these seriously disturbed people were involved in a process of idealizing their parents at their own expense. When we challenged the idealization of the parent with these patients, we noted that there was considerable resistance to changing both the idealized image of the parent and the negative image of self, and that the two processes were interrelated. In fact, when this idealization process was challenged directly in sessions where the patient was instructed to express negative ideas and critical comments about the parent image, there was a significant reduction in bizarre symptomatology and thought disturbance.[1]

Later, in applying this concept of the idealization of parents and family in an enlarged perspective, I began to comprehend its central role in psychopathological phenomena.

To illustrate, a patient recalled that when she approached adolescence, her father began beating her at night. At frequent intervals, he would come into her bedroom, wake her up, and physically abuse her. She said that at the time she "knew" he was right in punishing her, that she must have done something to make him angry. In the morning, in spite of her innocence, she would invariably apologize to him for causing trouble and being a problem child. If the patient had not assumed the blame for the beatings and instead had seen her father as being in the wrong, then she would have felt the full brunt of being in the hands of a highly disturbed, irrational, or even potentially murderous person who was out of control. It was the lesser of two evils for her to make his actions appear of rational character.

In my work with children ages 10 to 15, as well as with adults in a feeling release therapy, I was impressed that they all possessed a deep-seated conviction that they were "bad." When asked to make positive statements about themselves with feeling, strong primal emotions were induced, manifested by extreme sadness and sobbing. Statements such as "I'm not bad," when spoken sincerely

---

1 This technique was used while working with schizophrenic patients under the auspices of Dr. John Rosen. Our results were impressive with very regressed patients. Rosen's (1953) therapeutic approach is described in his book *Direct Analysis*.

by the patient in an accepting atmosphere, were accompanied by intense pain. Other positive statements, that is, "I'm good" or "I'm lovable," brought out similar outbursts when expression of the associated affect was encouraged. I concluded that this core of negative feeling toward self was an important dynamic in neurotic symptomatology and inimical lifestyles and was at the core of resistance to therapeutic change.

In my early work with schizophrenic patients and later in my office practice, I was progressing in my understanding of the dimensions of these self-destructive processes, but important aspects were missing. My associates and I were excited when we came upon several new developments in the early 1970s.

Early Investigations of the Voice

At that time, I was focusing on the emotional pain that patients experienced in group psychotherapy situations when they were confronted with certain types of verbal feedback or information about themselves. They would have strong negative responses to selective aspects of this information and would feel bad or depressed for long periods of time. Initially, I considered the old adage, "It's the truth that hurts," but then I realized that evaluations from others, regardless of accuracy, that support or validate a person's distorted view of him- or herself, tend to arouse an obsessive negative thought process.

From these observations, I discovered that most people judged and appraised themselves in ways that were extremely self-punishing and negative. Thus their reactions to external criticism were usually out of proportion to content, severity, or manner of presentation. I thought it would be valuable for people to become aware of the areas and issues about which they were the most sensitive, so I began to study this phenomenon with my associates and patients. In 1973, we formed a therapy group, made up of a number of psychotherapists, to investigate this problem and pool our information. This group became the focal point for my ongoing study of the specific thought patterns associated with neurotic, repetitive behaviors and later with self-destructive actions and lifestyles. Their observations corroborated my early hypotheses about a well-integrated pattern of negative thoughts, which I later termed the "voice." These preliminary explorations captured our interest and led to further investigations of the mechanism of self-attack.

Concurrently with the ongoing therapists' group, we began studying the manifestations of this hostile thought process in our patients. While saying their self-critical thoughts out loud, they learned that it was not so much the adverse circumstances or events in their lives that caused them discomfort; rather, it was their interpretation of these events. In these early sessions, we were surprised at the ease with which these patients not only grasped the idea of an internal self-attacking thought process but applied this idea to their everyday lives. Once they caught on, they seemed very familiar with the countless ways that they habitually reproached themselves. However, they were shocked to discover the degree to which this process of running themselves down had undermined their ability to function effectively and limited their satisfaction in personal relationships.

After isolating the content of their angry thoughts, patients and participants in my associates' group began to separate these antagonistic attitudes from a more realistic view of themselves. They found that it felt more natural to articulate their self-accusatory thoughts as statements spoken in the second person: *"You're* this or that" rather than "I'm this or that." They began to adopt this manner of verbalizing their thoughts without any prior instruction or suggestion. Later, we suggested that participants state their self-attacks in this dialogue format as though they were addressing themselves as an outside person.

At first, participants brought out the content of their self-attacks in a rational, cognitive, or discussional style. Soon, however, they began to spontaneously express emotion as they verbalized the contents of the voice. We were astounded by the malicious tone in which both patients and therapists attacked themselves when there was a free flow of thoughts and emotions. We became painfully aware of how angry people were at themselves, how divided they were, and how much they sabotaged their efforts to cope in their daily lives.

In one of our first sessions, a 30-year-old colleague, S. A., father of two young children, reported feeling increasingly anxious and self-doubting after taking over a supervisory position at a mental health clinic. His sense of discomfort had escalated to the point where he was thinking about leaving clinical practice and shifting his attention to research or returning to teaching. I wondered what destructive things he was telling himself about his new responsibilities at the clinic. I had the idea that he should reveal his self-attacks in the form of a dialogue or voice.

S. A. agreed to try the technique and began the exercise in a calm voice: "I'm not the right person for this job. I don't know the first thing about directing other people and I'm afraid I'll really mess up."

I asked him to try to say his self-attacks in a dialogue as though he were talking to himself. S. A. started off in a hesitant voice, saying, "You should just go back to the classroom where you belong," and then gained in momentum.

Don't try to be different. Don't try to be better than you are. You know you can't really do the job. And you'll find out later, because the interns really can't stand you. Nobody can stand to be told what to do by someone like you. You're such a creep! You have no awareness of people. You're insensitive to your patients. What makes you think you can help other people with their patients? You're just fooling yourself.

As S. A. expressed these self-attacks, his tone of voice and speech patterns changed dramatically and he sounded more and more like his father. It was startling to several of his associates (who knew S. A.'s father) to see this transformation.

> "You shouldn't have taken this position. You don't deserve it. You're just a quiet creep. You shouldn't be around people at all, much less try to give advice. You drive people crazy, the way you come across."

By this time, S. A.'s body language and his expression of the voice revealed a combination of rage and grief as he exploded with the torrent of emotional abuse:

> "You're really just second class. You're just worthless. You're not fit to be around people, and you should really hide it. Just be quiet! Shut up! Stay in the background, because when people really get to know you, you are shit to be with. You're just a shit person. Everything about you is shit."

S. A. paused for a moment to describe how this self-degrading voice affected his relationship with his children.

> So if anyone says anything even slightly critical about my children, I feel like they're criticizing me. I think the basis of the attack comes from things that happened in my own family when I was growing up. It's like they're saying to me, "You're just like us!"

His voice grew louder and angrier.

> "What makes you think you're any different? What makes you think you're any better? You're just a crazy, scummy person."

At this point, S. A. broke into deep sobs. Later, after regaining his composure, he said,

> I really started feeling a lot when I thought about my children, and how strongly I didn't want them to have this feeling about themselves. I can see that the way I believe this about myself and the way I live my life has probably already given that feeling to them, in some way. I know how important it is for me to change this for myself, but also for them, because I felt so bad when I said that, when I put words to that feeling that they were shit because I was shit.

S. A. had a better understanding of the destructive elements in his personality after the brief exercise. Before the experience with Voice Therapy, he had little awareness about why he was having an adverse reaction to his new position at the clinic. When he finished the exercise, he was alert to malicious negative thoughts that punished him for competing with his father, who had a serious drinking problem and had experienced repeated business failures throughout S. A.'s childhood. More important, he learned that he had internalized his father's aggression toward him as a child and had come to see himself as worthless and undeserving of any career success. In the weeks that followed, S. A. reported a growing sense of self-confidence and a significant decrease in anxiety related to assuming the additional responsibilities in his psychotherapy practice.

What my associates and I witnessed that day was a Voice Therapy session that would later be duplicated many times over by others. The new methodology was an important discovery. We realized that people's strong destructive propensities toward self could be accessed with the new procedure, and that this exposure had profound implications in terms of advancing our knowledge of psychopathology and human behavior. The spontaneous flow triggered by the new format not only illuminated the content of self-attacks and permitted a feeling release of considerable magnitude, but also shed light on the source of negative introjects.

The therapists in the group were excited as they became aware of the implications of this new procedure. We quickly discovered that formulating our harshly judgmental thoughts in the second person, as S. A. had done, had considerable emotional impact and led to valuable insights. Verbalizing the voice in this format not only brought out deep feeling but helped people separate it from their own point of view. We found that, once articulated through this mode of expression, the specific thoughts could be effectively evaluated and countered.

Findings From Early Investigations of the Voice

As various dimensions of the voice process were brought to the foreground in both groups of individuals (patients and colleagues), my thinking about this destructive force in people's lives gained importance. I expanded my study of this phenomenon and began to systematically examine a variety of procedures that could be used to elicit the voice.

Since 1976, my associates and I have conducted more structured investigations of the voice process. A number of volunteer "subjects," including my professional associates, continued to meet on a regular basis to examine negative attitudes toward themselves and others. As the participants in this new group expressed their self-attacks, they often launched into angry diatribes against themselves that were reminiscent of specific experiences within the family. They uncovered core defenses and well-established habit patterns that clearly originated in traumatic circumstances. Some identified their self-criticisms as statements they had heard one or both parents make to them during their developing years. Others recalled parental attitudes they had picked up in their parents' tone of voice, body language, or other behavioral cues—attitudes that appeared to be directly related to the subjects' self-attacks.

One woman who was abnormally reserved and reticent reported that she "heard" a voice that told her to be unobtrusive in social interactions.

> In social situations, I tell myself: "Just be quiet. Nobody wants to hear what you have to say. Don't bother people. Just stop talking. Don't say anything more. *Just shut up! [Spoken loudly with intense anger]* Don't talk to me, don't bother me! I never wanted you, you little bitch!"

The subject reported that she had always held a deep conviction that she was undeserving of love or respect, a belief that corresponded to the suppressed anger she had turned against herself. She became aware that she had incorporated extremely rejecting attitudes toward herself based on being seen as an unwanted intrusion by her parents.

Volunteer subjects arrived at their own interpretations of the clinical material. Their conclusions about the sources of their derogatory self-statements did not reflect an a priori interpretation of the material by the therapists. As we uncovered these voices, we found that there was considerable commonality in the content of negative thinking expressed by the subjects. Each individual could identify strongly with every other person in the group situation.

In our patient population as well as in the experimental group, we observed that remarkable changes were manifested in an individual's physical appearance and expression during voice sessions. These changes were particularly notable when there was a powerful cathartic release of feeling during verbalization of these self-disparaging thoughts. The subjects' bodies assumed postures and mannerisms that were uncharacteristic of their own style.

Subjects began to blurt out intense, vindictive statements against themselves in powerful, passionate language and with strong negative affect. For example, one subject loudly condemned herself for being overweight with this bitter diatribe: "You're disgusting! Look at yourself in the mirror! You pig! No one can stand you. You'll never lose weight. You have no willpower! You're a failure, do you hear, a total failure!"

Following this outburst, the woman recognized that she expended a great deal of energy in an internal dialogue consisting of a rapid succession of self-admonitions similar to the vicious self-attacks she had just verbalized. In subsequent meetings, she expressed this material in a sarcastic tone of voice quite unlike her usual mode of expression. She assumed a style that could be described as lecturing or sermonizing, together with snide innuendos and name-calling, a style she immediately identified as her mother's style of addressing her.

In general, when we scrutinized subjects whose families were familiar to us, we noted that the expressions we observed during the group experience were similar in style to their parents' mannerisms—in particular, to those of the parent of the same sex. It was as though the parental figures lived inside the subjects and could be brought out by this method. Phrasing and speech intonations underwent basic transformations and often took on the regional accents of the parents. This was especially obvious when the subjects' parents happened to be of foreign background. At this stage in our studies, we began to videotape sessions of our experimental groups to document these dramatic changes in subjects' appearance, mannerisms, and speech patterns.

We hypothesized that we were witnessing manifestations of parental warnings, directions, labels, definitions, and feelings. The hostile attitudes toward self expressed by individuals appeared to have been incorporated into their own thinking process during the formative years. The group meetings with my associates had an important impact on us. As we became familiar with the process of identifying negative thought patterns, we were better able to control the maladaptive behaviors that were regulated by the voice.

In the office setting, patients discovered the thought content of their depreciating, angry point of view toward themselves and expressed outwardly some of the repressed rage they had turned inward. They became aware of the extent to which they had accepted these at face value. They became cognizant of how they maintained certain undesirable behaviors to validate the "bad child" image they had assimilated originally in their family constellation. The release of affect that accompanied these penetrating exposures of the voice process relieved patients of the tension and anxiety caused by suppressing intense emotions. Afterward, patients reported feeling much more relaxed and at ease.

The technique of expressing the voice and the intense emotion that accompanied it became an important part of our procedure as it represented a more direct pathway to deeply repressed material in the unconscious. Moreover, we felt that this method had potential as a valuable research tool with which to study the unconscious cognitive processes involved in neurotic disorders, depression, and self-destructive or suicidal behaviors.

As our patients and subjects became more familiar with verbalizing their self-accusations, they were able to make connections between undesirable behavior and negative thought patterns. It became clear that voice attacks not only affected people at times of stress but could cause them discomfort in a variety of circumstances. Predictions of personal rejection, worries about competency, negative comparisons of themselves with rivals, and guilty self-recriminations for failures and mistakes were common "voices" reported by individuals as they became acquainted with the concept.

As material of this nature accumulated, it became a logical extension of our work to study this voice process in more depressed patients and in those who had a history of suicidal thoughts and attempted suicides. Our subsequent investigations indicated that this subliminal thought process underlies depressive states and strongly influences the acting out of self-destructive patterns. Although the voice has been observed to varying degrees in "normal," neurotic, and psychotic populations, it reaches life-threatening proportions in suicidal patients.

THE CONCEPT OF THE VOICE

Definition of the Voice

The "voice" is the language of the defensive process. It is defined as a well-integrated system of thoughts and attitudes, antithetical toward self and cynical toward others, that is at the core of an individual's maladaptive behavior. The voice process should not be confused with a conscience, superego, or value system (Endnote 1). The negative thought process or voice functions as an antifeeling, antibody process, comparable to obsessional thinking, wherein people live primarily in their heads, cut off from their emotions and bodily sensations. Even so-called positive voices of approval and seeming self-interest are indications that people are fragmented and removed from themselves.

I conceptualize the voice as being an overlay on the personality that is not natural or harmonious, but is learned or imposed from without. The voice may at times parallel one's value system or moral considerations. However, rather than motivating one to alter behavior in a moral or constructive manner, the voice process tends to occur *after* the fact and is generally harsh and judgmental. The definition of the voice excludes those thought processes concerned with values or ideals, as well as those involved in creative thinking, constructive planning, and realistic self-appraisal. It does not refer to mental activity that is generally described as fantasy or daydreams. To fit our criteria of the voice, the patient's thoughts must be identified as an incorporated external attack on the self.

Voice attacks are sometimes experienced consciously, but more often than not they are only partially conscious or even totally unconscious. The average person is largely *unaware* of his or her self-attacks and of the fact that much of his or her behavior is influenced and even controlled by the voice. Indeed, "listening" to the voice predisposes an individual toward self-limiting behavior and negative consequences. In other words, people make their actions correspond to their self-attacks.

Defensive Functions of the Voice

Later in our investigations, we discovered that there seemed to be two important aspects of the voice process: a protective, parental quality that acts to stifle one's enthusiasm, spontaneity, spirit, and sense of adventure, and a malicious or hostile quality that issues directives to mutilate the self emotionally and/or physically.

1. We noted that the voice had overtones similar to those of an overprotective parent, cautioning, directing, controlling, and advising people in a manner that seemed at first glance to have their best interests at heart. For example, the following was a common "advisory" self-attack: "Don't get too hooked on her (him). What if he (she) breaks up with you? Why go through all that agony just for a few weeks of happiness?"

In contemplating pleasurable activities, many people warned themselves about possible dangers: "Why blow so much money on this trip? You can't trust the brochures. Your French is hopeless. What if the plane gets hijacked? With the shape the world's in, why go anywhere?"

Even in situations where caution is advisable, we determined that the voice functions to stifle a person's enthusiasm and spontaneity. It is this factor, rather than the specific warnings of the voice, that damages people's spirit and sense of adventure. Indeed, many subjects reported "listening" to a voice that ridiculed them for being excited. They remembered being subdued as children by parents who made fun of their youthful exuberance. The derivation of this self-protective function of the voice became apparent when subjects repeatedly connected their derisive internal warnings to parental attitudes.

2. In our investigations, we observed that what initially appeared to be an abnormal defensive process soon became, when carried to its limits of expression, a powerfully hostile force, even in comparatively normal subjects. The pronouncements of this voice, even when self-protective or accurate, were malicious in their attitude toward the individual. As our subjects explored this process in greater depth and fully expressed the intensity of the negative affect associated with their self-critical thoughts, they discovered that their voices were sneering, sarcastic, and even savagely angry.

A number of subjects revealed extremely vicious voices commanding them to mutilate themselves or perform careless acts that could lead to accidents. For example, one man, whose father had been blatantly rejecting and at times physically abusive, expressed this attack on himself: "You're not that good a person, you know; you don't amount to much. What have you got to show for your life?"

He spoke slowly at first and without emotion but gradually his attacks intensified: "You know, no one would miss you if you weren't around. You don't have a wife or girlfriend like other guys. You're a nobody, that's all you are!"

In relation to his work as a carpenter, he revealed voices that taunted: "Go ahead, just put your finger closer to the saw blade; just stick it in there! Move a little closer, you bastard, just shove it in there!"

His voice grew louder and more savage: "Ram it in there, you cowardly bastard. You don't deserve to live! You worm, you cowardly piece of shit!"

This man bore no conscious malice toward himself when he began the exercise. He was not in a depressed mood or particularly upset. After expressing this powerfully spoken assault, he broke into deep sobs. Months later, he reported that prior to that session, he had often hurt himself in his job, but since this insight, he had become aware of the self-attacks and had adjusted his behavior by being particularly careful at those times. Malicious commands like the thoughts that tortured this man during his work no doubt contribute to accident-proneness in many people.

When we first heard subjects verbalizing these injunctions to harm themselves, we were shocked by the unexpected depth and magnitude of the rage they expressed. We were disturbed by the violence and the range of the voice's destructive commands, as were the participants in our group. It was difficult to believe that relatively well-adjusted individuals could harbor this degree of intense anger toward themselves. It was obvious to us that the murderous rage that we were tapping when our subjects dramatized the voice typically remains below the level of awareness in most people.

The connection between this internalized hostility, as exemplified in the case above, and in destructive acting-out behavior such as substance abuse, accident-proneness, or withdrawal from social contact, became more obvious. Indeed, we observed that several of our apparently "normal" subjects at times did behave in ways that were potentially dangerous or detrimental to their physical health. Many others tended to turn to isolated activities whenever their actions were being influenced by a voice "telling" them to stay in the background or to be unobtrusive. We learned that, as a result of "listening" to the voice, an individual tends to deny his or her wants and turn against important goals and priorities. I concluded, based on these observations, that the voice functions as a regulatory mechanism, mediating self-destructive behaviors and self-limiting lifestyles.

Negative Events That Arouse Self-Attacks

Financial setbacks, academic failure, criticism, rejection by a loved one, the death of someone close, and illness are all stressful events that activate thoughts of self-recrimination and associated feelings of self-hatred.

Failure. Academic and vocational failures are often precipitating factors in self-destructive thinking. Patients who had experienced business failures or setbacks reported telling themselves: "You're a total failure! You'll never get anywhere in life. You always mess up. Everybody hates you—you might as well give up."

Over an extended period of time, this kind of thought process can lead to serious states of depression and ultimately to suicidal behavior. It appears that individuals who are perfectionistic and are driven to maintain high levels of performance are exceptionally susceptible to this form of self-attack.

Rejection. Rejection activates the "bad child" image wherein a person assumes that he or she is at fault and therefore deserves to be excluded. In this situation, it is difficult to remain objective in one's self-appraisal and maintain good feelings about oneself. Thus negative experiences and interpersonal hurt cause most of us to feel unlovable. Individuals frequently interpret rejection as concrete evidence that they are undeserving of love, inferior, boring, sexually unattractive, or afflicted by myriad other undesirable qualities attributed to them by the voice.

Contact with people who are critical, dismissing, or insensitive can catalyze an individual's own self-attacks. Certain people or personalities have a toxic effect, while others who are compassionate and accepting tend to have positive effects. Having one's motives misunderstood or actions misconstrued by paranoid individuals validates one's voice. It is hard to remain unaffected by individuals who maintain disapproving, judgmental views of us. Often a person will choose to accept the negative evaluations and bad treatment to hold on to the relationship.

Illness. Poor health and illness tend to activate self-critical thoughts about one's body integrity. Even people in good health, facing yearly physical checkups, frequently torment themselves with hypochondriacal thoughts: "The doctor is going to find something terrible this time. You probably have cancer and he'll have to break the news to you. Why go, anyway? It's better not to know."

Illness can also trigger morbid ruminations about death. Thoughts such as "Life isn't worth living if you have all this pain" or "Nothing matters anyway if you don't have your health" increase one's feelings of despair and futility about life.

Positive Events That Arouse Voice Attacks

Paradoxically, positive as well as negative experiences can activate a self-destructive thought process.

Many people feel anxious or nervous when they receive acknowledgment for an unusual accomplishment. For example, many patients who had assumed positions of leadership as well as those who had achieved a significant success in their field of endeavor reported that they subsequently behaved in ways to undermine these achievements. In their sessions, they were able to trace their self-defeating actions to thought patterns that had made them self-conscious about their position or success.

Individuals often experience feelings of guilt when they attain a greater degree of success than friends, associates, or particularly their parent of the same sex. Their guilt reactions usually involve some form of giving up their new success by sabotaging their achievements. Similarly, many men and women reported voices following success in their personal relationships that contributed to a deterioration in their positive feelings. These events precipitated a flow of negative thoughts, some self-critical and others critical of their partner. One woman revealed that she "listened" to an angry voice that told her: "Why spend all your time with him? What about you? You need some time to yourself." She subsequently backed away from a satisfying, loving relationship and rationalized her retreat. My associates and I observed that fault-finding, "picky" thoughts and misperceptions of one's mate were more intense following times when the partners had been especially close, both sexually and emotionally. Happiness and loving times were often short-lived because of voice attacks.

Vanity as Compensation
for the Negative Self-Image

The voice functions to build up an individual's self-importance and supports an inflated self-image. It tells the person that he or she is exceptional and special and able to perform at unrealistically high levels. Later, the voice severely condemns him or her for falling short of these standards of perfection. Vanity predisposes gratification in fantasy followed by intense self-attacks when failure occurs.

Henry, a 45-year-old long-distance runner who had previously been able to run 12 miles, set a goal for himself of completing a 26-mile marathon. He trained for months, telling himself, "You're really good. You can do *anything* if you really want to." When he was forced to stop at the 20-mile marker because of exhaustion, he sank into a deep depression that lasted several weeks. Later, in exploring the sources of his "bad mood," he reported thinking extremely self-depreciating thoughts: "You quitter! You can't finish anything! You didn't have to quit. You could have seen it through to the end. You didn't have to stop, but you quit, just like you do in everything else you try!"

Although he was 45 years old, he compared himself unfavorably with teammates half his age and thought: "They finished the race, but not you. You trained longer and harder than they did, but you quit. You just don't have the guts, the motivation, the right stuff. You *could* have done it, you quitter!"

Still later, in analyzing the event, he realized how ridiculous this comparison was. In a session, Henry recalled how he had been built up by his father to compensate for his father's lack of real interest in him. He became painfully aware that much of his effort in relation to running and, indeed, to other endeavors, had been for his father's benefit, as an attempt to earn his approval, and therefore his real achievements brought him no pleasure.

The Voice and Withholding Behavior

Many of our patients described a voice urging them to hold back their performance at work, especially when they perceived, rightly or wrongly, that their efforts went unrecognized by management. They reported self-statements like the following: "Why should *you* do all the work, while *they* get all the credit? Why didn't *you* get a raise instead of so-and-so?"

These voice attacks make people overanxious or cautious and may actually interfere with their productivity. In general, the voice plays a prominent part in maintaining a posture of withholding. In all areas of endeavor, the voice warns people against being spontaneous and enthusiastic in the same derisive tone that their parents once used, for example, "Don't get so excited. What's the big deal anyway? Don't make a fool of yourself."

In personal relationships, the voice has been found to be influential in maintaining a posture of pseudoindependence and aloofness in each partner: "Don't get too involved. Don't get too attached to him (her). Keep it casual. What do you need a relationship for anyway? You were okay before he (she) came along."

The fear of being depleted or drained, both physically and emotionally, can be aroused in patients suffering from the effects of severe emotional deprivation in childhood. Enthusiasm, vitality, and spontaneity are dampened or totally stifled in those individuals whose behaviors are regulated by too many of these seemingly self-protective thoughts. When people have generous impulses, they frequently tell themselves: "Don't get carried away. They don't want (need) anything from you!" or "What did he (she) ever do for you?"

THE DUAL FUNCTION OF THE VOICE

As noted, both contradictory viewpoints—toward self and toward others— are symptomatic of the deep division existing within all of us. At times we view our loved ones with compassion and affection, while at other times we think of them in cynical or disparaging terms.

In sessions, patients often alternated between expressing self-attacks and verbalizing harsh or suspicious attitudes toward others. In their everyday lives, people tended to vacillate between criticizing themselves for failures and blaming someone else. It became increasingly evident to us that hateful, judgmental views of other people were inextricably tied to self-attacks by the voice.

Patients and subjects anticipated rejection based on these two aspects of the voice. In the first instance, they reported statements such as these: "He has no interest in you. Why should he want to be *your* friend? *You're* not attractive or intelligent like his other friends." In the second case, they had thoughts condemning others: "*She's* no damn good. Who wants to be with her, anyway?" and, more generally, "People don't really care. *They* don't understand. You can't trust women. They're fickle." Both types of voices, belittling self and others, predispose alienation.

THE VOICE AS DISTINGUISHED FROM
HALLUCINATED VOICES IN PSYCHOSIS

The hallucinated voices in schizophrenia are exaggerated manifestations of the voice in neurotic disorders. In psychotic states, the voice has been externalized and is experienced as real sensation, seemingly originating in the outside world. The psychotic patient actually hears commands, directions, criticisms, and judgmental pronouncements as in a real conversation. The schizophrenic patient's ego is in an extremely weakened state, and he or she will frequently act upon these commands in a maladaptive fashion, regardless of the consequences. The patient is almost totally at the mercy of, or completely "possessed" by, this alien point of view. Bizarre behavior, neologisms, paleologic connections, delusions, hallucinations, and idiosyncratic symbolism indicate the profound intrusion of the voice into the patient's cognitive processes.

The basic character of the "voices" or auditory hallucinations in psychotic disorders is similar in many respects to the tone and quality of the inner voice in neurotic disturbances. The hallucinated voices heard by schizophrenic patients have a parental quality that is similar to the judgmental character of the neurotic patient's self-critical thoughts and negative self-appraisals. Both self-attacking thoughts and auditory hallucinations are indications of a self-parenting process that undermines the personality.

ROLE OF THE VOICE IN THE
INTERGENERATIONAL TRANSMISSION
OF NEGATIVE PARENTAL TRAITS AND BEHAVIORS

Voice Therapy theory reveals how negative parental attitudes and even unconscious malice are incorporated by the child. These introjects or internal representations, similar in some respects to Fairbairn's (1952) and Guntrip's

(1969) concept of the antilibidinal ego, seriously restrict the child's natural development as a unique individual.

The voice originates in the abuses of childhood: Its primary source is the incorporation of an attacking, condescending parenting process, acquired in the social matrix of the family. The voice is the unconscious or partly conscious mechanism primarily responsible for the transmission of negative parental qualities, behaviors, and patterns of defense from one generation to the next. Its function in perpetuating mental illness, self-destructiveness, and child abuse through succeeding generations may be as significant to human development as the transmission of parents' physical characteristics through the DNA molecules carried in the genes.

The power of the voice lies in the fact that most people are unaware that they are following its dictates because it is largely unconscious. However, most people do follow the prescriptions of this internal parent to their own detriment, with significant negative consequences in their everyday interactions with their offspring.

In one group meeting,[2] Gordon verbalized voice statements that chastised him for the way he was talking:

> "You'd better say it right, buddy! Just say it right or don't say anything! If you can't say it right, just shut up! You'd better talk better next time!"
>
> There's a lot of pressure that I put on myself. It all comes down to this fury that I feel against myself—and I feel it against my son. [*Sad*] I don't want to.

Gordon's son, Jimmy, had introjected the same demanding voice that plagued his father. Because of it, he was hypersensitive to criticism and found it difficult to take suggestions. He tended to react angrily and defensively to relatively minor events or slipups that might detract from a perfectionistic view of himself. In a family session, Jimmy spoke of this internalized anger:

> In sports, I have to be the best or I'm just nothing. I can't just be average. In baseball, if I make an error, I just tear into myself. I call myself an idiot a thousand times. It's like I'm screaming at myself inside my head. Or if I'm losing a tennis match, I tell myself: "If you can't beat him, you're a jerk!"

The clinical data documented here suggest that the voice is a representation of negative parental introjects that significantly affect our perception of ourselves. Thereafter, the voice functions to tie individuals to their parents in the sense that, even though physically separate or geographically distant from the family, adults still possess an internal parent that directs, controls, and punishes

---

2 This excerpt is taken from the video documentary, *The Inner Voice in Child Abuse* (Parr, 1986).

them. These voices, albeit unpleasant, serve the function of maintaining the fantasy bond and shield the individual from experiencing his or her aloneness, sense of separation, and death anxiety. In one of his last writings, Sigmund Freud (1926/1959) commented on the security provided by the "introjected parents":

> I am therefore inclined to adhere to the view that the fear of death should be regarded as analogous to the fear of castration and that the situation to which the ego is reacting is one of being abandoned by the protecting super-ego [introjected parents]—the powers of destiny—so that it has no longer any safeguard against all the dangers that surround it. (p. 130)

The patient is terrified of losing the internal parent represented by the voice. The irrational fear of disrupting the illusory connection or fantasy bond with the family and the dread of reexperiencing feelings of infantile frustration and a primitive sense of helplessness are at the core of resistance.

CONCLUSION

Voice Therapy addresses the critical function that predisposes self-destructive, self-limiting lifestyles. It attempts to disrupt the intergenerational transmission of negative thought processes. The methodology is a broadly based therapy technique with an emphasis on both cognitive and affective components (Endnote 2). It is derived from a systematic theory of neurosis, based on the conceptualization of the fantasy bond as a core defense that underlies an individual's fundamental resistance to change or progress. The rationale underlying Voice Therapy is that recognition of one's internal enemy can help free one from its tyranny. It brings to the surface patients' negative thoughts and accompanying affect, helps them form insight into the sources of their discomfort, assists them in gradually modifying behavior in the direction of their stated goals, and aids them in opposing the dictates of the negative thought process. Ultimately, progress depends on breaking away from fusion or fantasies of connection and moving toward individuation, self-sufficiency, and autonomy.

ENDNOTES

1. Freud used the terms *superego* and *conscience* interchangeably in many of his writings ("The Ego and the Id," 1923/1961). Another example can be found in Freud's (1940/1964) last work, "An Outline of Psycho-Analysis," in which he stated,

> The torments caused by the reproaches of conscience correspond precisely to a child's fear of loss of love, a fear the place of which has been taken by the moral agency. . . . The

super-ego continues to play the part of an external world for the ego, although it has become a portion of the internal world. (p. 206)

In "The Concept of Superego," Joseph Sandler (1960/1987) traced the progression of Freud's thinking related to the superego and the ego ideal. According to Sandler, the functions of a "conscience" were ascribed to the superego by Freud, and the superego "exercises the 'censorship of morals' " (p. 20).

Loewenstein (1966) clarified the distinction between the superego and conscience in his essay "On the Theory of the Superego: A Discussion":

One characteristic of the superego is today often neglected: namely, the fact that . . . its contents and functioning often differ widely from the consciously adopted moral code of the individual. (p. 300)

In *The Ego Ideal,* Janine Chasseguet-Smirgel (1975/1985) discussed the views of several authors about distinctions between the superego and the ego ideal. She summarized her views regarding the origins of the ego ideal as follows:

The primary loss of fusion . . . leads both to a recognition of the object, of the not-me, and to the creation of the ideal from which the me, the ego, is then cut off. The gaping wound thus created in the ego can only be closed by a return to the fusion with the primary object. (p. 191)

2. Voice Therapy procedures are similar in some respects to Aaron Beck's (Beck, Rush, Shaw, & Emery, 1979) Cognitive Therapy and Albert Ellis's (Ellis, 1973; Ellis & Harper, 1975) Rational-Emotive Therapy; however, there are a number of basic differences. I strongly disagree with Ellis's primarily biological viewpoint that human beings have powerful innate tendencies to think irrationally; instead, I believe that disordered thinking is a function of deficient child-rearing practices.

Beck's and Ellis's reports, describing "automatic thoughts" and "irrational beliefs," appear to coincide with certain aspects of the voice process. My perspective, however, is at variance with Cognitive Therapy and Rational-Emotive Therapy in that I am concerned with the dynamic origins of the voice rather than attempting to argue the patient out of his or her false beliefs using logic, humor, questioning, or negative imagery of the "worst situation."

10

Approach to Psychotherapy

> The criterion of mental health is not one of individual adjustment to a
> given social order, but a universal one, valid for all men, of giving a
> satisfactory answer to the problem of human existence.
>
> *Erich Fromm (1955, p. 14)*

Psychotherapy represents a powerful personal interaction wherein a trained person attempts to offer psychological assistance to another. There is a renewed opportunity for personality development on the part of the patient that exceeds and transcends virtually any other mode of experience. The techniques or treatment strategies used in rendering aid are based on implicit and explicit assumptions held by the therapist about human beings and their institutions. A comprehensive theory of psychopathology and a comparative mental health model help the clinician to develop a treatment strategy. As Robert Langs (1982) stated,

> The nature of this therapeutic relationship, and of the transactions between the two participants, is structured and *shaped by the implicit and explicit attitudes*

AUTHOR'S NOTE: The substance of this chapter is taken primarily from an article titled, "Prescription for Psychotherapy," *Psychotherapy, 27* (1990), pp. 627-635. Used with permission.

and interventions of the therapist [italics added]. . . . The treatment is designed to offer the patient the best possible means of relief or cure. (p. 3)

Langs's statement raises a number of important questions. What are the criteria for mental health? What procedures are effective in relieving emotional suffering and fostering behavioral change? Is the reduction or absence of neurotic symptomatology on a clinical level sufficient indication of a successful outcome to therapy?

This chapter addresses these fundamental questions. My theoretical position is based on a unique and definitive view of human experience. The steps in the therapeutic process reflect basic attitudes toward patients' individuality as contrasted with their role in family and society, as well as a conception of the structure and function of their psychological defenses.

NEUROSIS AND MENTAL HEALTH

Human beings exist in a state of conflict between the active pursuit of their goals in the real world and an inward, self-protective defense system. As noted, the resolution of this conflict in the direction of a defended lifestyle has a profound negative effect on an individual's overall functioning. The defended person's life is significantly distorted by a desperate clinging to addictive habit patterns, strong guilt reactions, low self-esteem, and a distrust of others, whereas ideally an undefended or mentally healthy individual exists in a state of continual change, moving toward increased autonomy and enjoying more satisfying relationships.

Both approaches to life have advantages as well as disadvantages. The "adjusted," albeit defended, person may feel less anxious and on the surface more secure; nevertheless, his or her adaptation has negative consequences in a loss of freedom and feeling and a constricted life. Moreover, this condition often leads to maladaptive behavior patterns and neurotic symptom formation.

The comparatively less defended individual feels more integrated, has a stronger identity, a greater potential for intimacy, and is more humane toward others. However, the mentally healthy person, who is relatively free of symptoms and the compulsion to repeat familiar destructive patterns, must live with a heightened sense of vulnerability and sensitivity to both joyous events and emotionally painful situations. Individuals who are open and less defended have more integrity and appear to be *more* responsive to circumstances in their lives that impinge on their well-being. They feel sad in relation to life's tragic aspects and are aware of its temporal quality. This type of person is investing in a life he or she must certainly lose, and there are poignant reactions to core existential issues. As mentioned previously, the choice to live nondefensively is partially an ethical one because the inherent damage caused by defenses inflicts corresponding damage on loved ones, especially one's children.

The dilemma facing both therapist and patient brings these two alternatives to the foreground. Ideally, an effective psychotherapy would enable the patient to discover a truly moral and compassionate approach toward him- or herself and others. My basic philosophy stresses the primary value of the unique personality of the patient and his or her personal freedom and potential for self-realization. There is an important emphasis on each person's sense of self in opposition to the invalidation of self caused by maintaining defenses.

THE BASIC PRESCRIPTION

> The cumulative effects of interpersonal relationships . . . typically in childhood—has made the patient "ill" and . . . another human relationship, with a professionally trained person and under particularly benign circumstances, can provide corrections in the patient's self-esteem and in the quality of his or her interpersonal relationships with significant others. (Strupp, 1989, pp. 717-718)

The steps in the therapeutic process that lead to basic character change and to a nondefended existence necessitate incisive therapeutic inroads, not merely symptom reduction or minor shifts in defense mechanisms or addictions. Moreover, the therapist must be sensitized to, and able to access, patients' special points of identity to help them give value to themselves.

As discussed earlier, my approach to psychotherapy has a twofold aspect: (a) to challenge addictive attachments and self-parenting habit patterns and (b) to encourage movement away from fantasy toward gratification and real personal power in the external environment. Addictive behaviors and attachments act like a drug to cut off feeling responses, thereby seriously impeding the development of self. They must be dealt with or there cannot be fundamental change. Yet there is strong resistance to altering character defenses, because intense anxiety and even terror is aroused in moving toward separateness and independence. People are fearful of giving up passive, dependent machinations, reliance on fantasy, and addictive attachments. Resistance to a better life is at the core of the neurosis itself and is expressed in every aspect of the defended person's lifestyle.

HISTORICAL DEVELOPMENT
OF METHODOLOGY

My theoretical position underlying this treatment strategy is based on a 35-year study of resistance to change or progress in psychotherapy. Working with schizophrenic patients under the auspices of John N. Rosen (Rosen, 1953), I developed the basic concepts of my theoretical approach to schizophrenia. Later, I extended and applied these concepts to the neuroses. In my doctoral dissertation, *A Concept of the Schizophrenic Process* (1957), I described the dimensions of the fantasized, "self-mothering" process that the schizophrenic patient relies on for gratification at the expense of interpersonal relationships. Schizophrenic patients in effect "mother" themselves; that is, in their imagination they are joined or connected to the image of the "good," powerful mother. They are split between being the powerful parent and the weak, helpless child, and there is a certain amount of ego fragmentation (Endnote 1).

To counteract the self-parenting process, my colleagues and I provided an interim form of parenting that helped to compensate for the earlier emotional deprivation. Our therapy was a direct attack upon the patient's internal source of gratification through fantasy while at the same time an attempt to make reality more inviting. The methodology challenged patients' idealization of the mother and provided emotional support that enabled them to progress through the early stages of development at which they had been fixated.

Rosen's treatment of patients in a noninstitutional atmosphere, where they lived with their therapists, as well as the wealth of information about the patients gathered in this setting, left a lasting impression on me. My attitude toward the patients with schizophrenia was one of respect for their attempt to maintain some form of integrity in the face of severe trauma, and support for the fact that their symptoms made logical sense. I believed that these people had come by their symptoms honestly; that is, I felt that real events harmful to their psyche had occurred to foster this level of regression.

In a videotaped interview (in 1988), I described my experience at Rosen's residential treatment center:

> It was an enlightening experience. The way the patients related to us at very close quarters and the tension, the excitement, the investment of ourselves all combined to lead to very important discoveries.
>
> I realized how closely the pathology was to the deprivation and to the painful experiences that these people had suffered, and that there was plenty of justification for their symptom formation. They were compensating for a situation that was truly horrible. I believed in their integrity in that sense. I believed that they had actually experienced the tormenting events or trauma that led up to their withdrawal and their dependence on fantasy, and that using that mechanism further debilitated them. It gave them an illusion of being powerful while they were surrendering and giving up aspects of reality that weakened them and made them helpless, dependent, and finally institutionalized.

Later, in private practice, my associates and I worked with over 200 patients and subjects for a period of 4 years, using the techniques of an intense feeling release therapy. Our experience with this form of psychotherapy, together with our ongoing investigations into destructive thought processes, led to the formulation of the elements essential for maximizing positive therapeutic outcome.

The ultimate goal of my therapy is to help patients move away from compulsive, self-limiting lifestyles so that they can expand their lives and tolerate more gratification in reality. We hope to help individuals achieve a free and independent existence, remain open to experience and feelings, and maintain the ability to respond appropriately to both positive and negative events in their lives. To this end, the process of identifying the "voice" and the associated feelings of self-hatred and rage toward self, combined with corrective strategies of behavioral change, significantly expand the patient's boundaries and bring about a more positive sense of self.

STAGES IN THE THERAPEUTIC PROCESS

Voice Therapy, the multidimensional approach that has proved most beneficial in overcoming resistance and promoting behavioral change, is composed of the following techniques.[1]

Intense Feeling Release

This first method is primarily affective. Prior to the sessions, individuals are asked to avoid painkillers—cigarettes, alcohol, and other self-feeding habits—and encouraged to spend time in isolation and self-contemplation while developing a written case history.[2] The prohibition against the use of substances and the interruption of routines have the effect of creating an immediate state of heightened tension and deprivation. The warm-up period generates anxiety, and feelings tend to surface.

In the sessions,[3] patients are encouraged to breathe deeply, to allow sounds to emerge as they exhale, and to verbalize any thoughts that come to mind. As powerful feelings are released in this manner, patients form their own insights and spontaneously relate irrational or primitive emotional responses, as well as present-day limitations, to early negative experiences in the family. Most individuals describe their memories with unusual clarity and appear to genuinely relive events and feelings from early childhood. Patients generally interpret their

---

1   The three procedures do not necessarily follow in a sequential pattern, and the methods are adapted to the specific requirements of each patient.

2   This methodology is based on Arthur Janov's (1970) technique for eliciting primal feeling.

3   It is preferable to conduct feeling release sessions 1-1/2 hours per day, five times a week, for a period of four to six weeks. These sessions are generally followed by several months of once- or twice-a-week sessions.

own material and integrate it without assistance or intervention from the therapist; thus transference reactions tend to be minimal during this phase.

Janet, 35, and the mother of three, had lived a complacent and safe existence for the better part of her life, subordinating herself to her husband and living her life through his accomplishments, to the detriment of her own capabilities and intellect. She had hoped to gain a greater sense of self through the therapy and to become more independent in her relationship with her husband. In her first sessions, she recalled vivid scenes of her early years spent in a large lonely house on a ranch in the Southwest. The following are excerpts from her journal:

Session 3: Why am I such a coward? What am I afraid of? Of him, my father. Why? I see him with his hand raised (often I picture him that way)—he is going to hit me. Why? Then I see an awful veiny thing hanging down between his legs at my eye level. I feel disgusted. It's red and veiny and I don't seem to know what it is. It is dripping a sticky, colorless liquid. He has been fucking someone! Then I see two bodies on the bed, very clearly, from the rear—I see his behind. I walk into my father and mother's room. He is screwing and then I see her lying on the bed. I don't want to look, but I see that it is the Hispanic maid in our house. She is young and slight, slim and thin. (My mother is fat and ugly—I always feel fat. I always feel awkward around women shorter than I, especially if they are slim.) My father raises his hand to me and chases me back to my bed in my own room. I cower on the bed and let him hit me! I feel like a coward, but I got his attention away from her! (I get Bill's attention by provoking him to be angry, and one time I even managed to get him to strike me. Then he doesn't have any heart for anyone else, even though the attention focused on me is negative attention.)

Session 9: I was a baby calling for mommy to come and pick me up. After many screams, she came! She put something in my mouth—I didn't want it (a bottle?)—I felt smothered. I imagined what it would be like to be held in someone's arms, and felt warm and safe. I liked it so much and felt it for a long time. Then I remembered what it was really like. I felt lost, held myself, tried to comfort myself and could not keep myself warm, it was a cold feeling, I was anguished. I am still trying to care for myself by stuffing myself with food or indulging myself by buying things for myself. When I was ungenerous about serving people in my house, I remember an irrational feeling that there would not be enough food left for me—I would starve.

Despite her regression within the sessions themselves, Janet functioned in an adult and rational manner during her everyday life. Other sessions, similar to session 9, touched on themes from a primitive stage of development, where the patient relived memories pertaining to the frustration of her needs on an oral level. She became aware that this was the source of her current underlying dependency on her husband. Direct oral material of this nature, such as memories of frustration at the breast, are usually not accessible in traditional insight therapy to a person with the ego strength of this particular patient.

The knowledge of self and personal understanding gained through feeling release sessions are unusually direct and pure. It is as though patients are able to envision their childhood situations, "seeing through" their present-day problems rather than intellectually "figuring them out" or analyzing them.

Our results confirmed the findings of Arthur Janov (1970) as well as his view that defenses are basically a protection against feeling primal pain. In contrast to Janov, however, who felt that repeated expression and release could empty the reservoir or "pool of primal pain" and lead to a "cure," our investigations showed that this "pool" cannot be emptied as such. If defenses formed early in relation to interpersonal traumas stood alone and were not reinforced by reactions to death anxiety, Janov's assumptions and hopes might have been realized.

Moreover, I found that the techniques of feeling release were not sufficient to alter an individual's basic attitude or defense. As important as it is for patients to understand the connection between their current behavior and past trauma and have access to their deepest feelings, this methodology in and of itself does not necessarily change the compulsive reliving of destructive patterns, restricted lifestyles, and the preference for fantasy gratification and self-parenting defenses.

In conclusion, feeling release sessions offer a heightened awareness of those childhood experiences that affect current behavior. They help a person become far less defensive, and there is often a significant reduction in tension and anxiety associated with repressed feeling. In addition, feeling release sessions help a person to cope with the intense emotional reactions linked to the verbalization of negative thought patterns in the next phase of treatment.

Verbalization and Identification of Negative Thought Patterns

As described in Chapter 1, patients in Voice Therapy sessions learn to verbalize their self-critical thoughts in the second person, as though another person were addressing them, for example, in the form of statements *toward* themselves, rather than making statements about themselves. Expressing voices in the second person format facilitates the process of separating the patient's point of view from negative thought processes antithetical to self and hostile toward others that had been incorporated during the developmental years. It also serves to facilitate the expression of affect associated with negative introjects.

The process of identifying the contents of self-critical or hostile thought patterns can be approached intellectually as a primarily cognitive technique or more dramatically using cathartic methods. In both procedures, the patient attempts to identify and analyze self-attacks and defensive negative prescriptions and learns to restate negative thought patterns in the second person, as described above. In the latter technique, there is an emphasis on the release of affect accompanying the expression of self-destructive thoughts. In this abreactive method, patients are asked to bring out their negative thoughts and express them more emotionally, with instructions to "say it louder" or "let go and say anything that comes to mind." Many patients voluntarily adopt an emotional style of expression when "saying" the voice. They often release intense feelings of anger and sadness as they reveal the self-derogatory thoughts and attitudes that hold special meaning for them. When patients verbalize the voice in this form, it is remarkable to witness the scope and intensity of angry affect directed toward self that is so close to the surface.

Identifying the contents of the patient's negative thought process is the first step in a three-step procedure in which patient and therapist collaborate in understanding the patient's distorted ways of thinking. To illustrate the first step, a 25-year-old male subject in a group session verbalized his voice about his relationship to women:

"You are so despicable. You are so low. No woman could ever feel anything for you. And you don't have any feelings for them! You're just not an attractive-looking person. You're not masculine, you're just not like other men."

In this example, note that the subject brought out his hostile self-attacks in the second person. Later in the same session, he expressed considerable anger at being limited by this destructive form of thinking about himself.

In the second step, patients discuss their spontaneous insights and analyze their reactions to verbalizing the voice. Then they attempt to understand the relationship between their voice attacks and their self-destructive behavior patterns. They subsequently develop insight into the limitations that they impose on themselves in everyday life functions. Incidentally, becoming aware of one's self-imposed restrictions reduces paranoid reactions to others and feelings of victimization.

Here, the same subject discusses his reactions to the self-attacks he had just verbalized:

Immediately after I finished saying my voice, I had another quick thought, a voice that said:
"Okay, so now you've said your voice, but what difference is it going to make in your life? It isn't going to change anything."
I didn't really go with that feeling. I realized what it was—that it was a voice attacking what I'd just said, and I didn't think it was a real point. But I *did* notice how quickly it came up, trying to invalidate everything I'd just said.

I also realized that since the session last week, I've generally felt better. I felt like taking more positive steps in my life, and it always seems like when I feel that way, positive things tend to happen. I had more to do with women, and I felt I was making more friends in general. I just felt more alive overall.

Third, the therapist asks the patient to formulate an answer to the voice. In the analytic approach, the patient is asked to respond with a more realistic, objective self-appraisal. In the cathartic method, patients are encouraged to talk back to the voice and challenge it directly as though they were addressing an actual person. Because people tend to identify the voice in relation to parental figures early on, many times they end up talking back directly to their parents in a form of psychodrama.

In the following segment, the same subject articulated his response to the voice attacks concerning his feelings about women. In the course of separating and strengthening his own point of view, he clearly differentiates between his view and that of his parents. It is important to note that the subject responded to his voice with considerable forcefulness, mobilizing deep feelings of anger and sadness as he answered back:

"I'm not that way. I'm not that person you're talking about. I care a lot for women."

Another thought that comes to mind:

"I'm not like you! [*Loud*] I've got some feelings. I care! I want something. You never wanted anything. [*Mournful*] I want something in my life." [*Angry*]

Defending one's own point of view in contradiction to voices represents an attack on the introjected parental images, only one step removed from attacking parents themselves and, as such, can cause considerable tension and self-recrimination. Voicing these angry, hostile feelings toward parental introjects in a session tends to disconnect a person from imagined or symbolic sources of security, and regressive trends may follow. Therefore, I tend to *discourage* dramatic answers to voice attacks for patients who appear to lack sufficient ego strength to cope with the resultant guilt and anxiety. In these cases, a nondramatic evaluation of voice attacks on a cognitive level is less threatening and partially serves the purpose of separating out destructive elements and improving the patient's self-concept.

Evaluating the truth of the patient's self-criticisms, that is, subjecting the content of voice attacks to a process of reality-testing, is an important part of the procedure. Although in many cases, patients' negative thoughts toward themselves are made up of real components regarding undesirable behaviors or personality traits, angry affect and malicious attacks on the self are always unjustified. Self-evaluations that are realistically negative, yet objective, based on the underlying premise that a person can change long-standing character traits are very different from voices that categorize the patient as inherently defective. During this phase of therapy, patients learn that it is not appropriate to attack themselves for shortcomings or weaknesses; rather, it is more productive to work on modifying behaviors they dislike.

My approach to eliciting and identifying the contents of the voice is *not* didactic, that is, I do not directly persuade people to think or behave rationally; rather, I help them discover what they are telling themselves about important situations in life and attempt to assist them in moving away from negative attitudes and prohibitions.

In summing up our investigations working directly with voices or negative thought processes, my associates and I were surprised to discover the degree to which individuals were divided within themselves. As described earlier, we were shocked at the intense rage and hostility underlying self-critical and self-punishing thought processes, even in clinically "normal" individuals. In addition, we became aware of patients' strong resistance to experiencing their internal conflict. People are understandably disconcerted and frightened to feel the depth of their animosity toward themselves. In an effort to achieve integration and appear more consistent in their behavior and attitudes, they frequently side with the alien point of view represented by the voice and accept this negative identity as their own. Helping patients externalize negative thoughts enables them to cope more effectively with self-defeating, self-limiting, and self-destructive tendencies. Finally, by identifying the destructive effects of internalized voices, discovering their source, and understanding the role they play in restricting one's current life, a person can separate from the dictates of the voice and move on to corrective experiences.

Corrective Suggestions

In this phase of treatment, patient and therapist attempt to interrupt maladaptive behavior patterns through collaborative planning and suggestions for behavioral change that are in accord with each individual's personal motivation. Plans for behavioral change fall into two categories: (a) corrective suggestions that help control or interrupt self-feeding habits and disrupt dependency bonds and (b) corrective suggestions that expand the patient's world by taking risks and gradually overcoming fears related to pursuing wants and priorities. First, patients formulate the unique values that give their lives special meaning; second, they plan, with the therapist, means of supporting these goals; last, as they move toward risk situations and a new level of vulnerability, they learn to tolerate the anxiety involved in positive changes. The overall procedure has an experimental flavor and is undertaken in a cooperative spirit.

It is important to reiterate that the steps or methods in this treatment strategy are not discrete but overlap one another. Even in the beginning phase, corrective suggestions are used in preparation for feeling release sessions, that is, encouraging patients to avoid the addictive substances and habits they use to suppress feeling. Similarly, during their involvement with Voice Therapy procedures, patients make their own choices to "defy" voice commands and alter behaviors.

By the time patients reach the ending phase, their personal goals have become very clear and self-evident; they are acutely aware of limiting factors in their freedom and have compassion for themselves, and there is a concerted focus on action.

Corrective suggestions, if consistently followed, bring about changes in the emotional atmosphere that lead to a corrective emotional experience (Endnote 2). For example, as a patient alters offensive, provoking behaviors that alienate others and keep them at a distance, he or she is generally responded to with more warmth and affection. In a therapy group, one patient, a lawyer, was asked to refrain from making "courtroom rebuttals" and condescending statements to other members who had things to say to him. He stopped this style of defensiveness and found that they were far less put off by him. He began to be likable and evoked less negative feedback.

The new set of circumstances, albeit more positive, is unfamiliar and initially leads to anxiety. Resistance may be encountered when a particular suggestion affects a well-established defense even when instituted by the patient. For this reason, special attention must be paid to the proper timing of suggestions, and careful follow-up is needed of the patient's reactions.

Patients report that, although there often are strong voice attacks after significant movement, these self-attacks gradually diminish after the new behavior has been maintained over an extended period of time. The importance of teaching patients to "sweat out" important changes in their style of relating cannot be overestimated. In this sense, patients must relinquish their crutches *before* they learn that they will not fall without them. Only by coping with the anxiety generated by positive changes can a person hold on to the psychological territory he or she has gained. Corrective suggestions teach patients, on a deep emotional level, that by using self-discipline, they can gradually increase their freedom of choice without being overwhelmed by primitive fears and anxiety states.

In regard to the final phases of psychotherapy, working on termination represents a form of corrective experience that addresses transference reactions, resolves the dependency bond between the patient and therapist, and establishes equality between the two participants. Positive therapeutic outcome involves successfully coping with the anxiety of separation, which signals an end to the need for office visits and indicates the patient's potential for a self-support system.

RESISTANCE IN VOICE THERAPY

Resistance occurs in all forms of therapy and is indicative of an underlying fear of and aversion to change. Although most patients are dissatisfied with their present-day lives and desire to feel better, they are heavily invested in an inward, defended lifestyle that precludes "the better life." Movement toward fulfillment, independence, freedom, and happiness is threatening and arouses considerable guilt.

Resistance can take many forms: Patients may come late for appointments, act out self-nourishing or self-destructive behaviors outside the session, manifest hostility toward their therapist, or become delinquent in paying for their sessions. Resistance as manifested by patients in Voice Therapy centers on maintaining and protecting the fantasy bond or core defense. Preserving a fantasy of connection with one's parents, and symbolically parenting oneself, offers an illusion of protection and security. The primary defense derives from the fantasy that the individual can nurture him- or herself, thereby avoiding the risk involved in real wanting and possible frustration in relation to others.

Each aspect of the patient's resistance can be examined and understood in terms of how it functions to protect the fantasy bond or core defense. Generally, it can be determined that a direct relationship exists between the types of voice attacks identified by the patient, the behaviors he or she elects to change, and the particular aspect of the defensive process being challenged. Resistance can be expected to occur at those points where core defenses are challenged by Voice Therapy procedures. The therapist who understands the theoretical basis of Voice Therapy can be alert for signs of resistance and negativity as the patient's progress encroaches on specific defenses.

Patients are resistant to changing negative, hostile perceptions of themselves and cynical views of others, causing them to relive maladaptive, self-defeating patterns of the past. At the same time, they tend to avoid positive experiences with potential for *real* gratification from the interpersonal environment. Every aspect of this secondary line of defense functions to protect the core defense— the fantasy that they and only they can feed and sustain themselves.

When therapists view resistance in terms of protecting the primary defense or fantasy bond from intrusion, they are better able to predict the points at which the patient's anxiety will be aroused. Negative reactions can be anticipated whenever there is any change in the patient's cognitive, behavioral, or affective state that threatens either the self-nourishing process or object dependency.

Keeping this relationship in mind, let us examine the kinds of resistance typically encountered in Voice Therapy. Important areas of resistance may be catalogued as follows:

1. Resistance to using specific Voice Therapy procedures
2. Resistance to changing one's self-concept
3. Resistance to formulating personal goals and corrective suggestions

4. Resistance and regression after answering back to voice attacks

Resistance to specific procedures. People are reluctant to recognize the presence of an alien, hostile, or destructive point of view toward themselves and experience the accompanying sense of fragmentation. For this reason, they may become resistant to learning or following Voice Therapy procedures that separate out discordant elements of the personality. In the analytic method, patients or subjects may be hesitant to verbalize what they are telling themselves about the negative events in their lives or their basic problems. They may refuse to state their self-attacks in the second person as outside attacks or voices. In the abreactive method, they may refuse to participate in the dramatization process or hold back significant feelings.

Sometimes patients irresponsibly use Voice Therapy procedures to rationalize negative feelings and attitudes toward self and others. They attempt to distance themselves from or disown responsibility for the negative viewpoint, saying, in effect, "That's just my voice." They continue to act out behavior based on the voice while refusing to give it away or separate it out, even *after* they have identified the specific thoughts influencing their actions. Their resistance or refusal to apply their new knowledge of self masks a need to maintain a childish, provoking mode of interaction with significant others, a posture repetitive of the fantasy bond with their families.

Resistance to changing one's self-concept. There is fundamental resistance in Voice Therapy to identifying voices and self-attacks that challenge the basic self-concept. One would imagine that people would be happy to see through and modify negative views of themselves that make them feel bad. Surprisingly, this is most often *not* the case because to accept changes in one's identity implies a disruption of the self-parenting process and one's negative identity formed within the family. It interferes with the idealization of the family necessary for successful self-parenting and therefore threatens one's sense of security. One cannot effectively parent oneself with an inadequate, weak, internalized parental image. In this sense, positive changes in self-concept are linked to the exposure of parental weaknesses, and this exposure threatens one's sense of security within the family constellation.

Altering one's basic self-concept to a more positive outlook implies changes in behavior and in the style of relating to the important people in one's current life. Valuing oneself and increasing one's sense of personal worth will have an impact on such divergent aspects of living as asking the boss for a raise, refusing to accept personal abuse or submission to another, leaving an unsatisfying relationship, or other symbolic acts asserting one's point of view and independence. Because there may be considerable anxiety in asserting one's belief in oneself, many people prefer to hold on to and preserve a static, albeit negative, view of themselves.

Resistance to formulating personal goals and corrective experiences. Most people are reluctant to formulate definitive goals and to choose specific actions appropriate to working toward them. Strong voices are aroused when individuals take bold steps to pursue their own lives in a manner that is free, nonconforming, or independent. Although corrective suggestions are generally initiated by patients and develop out of their own motivation to alter self-defeating behaviors, the situation still lends itself to the arousal of strong feelings of resistance.

Intrapsychically, corrective suggestions for behavioral change represent a separation from parental introjects and prescriptions for living. Interpersonally, patients usually institute specific changes to break habit patterns that have been modeled after undesirable behaviors displayed by their parents. The subsequent differentiation from parental figures and symbolic separation from the family bond frequently bring the patient to a crucial point in his or her therapy.

Although initially collaborating on the suggestion as an equal partner with the therapist, a patient may subsequently reverse his or her point of view concerning the desire to change. At this time, patients tend to distort the situation and deal with it in a paranoid manner. For example, they may believe that the therapist is telling them how to run their lives, or accuse the therapist of making decisions for them. They project their desire to change onto the therapist and perceive the therapist as having a stake in their progress.

Subsequent negative transference reactions may include childish, dependent ploys for help or, on the other hand, attempts to provoke anger and rejection from the therapist. Resistance functions to disrupt the patient's active and equal participation in the therapy process and therefore acts to establish a fantasy bond with the therapist.

Unfortunately, during the cooperative planning of corrective experiences, many patients tend to respond to the "inner experience" of being a separate decision-making individual by attempting to form a connection with the therapist with renewed efforts to extract parental or caretaking responses. Others maintain their independent point of view, take responsibility for their actions, and progress to new levels.

Regression and resistance after answering to voice attacks. Regressions in Voice Therapy are not fundamentally different from those in other therapies and arise from two principal but divergent sources: (a) unusual positive developments, acknowledgment, and personal achievement, or (b) negative events, that is, guilt reactions, rejection, or frustration in relation to goal-directed activity. One interesting, albeit painful, source of regression is the guilt reaction caused by the breaking of fantasy bonds and moving away from destructive relationships and ties (Endnote 3). Contact with family members also tends to reinforce parental introjects and voice attacks, precipitating regression, even when the interaction is uneventful or even positive on the surface.

Becoming aware of this situation causes a conflict for patients who have no desire to hurt their families yet would tend to avoid them because the patients recognize that they feel bad after contact. Social pressures to conform and prescriptions against choosing a unique or original lifestyle also militate against constructive change and personal development.

Resistance is often encountered following sessions where patients directly challenge the voice. In attempting to counteract the effect of the voices on their lives, behavior, and emotional states, patients may elect to answer the voice dramatically with strong anger. "Yelling back" even at *symbolic* parental figures unleashes feelings of hatred for which one may feel tremendous guilt. We have observed that many patients, after responding angrily to voice attacks and differentiating themselves from their parents—for example, "I'm not like you, you bastard," or simply "I'm different"—subsequently reverted to the very behaviors they were challenging.

Although in my application of Voice Therapy, I have not experienced severe regressive reactions, suicidal behavior, or psychotic episodes, my methods have been applied with care and respect both for patient selection and alertness to the dynamics involved. It has been my concern that moving too quickly toward behavioral suggestions or expressing too much aggression in answering back can lead to significant problems.

The Problem of Anger in Psychotherapy

In general, the problem of voicing aggression toward parents and parental introjects in sessions is a serious issue in any therapeutic endeavor. When patients become aware of the damage they sustained in their early development, they experience a good deal of pain and sadness. These memories and insights give rise to primitive feelings of anger and outrage. Feeling their murderous rage is symbolically equivalent to actually killing, or expressing death wishes toward, the parents. Therefore, patients often experience intense guilt reactions and anxiety when they mobilize these emotions. To compound matters, the symbolic destruction of parental figures leaves the patient fearful of object loss.

The combination of the two emotions, guilt and fear of losing the object, can precipitate regressive trends in any therapy. Intense negative transference reactions in psychoanalysis usually indicate the presence of strong death wishes toward parental figures. Often there will be a breakdown in the therapeutic alliance at this stage. Similar problems may be encountered in feeling release therapy when patients progress steadily until they uncover intense rage reactions about the abuses they suffered. Because of their guilt and fear, they often turn the anger against themselves, taking on the parental point of view, and generally regress to a more childlike mode of interaction. In many cases, the patients never fully work through their aggression, and the therapeutic process from then on may lack the energy manifested in earlier sessions. In conclusion, much attention must be paid to the possibility of negative trends in psychotherapy directly following the patient's expressions of intense angry affect toward either parents or parent symbols.

THE ROLE OF THE THERAPIST

It is not difficult . . . to visualize the *Ideal Therapist* as one who is able to function as a professional depth therapist to any patient. Rarely, someone develops this degree of maturity; but if he does, he usually becomes so out of synchrony with the culture that he is unacceptable in it. If psychiatry could offer the young therapist adequate enough treatment for himself, he might become so mature that he could live beyond and above this rejection by the culture. (Whitaker & Malone, 1981, pp. 136-137)

The personality of the therapist sets the tone and the emotional quality of the therapy process and therefore cannot be divorced from the prescriptive interventions I have delineated. The therapist should ideally be a person of integrity and personal honesty, uncompromising in his or her approach to defenses that limit and debilitate patients. The therapist as a catalyst and facilitator must be sensitive to the wide range of addictive patterns manifested by the patient and have the courage to help expose and interrupt these patterns.

Effective therapists do not fit their patients into a particular theoretical framework or model. Instead, they are willing to experience the painful truths their patients reveal over the course of treatment and respond as patients' individual needs dictate. Because they are cognizant of the inherent destructiveness of defenses and their projection or imprint on society, therapists ideally would refrain from placing social conformity above the personal interests of their patients.

Many therapeutic failures can be attributed to limitations imposed on the patient by the therapist's own defense system. Therapists often fail to recognize the serious restrictions imposed on the self by internal forces and external social pressures. The fact that the resultant impairment in functioning may fall within the range of statistical normalcy does not necessarily signify that it is mentally healthy. The majority of people in our culture suffer from disturbances in their psychological functioning. This fact can obscure pathological manifestations, causing both patient and therapist to overlook dysfunctional behaviors and symptoms. If therapists fail to help their patients learn to value themselves as individuals, they will have encouraged them to surrender to a progressive obliteration of the self through conformity.

In an important sense, the therapist can be conceptualized as a "transitional object" in that he or she provides an *authentic* relationship for the patient during the transition from depending on self-nourishing processes to seeking and finding satisfaction in genuine relationships in the world outside the office setting. As such, therapists must remain human (be interested, warm, caring, and empathic as well as direct and responsible) to temporarily "hold" or sustain the patient as he or she moves away from sources of self-gratification toward real relationships.

The good therapist anticipates the termination phase by continually encouraging the independent development of healthy ego functioning in the patient. Excessive dependence on the therapist and attempts to seek fusion are discouraged; instead, transference reactions are interpreted and worked through with sensitivity and proper timing.

Finally, my approach to psychotherapy is based on an understanding of the conditions that hurt the child originally and continue to detract from his or her humanness as an adult. Viewed from this perspective, the goal of therapy and the therapist's task are self-evident. The therapist must be exceedingly skillful in helping the patient reconnect to him- or herself and to his or her life. To move toward this goal, the therapist, like an artist, must be sensitive to a person's real feeling, qualities, and priorities, and distinguish them from the overlay on the personality that prevents the patient from reaching his or her full potential for living.

CONCLUSION

Voice Therapy procedures are not used as a rigid system applied to all individuals seeking therapeutic intervention. All of the procedures may not be included in the program where there are time constraints or other diagnostic considerations. In other words, they are applied as necessary in a therapeutic program tailored to the specific patient. Moreover, the therapist applying these techniques must come to understand each individual's particular areas of resistance. Each aspect in our treatment plan exposes and challenges basic character defenses and inner processes of fantasy gratification. Therefore, resistance may be encountered at any phase of treatment.

As patients break addictive patterns and separate from destructive ties with parents and parent substitutes, they anxiously anticipate feelings of helplessness, abandonment, and rejection. It is the therapist's task to help patients realize, on an emotional level, what they know intellectually: that as adults they have substantial control over their lives, and that their fears in interpersonal relationships can never realistically be of the same magnitude as those that overwhelmed them when they were powerless children.

For the patient to have the opportunity to approach his or her true potentiality, powerful inimical forces within the personality must be exposed and countered. If these forces are *not* dealt with successfully, the therapeutic endeavor, in much the same manner as the original parenting, may inadvertently deprive the person of his or her capacity to live fully.

Treatment is generally long-term (1½ years or longer). The patient's movement toward individuation is undertaken with care and diligence as well as with a deep understanding of personality dynamics. Brief or short-term psychotherapy based on our techniques can be accomplished by a skillful therapist. Indeed, Voice Therapy techniques are as effective as other forms of psychotherapy used as brief interventions for alleviating depressed states and other forms of psychological distress. However, the person's potential for future development should not be compromised by treatment processes that focus only on the amelioration of symptoms and relief of anxiety. Therapeutic shortcuts usually deal only with pieces of the problem and not with the total person. Nonetheless, the methods described here *can* be used as an adjunct to other approaches. Even when these procedures are not the treatment of choice, the theory and methodology have value in understanding the core of resistance to any form of psychotherapeutic endeavor.

Voice Therapy techniques have been valuable in helping individuals in all states of depression. My associates' and my clinical experience has shown that the depressed patient reaches a stage where the balance has shifted in such a way that the alien point of view represented by the voice actually becomes the patient's own point of view. In other words, the depressed person adopts the voice—its constructions, commands, and directives—as his or her own.

Although depression may have physical components, in most cases patients are exceptionally responsive to Voice Therapy. Being allowed to express the negative parental introjects in the session helps the depressed person to perceive these cognitive distortions as coming from an external source, and he or she can begin to question or challenge their validity. We have found that Voice Therapy methods separate out self-critical, self-attacking thoughts more effectively than other methodologies. The techniques break through the resistance with which the depressed patient is holding on to self-depreciating attitudes and ideologies. Moreover, depressed patients report unusual familiarity with destructive voices, whether on a neurotic or psychotic level (as auditory hallucinations). They feel immediately understood by therapists using Voice Therapy methodology.

To summarize, Voice Therapy is a broadly based methodology derived from a systematic theory of neurosis. My approach challenges defenses and supports the individual's gradual relinquishment of the authority of the voice as an antifeeling, antilife, regulatory mechanism. The improved patient becomes an investigator, an explorer uncritically accepting and examining his or her most irrational thoughts and feelings. He or she attempts to live life as a continuous process of discovery and adventure while respecting the boundaries and freedom of others. The therapeutic venture, through counteracting the dictates of the voice and disrupting fantasies of connection to introjected images and external objects, offers the opportunity to fulfill our human potentialities.

ENDNOTES

1. At Rosen's residential treatment center, I was presented with a unique opportunity to develop and expand my ideas about schizophrenia. I had a chance to work independently and relished this opportunity, although it was emotionally painful to be living with patients, surrounded by this illness and with the threat of violence. During the year spent working with these patients, I evolved my ideas of the "self-mothering process," which I later refined and generalized to a theory of the neuroses.

2. The term *corrective emotional experience* was first used by Franz Alexander (1961) in his application of psychoanalytic therapy to cases that had been generally refractive to treatment. Alexander's emphasis was on experiencing emotionally the discrepancy between transference reactions and the analyst's actual behavior and personality.

3. Murray Bowen (1978) discussed the issue of breaking destructive emotional ties with one's family in his chapter, "Toward the Differentiation of Self in One's Family of Origin." Bowen stresses that patients (family members) who focus on differentiating themselves from their families of origin "make as much or more progress in working out the relationship system with spouses and children as families seen in formal family therapy in which there is a principal focus on the interdependence in the marriage" (p. 545). However, Bowen also notes, "One never becomes completely objective and no one ever gets the process to the point of not reacting emotionally to family situations" (p. 541). Bowen's therapy focuses primarily on the patient's differentiation of self from the "external" family. Voice Therapy techniques focus on helping the patient in the differentiation of self from the "internal" family, that is, from the negative parental introjects.

11

Application of Voice Therapy to Couples and Parenting Groups

Voice Therapy is both a unique laboratory procedure and a psychotherapy technique. In the laboratory setting, it has provided the means for eliciting and identifying partly conscious or unconscious negative thought patterns that impair personality functioning and damage relationships. The techniques have been effectively applied to evaluating suicide potential, individual therapy, group therapy, couples therapy, problems in sexual relating, and specialized parenting groups as a form of preventive psychotherapy.

APPLICATION OF VOICE THERAPY TO COUPLE RELATIONSHIPS

In couples therapy, partners progress through the following steps over the course of treatment: (a) formulating the problem each individual perceives is

168

limiting his or her satisfaction within the relationship, (b) learning to verbalize self-critical thoughts and perceptions of each other in the form of the voice and release the associated affect, (c) developing insight into the origins of the voice and making important connections between past experience and present conflicts. They learn to take back their projections, and this process helps them to avoid focusing blame on the other.[1]

In the following pages, I describe clinical material gathered during a series of group meetings in which Voice Therapy procedures were used to elicit and identify the contents of internalized prescriptions regarding participants' personal relationships.

Clinical Material

Our results, based on this series of meetings, were divided into four principal categories from which we derived the following hypotheses: (a) Individuals have varying degrees of animosity toward self and experience feelings of worthlessness and unlovability that foster desperation in interpersonal relationships. These thought processes and feelings can be elicited in a "voice" group situation. (b) Personal relationships characterized by complementary or opposite traits that are based on deficits within each partner's personality eventually lead to marital difficulties. The same qualities that were the basis of the original attraction often become areas of animosity later on. (c) People are following prescriptions based on their parents' defensive attitudes toward life; when they break with this programming, they experience considerable anxiety and intensified voice attacks. (d) The fear of rejection by objects masks a deeper fear from within, a fear of arousing one's own self-critical, self-destructive, or suicidal tendencies.

(1) Animosity toward self based on feelings of unlovability. In using Voice Therapy procedures with couples, it became apparent that each partner's internalized destructive voices significantly affected the quality of the relationship. To illustrate, one subject who had serious doubts about herself as a woman gave words to her self-depreciating thoughts. As she succumbed to the process and allowed her feelings to flow, her voice became louder and noticeably angry. Soon she gave vent to feelings of strong self-condemnation, attitudes she was largely unaware of prior to the meeting:

> "Nobody would ever choose you. You're never going to have anything, so you'd better call him. You'd better ask him out. You'd better go for it."

---

1 Each member of the couple verbalizes his or her negative feelings toward self and the other in each other's company. In a very real sense, they are sharing each other's individual psychotherapy.

"Look at you! You're going to be alone! [*Loud, angry voice*] What makes you think you can have anything? You're going to have nothing! If you just sit there, you're going to have nothing! nothing! nothing!"

At this point, the woman's voice took on an irate, parental tone:

"You're a measly little piece of garbage! What makes you think a man would ever choose you? What makes you think you could have anything? You're not any better than *me*. You're worse!"

Over a period of 10 to 15 years, the quality of this woman's relationships with men had gradually deteriorated and she had gained considerable weight. She experienced despair about her future. Much of her life was dictated by these voices and her overall lifestyle mirrored her self-attacks. Internal feelings of being unlovable led to desperation in her interactions with men, and her hunger and possessiveness tended to drive men away.

In another case, a man revealed a hateful, contemptuous voice that he recognized as reflecting his mother's spoken and unspoken expectations for him:

One of the things I'm embarrassed about is that my "voice" is more like my mother's than my father's. It's even embarrassing to say it out loud:

"That's what men are there for. You're supposed to take care of women. That's your job—and you're supposed to satisfy me! You're supposed to give me all the things that your father couldn't provide for me. [*Furious*] You! You! Not him! He can't do it! You are mine. You're supposed to take care of me. You're supposed to do well in school so that I can compete with my sisters."

[*Embittered tone of voice*] "You're supposed to be my pride and joy and you're *not* doing it. Your job is to take care of me. That's your job. You take care of me and you'd better do a better job because your father can't do it. So *you* do it! *You* take care of me. That's your job!

"You're here to take care of women. You're *nothing* except how you can take care of a woman. That's your job! That's what you're supposed to do. Do it!"

After he spoke, he reflected on the session:

So that's my standard for everything I do. Am I taking care of the woman? Am I treating her nicely, am I giving her what she wants rather than satisfying myself?

Because this man adopted his mother's negative point of view about men, he was confused about his sexual identification. In another episode, he elaborated his feeling that women did not see him as a real man and identified disparaging thoughts concerning his body, general appearance, and sexuality. Feelings of inadequacy and failure to meet his mother's demands contributed to a defeatist view of himself as a man and increased his passive-aggression toward women. In general, over the course of the sessions, we noted that critical voices expressing malicious attitudes toward self and antagonism toward one's mate reduced themselves to the same issue: Both predispose an alienated and defensive posture that has a destructive effect on relationships.

(2) Reciprocal voices based on personality deficits. A number of participants disclosed voice attacks that clarified the dynamics operating in their relationships that led to disharmony. We found that opposite or complementary characteristics in the partners and compensatory personality traits were based on internal voices. In many couples, both partners reported the same or equivalent voice attacks. The overlap or mutuality of self-depreciating thoughts in the partners was correlated with a negative prognosis for the relationship.

For example, after Andy and Dianne became involved sexually, they experienced many serious difficulties. Andy expressed the following thoughts regarding the situation:

> "You should be getting her things, you should be taking her places. Now that she's really given you something, you should give her something. You should take care of her. Give her what she wants. Be nice to her."

His expression of the voice also revealed his mother's, and incidentally his father's, derisive point of view about men:

> "Don't be like other men, mean, rough, aggressive. Don't be a prick. Be nice. Be a nice man. Give her what she wants even before she asks for it."

Later, he attacked himself more directly:

> "You're so lucky to be involved with her. You're so lucky to have her, you're so lucky to have a woman that likes you. You're just lucky, because you're really a piece of shit. You're really not much of a man, so you'd better hold on to her.
>
> "You'd better give her what she wants. You really better hold on to her. She'll see through you. Just give her what she wants. She won't see then. You better hold on to her."

At another meeting, he had verbalized the following voices regarding his physical appearance:

> "You're short, small. Women think of you as a boy, not as a man. You're soft. You're odd. You're different from other men. You're just not a real man!"

Dianne reported negative injunctions similar in content to those Andy had indicated.

> "You don't want to lose him. Give him whatever he wants, he may be the one. He's nice, see, he's really nice to you. He gives you gifts. He buys you all these things. You don't ever want to disappoint him because you may lose that. He's nice, he's successful, he'll take care of you.
>
> "You'd better just give him whatever he wants. If you don't, he's going to leave you, and you're going to be alone and you're never going to meet anybody. You don't want to be alone. You won't ever meet a nice guy again."

In a loud, angry voice, she said,

> "Men don't like you. You're lucky to have this one. You don't want to screw it up. You'll end up alone. You won't ever have anybody. One wrong step and you'll be all alone. Just stay in line."

Like Andy, Dianne later went on to report harsh attacks on her femininity:

> "You have a body just like a boy. Your breasts are small, too small to be like a regular woman. They don't look normal! What man would ever be attracted to you?"

Dianne's sense of being an incomplete person created a compelling need to find someone to fill the void. She felt flawed as a woman, and Andy had corresponding fears as a man, which heightened their sexual attraction initially but subsequently led to problems. Each partner revealed a similar pattern in previous relationships.

Andy revealed voices that he should take care of a woman, whereas Dianne reported voices indicating that she needed to be taken care of. One can observe the reciprocity of voice attacks in the expressions of each individual.

Andy and Dianne also disclosed attitudes indicative of a reversed sexual orientation or identity. Andy perceived strength in a man as harsh and aggressive and saw himself as more gentle or soft, like a woman, whereas Dianne experienced herself as more masculine than feminine. Unfortunately, the insecurity and confused sense of sexual identity in both people eventually led to the dissolution of a relationship that had started off with much promise.

Many men and women come together in an attempt to compensate for their deficiencies and self-attacks. The more rejection or deprivation an individual experiences during the formative years, the more he or she seeks security and a sense of wholeness through a fantasized connection with another. Eventually, these relationships develop into an addictive attachment in the sense that both individuals are using each other as an instrument to assuage feelings of insecurity. This misuse of the other leads to a deterioration of their original feelings (Willi, 1975/1982) (Endnote 1).

(3) Prescriptions for living based on defensive parental attitudes. Another significant finding was that sexual stereotypes, distorted perceptions of men and women so pervasive in our culture, are related to voice attacks. Defensive attitudes toward the opposite sex held by parents are passed on to succeeding generations. We found that the majority of women adopt their mother's point of view about men, while men are generally influenced by their father's attitudes toward women. Julia has recently separated from a strong dependency relationship and is currently pursuing an independent life in which she feels more self-possessed. In a discussion group, after becoming emotional, she exposed her mother's prescription for living, one that involved prejudicial attitudes toward men.

I know what my mother's voice is and it's like she's saying: "Let me tell you how it is. Let me tell you how it really is. Men don't have feelings. Men don't care about anything. They don't care about women and they don't care about children. But women need them and so here's how you do it. Here's how you go about it.

"You've got to make them interested and you've got to keep them interested and then you've got to keep control. And then you better take this lesson, you better learn it because you've got to keep a man and you've got to keep him under control because you need him to take care of you.

"You better find somebody and you better keep him close by and under control. You've got to build him up, you've got to make him think that you think he's good. You've got to make them seem strong, you've got to make them feel like they're really important. You've got to kiss up. You've got to do everything they want. And then you'll have them.

"But don't expect niceness. Are you crazy? Don't expect niceness. They don't have it in them! You better hang on. You better hang on because there's nothing like being taken care of. You can't take care of yourself."

At this point, the anger associated with her mother's point of view escalated:

"But have you ever blown it, my dear. Have you ever blown it! What is all this stuff about independence? What is this independence stuff? You didn't listen to me. You didn't listen to me! Are you ever going to be sorry! Are you going to be sorry at the end of your years."

[*With real fury*] "You'll be alone and you'll be cold and nobody's going to give a shit about you. You didn't listen to me. You idiot! I tried to tell you what to do. I tried to tell you to get somebody and hang on to him like I did!"

In another case, a man who mistrusted women and was reluctant to commit to a relationship articulated a voice that reflected his father's viewpoint:

"You better not trust her. She's just going to flip. You'd better be careful. You're going to be just like me. You're going to make her go crazy just like I made your mother. She's going to end up screaming at you and acting crazy if you don't act nice.

"If you ever get angry at her, she's just going to go crazy. She's just going to lose it and you're responsible for her. If she goes crazy it's on you. You, you caused it."

Breaking with parental prescriptions. When people move away from their parents' defensive lifestyles, there is a sense of disequilibrium. Positive movement in life can trigger anxiety and severe voice attacks. For example, Vivian described feeling closer and more open to her husband, who is genuinely kind and loving toward her. In the meeting, she exposed the following self-attacks:

I had a lot of different thoughts, but I felt like when I grew up my mother gave me a prescription for life; she told me how to be in relation to my father, in relation to her, in relation to life. The feeling is that my mother knows how to get by. The voice is:

"Just keep your equilibrium. Just keep your mouth shut, don't draw attention to yourself from him, but don't feel too bad. Don't get too depressed either, because then you'll draw negative attention. Just keep in the middle of the road."

Vivian became increasingly angry and emotional:

"Just put your blinders on, he [father] doesn't want to hear anything that you have to say about me or any opinions that you have about me or about what's going on. Just try opening your mouth around me."

Now she assailed herself more directly:

"You idiot, you're so stupid! Don't get happy from being with him [Vivian's husband]. Don't get happy because you'll be really disappointed because there's nothing for you there. There's nothing from a man. Don't get happy for a moment. Because he's just going to let you down.

"But don't feel too bad or he'll just go away. You may feel like shit but you better not show anyone because life is shit. It's a shithole out there and you're by yourself and you better believe it and you better just live and die the way I did! By yourself! I did it! I did it!

"I succeeded! I died without anyone, without you, without him. So don't you go getting your hopes up about anything, about having a man in your life.

"Don't threaten me because I'm way bigger and way meaner than you. And I'll put you in your fucking place and so will he [father], by the way. We'll both put you in your fucking place if you open your mouth. So just shut up!" [*Sobbing*]

After regaining her composure, Vivian spoke with deep sadness: "I feel like this is the way I've been living my life for a long time."

Separating out her mother's prohibitions and stereotypical views about men in terms of the voice, Vivian was attempting to break with generations of tradition. Until she began challenging this process, she was exceptionally quiet, reserved, and reluctant to reveal her innermost feelings, especially when she was troubled. In relation to her husband, she had felt victimized and misunderstood and had had difficulty getting along.

Vivian's continued progress in healthy relating depends primarily on whether she has the courage to stay vulnerable and open in her ongoing relationship. She must have the ego strength to tolerate the inevitable anxiety involved in fundamental character changes, to triumph over her voice attacks, and to gradually adjust to her new identity as a loving and lovable woman.

(4) Fear of rejection masks a greater fear of arousing one's self-attacks. Based on in-depth interviews, we conjectured that people do not fear the actual rejection or object loss as much as they fear the self-attacking thought process that will be triggered by the rejection. They are apprehensive about arousing their own internal malice. Even when initiating the separation, many individuals experienced self-attacks declaring that they were mean or bad. Some admitted that they were frightened of being left alone with their inner "demons."

Andrea, an attractive computer programmer, decided to extricate herself from a 3-year relationship with a man who was an alcoholic. When she confronted him and told him she was going to leave him, his response was at first angry, then cold and indifferent. Subsequently, she felt overwhelmed with anxiety and dread about her future prospects, and later renewed the contact. In a group discussion, she revealed the angry self-accusations that intimidated her, causing her to eventually go back on her decision:

At the time, I thought: "You can't do this to him. You have to make it right! Why are you doing this to him? Can't you see you're hurting him? Can't you see that you're giving up something that you should be keeping anyway? This is the right thing for you. You're supposed to get married. Give him what he wants.

"How can you leave him like this? You're hurting him. You're a bitch! Just go back to him. Make everything all right. Go back and make everything okay and be there for him."

After she released these guilt feelings, Andrea continued in a louder voice filled with fury:

"Don't you *dare* go away from him! He wants you and you *should* have him. He wants you and that's the way it's going to be. Sorry that you want something better. You can't have it! It hurts him! You're hurting him!" [*Angry and sobbing*]

"You're *supposed* to be with him. He's *supposed* to be with you and you can't screw it up. Don't fuck with it! Don't mess with it! Who cares about *your* feelings and that you feel like you're being held back? This is how it's supposed to be!"

Andrea then described her boyfriend's reactions and explained how they intensified her fear of being alone:

His coldness made me feel that I just couldn't stand it. When he walked out the door, I felt like saying to him, "I'm sorry, I'm sorry. Please come back. I take it all back. Please don't be angry. Please don't go away. I'll do anything. Only don't reject me. I need you. I need you to like me. Please don't turn away from me right now. I'll hurt so much. I'll hurt so bad." [*Agitated and crying*]

Later, when I was alone, I thought to myself: "You won't be able to stand it that you did a stupid thing like this. You've got to make it right, right now! You can't leave it like this."

Andrea's desperation to hold on to a harmful relationship with a man she did not love was based on a fear that losing it would validate her worst self-attacks and precipitate a self-destructive thought process. In general, the dread of arousing intense voice attacks and suicidal impulses causes many men and women to cling to negative relationships where they progressively give up their individuality and sense of identity.

Discussion

In this study, we found that the lifestyle of each partner in a couple directly followed his or her specific voices or parental prescriptions. Individuals who selected partners with opposite character traits based on similar or overlapping voices, as was true in the case of Andy and Dianne, were attempting to compensate for personality deficits (Endnote 2). In general, a sexually restrictive society laden with moralistic attitudes inevitably leads most people to confuse strong sexual attraction with love. However, an intense sexual attraction may mask destructive needs based on emotional hunger and desperation. The effort to become a complete person through connecting with another is ultimately doomed to fail.

In summary, it is valuable for individuals to challenge their negative voices in a psychotherapy that exposes core issues. They must learn to free themselves of self-defeating, restrictive behavior patterns that cause them so much distress in their relationships. Recognizing the enemy within enables people to broaden their experience in living and significantly improve their relationships. Indeed, there is no defense or "problem" that is impervious to change, providing the parties have the courage to risk vulnerability in their close associations rather than remain imprisoned by early programming and illusions of connection.

Voice Therapy procedures uncover major defenses that directly affect repetitive behavior and the compulsive reliving of the past with new objects in present-day relationships. In the context of couples therapy or marriage counseling, each partner has the opportunity to develop empathy for the other, because each partner is exposed to the other's psychotherapy experience. Understanding their self-attacks as the primary source of misery in their lives takes pressure off the relationship. Freeing this energy has a powerful effect on altering and improving attitudes toward their mates as well as enhancing each individual's own personal growth (Endnote 3).

VOICE THERAPY APPLIED TO PARENTING GROUPS[2]

In using Voice Therapy procedures in specialized parenting groups, my associates and I helped parents uncover the source of their ambivalent attitudes toward themselves and their children, which enabled them to gain control over destructive child-rearing practices. As noted in Chapter 4, the dimension of our parenting groups that differentiates them from other forms of group psychotherapy is their focus on (a) parents' attitudes toward their children and (b) the experiences parents went through in their own childhood. This twofold concentration helps parents have more compassion for themselves by developing feeling for what happened to them as children. The goal is for parents to develop an empathic understanding of the sources of their limitations and then to see their child from that same perspective, that is, to pass on this sensitive view to their offspring. Regaining feeling for themselves may well be the key element that enables parents to alter their child-rearing practices in a positive direction (Endnote 4).

---

2 The material in this section is taken primarily from an article titled, "Parenting Groups Based on Voice Therapy," *Psychotherapy, 26* (1989), pp. 524-529. Used with permission.

Steps in the Therapeutic Process

The format of the specialized parenting groups consists of the following steps.

Expression of ambivalent feelings and attitudes. Initially, parents presented problems about their children that disturbed them, complaints relating to a particular aspect of their child's life they had observed that caused them worry or distress. After this initial discussion, the first step was to bring out the negative attitudes that parents held toward themselves. For this purpose, we used Voice Therapy techniques. Parents were asked to bring out their self-attacks in the second person—"*You're* not handling things very well," "You're so impatient," "You're just not a very good mother (father)," "You never do things right."

After expressing their self-attacks, parents were encouraged to reveal their ambivalent reactions toward their children and to identify the specific circumstances, situations, and types of behavior in their children that aroused hostile feelings. Participants made connections between their self-attacks and the aggressive, resentful attitudes manifested toward their children.

Christopher, who was raised by a harsh, authoritarian father, spoke about the intense emotional reactions he had toward his son, Doug, whenever he sensed the youngster was frightened of trying something new.

> With Doug, it would be any situation in which I would want him to do something and he wouldn't want to do it. He would say either that he didn't want to do it, or that he didn't know how; he was scared about it—whatever it was. But I thought that he *could* and *should* do it. When he wouldn't do it, I would get so angry, because [*Pause*]—
>
> I know that I have this feeling in myself that if I feel like I'm supposed to be able to do something, then I've *got to do it*! [*Angry tone*] I think things like, "You've got to do it. Do it now! What's the matter with you?" Then if I didn't do it, I would feel extremely critical of myself for not doing it.
>
> I would feel exactly the same way with Doug. I would feel furious because he wouldn't do it, and then I felt like it was some basic failure in his life and failure in my parenting him—that I had to make him really do it.
>
> It became really crucial. Those were the most fierce times, things like, "Cut your meat the right way" or "You just climb the ladder, you can climb it." [*Yelling*] "*Climb the ladder!*" And he would be so afraid. [*Sad*] Thinking about it like this, I know I have exactly the same set of feelings toward myself.

While describing the turbulent feelings aroused in him by the boy's timidity, Christopher recalled feeling terrified as a child in similar situations with his own father. However, not until he talked about the specific characteristics and behaviors in his son that had triggered his fury did he develop insight into both himself and their relationship. Connecting his own self-censure with the harsh feelings he had toward his son led to a sense of kinship with the boy.

Participants reported experiencing a sense of relief from feelings of guilt after they expressed their negative attitudes toward children in the accepting, non-judgmental atmosphere of the group. They observed that others revealed similar feelings of resentment and anger toward their children and so began to feel less guilty about these feelings within themselves. Guilt feelings were further ameliorated by parents adopting a positive course of action rather than feeling depressed about the state of their child's maladjustment.

Recall of painful events. Parents were asked to remember and refer to experiences in their families that had caused them pain and stress. They were encouraged to recall the specific incidents of abuse, both verbal and physical, to which they had been exposed as children and to share their emotions. As the participants revealed traumatic incidents from their past, they became aware of almost uncanny parallels between the specific abuses they had suffered in their development and their own faulty patterns of child rearing.

One young woman described being abandoned by her mother when she was 2 years old. In a repetition of the mother's desertion, this woman had left her own son when he was a toddler, after she became frightened of the strong aggressive impulses that she felt toward him. At the time, however, she failed to connect the two events in her mind. Later, in sharing her experiences with others in the parenting group, she recognized the full impact of her mother's desertion and that she had unconsciously and compulsively repeated her mother's pattern. She also realized that she had somehow blamed herself for her mother's desertion and had experienced intense feelings of anger toward herself. When she became a mother, this repressed rage had emerged in relation to her small son, arousing anxiety reactions in her.

Release of repressed affect. From previous clinical work, we learned that most individuals tend to deny the validity of early trauma as well as minimize the emotional impact these incidents had on them as children. Therefore, we usually encouraged participants to express the feelings associated with the painful events they recalled from early interactions within their families. We felt that, in general, it was important for parents to experience these feelings to develop compassion for themselves and their children. The expression of emotion was facilitated by giving verbal support, that is, if an individual began to indicate affect, we would say, "Let it out," or "Don't hold back," or "Try to really feel that," or other supportive statements.

Because of the commonality of experiences that had occurred during people's formative years, one person's revelations had the effect of stimulating the recovery of memories in others. Parents strongly identified with the stories related by their fellow participants. Even individuals who were resistant to remembering events of their childhood were able to recall the incidents in detail and experience the deep emotions associated with them.

Connections between present-day limitations and early defenses. Although our specialized parent sample was primarily made up of well-adjusted individuals, through talking more openly about themselves, even they became cognizant of areas in their lives where they still felt limited. They brought up material relating to patterns of inwardness, passivity, paralyzing forms of withholding, and passive-aggressive responses that they had found difficult to overcome. They were able to link these habit patterns and behaviors to specific events in childhood or to the emotional climate that originally had caused them to construct nonfunctional defensive patterns. Consider the statements of one parent, an attorney, who tended to isolate himself because of extreme social awkwardness. He recalled his relationship with his mother:

> I was never hit or beaten ever, I mean, never—but I know that my mother took over my entire life from a very early age, and that I just became a performing object. I was 2, 3 years old and she was teaching me how to read and giving me dancing lessons and, I mean, my entire life was out of my hands, and I was always performing.
>
> If there was a party and I was asleep, I'd be awakened and called out of my bedroom into the living room. I'd have to read something or do a dance or whatever it was. I mean, it was an endless succession of performances.
>
> And I know that now, I can't go into a room with people in it without thinking about what I'm going to do. What am I going to do to please these people or what am I going to do to make people like me?

Following this insight and with further understanding of related feelings, this man felt relieved of the pressure to perform and found himself more at ease in social situations.

In learning how they had been limited in their early lives, these people could not help but recognize that they had also been implicitly taught to blame themselves for their inadequacies. As they came to a deeper awareness of the sources of their weaknesses, they began to adopt a more compassionate attitude toward themselves and their children.

Exposure of inadequacies in their families. As men and women developed more sensitivity toward themselves, it was inevitable that they would challenge the idealized images they held of their parents. Virtually all the participants noted strong tendencies in themselves to protect and excuse their own parents and to rationalize the abuses they had suffered as children. As they dealt with these issues on a more profound level, they began to feel the full brunt of the outrage and grief they felt in being limited by these early experiences. Their basic attitude was not one of blaming, but more one of accounting for what happened in their childhood and reacting appropriately to the discoveries.

Sensitive treatment of children. As the parents changed, they began to develop a new perspective on child rearing. They saw that they could be different from their own parents. Becoming sensitive to their children in ways their parents had not been sensitive tended further to break into the idealization of their families and the corresponding depreciation of themselves. People developed a new point of view concerning their parents, perceiving them more objectively as real people with strengths and weaknesses. In isolating the traumatic experiences that were harmful to them in their formative years, parents began to formulate positive attitudes and countermeasures that served as constructive guidelines to child-rearing practices, which in turn minimized damage to their offspring. In becoming more compassionate toward themselves, they developed a sensitive interest in their children and initiated steps to prevent their children from incorporating an image of themselves as "bad." They were more successful in avoiding negative or destructive interactions with their children, as well as offering them experiences that would enhance their self-esteem.

To illustrate, one father's change in attitude is apparent in the following transcription:

I've realized a number of things about the way I treat children and the way other people treat children since we've been talking about this subject. One of the things I realized was the frequency and the routineness of talking to children in terms of good and bad, that almost everything that a child is told is based on good and bad. Whether he obeys the parent or not, he's good or bad. "Are you going to be a good boy and do this?" or "You're bad when you do that." So I've made a real effort to talk to my daughter and other children in other ways.

I have developed resource material that resulted in a parent education program. This preventive mental health measure provides a comprehensive format based on Voice Therapy theory that is effective in parent training groups. The classes include videotaped excerpts from our specialized parenting groups (see the Appendix).

The type of group process delineated here may well be the most effective psychotherapy for parents. Consideration for their children's well-being acts as a strong motivating force. Taking advantage of the opportunity to modify damaging responses to their children helps them in their own healing process. It appears that only through understanding themselves can parents really change the destructive attitudes and feelings they express, overtly and covertly, toward their children.

CONCLUSION

The role of the voice in the cycle of physical and emotional child abuse is a three-step process: (a) To varying degrees, all children suffer trauma and rejection in their formative years. Particularly during times of stress, they incorporate an *internal parent,* represented by a destructive, self-critical thought process or voice. (b) Children retain this hostile voice within them throughout their lives, restricting, limiting, and punishing themselves. (c) When they become parents, they are compelled to act out similar abuses on their children, who, in turn, incorporate the punishing attitudes as a self-depreciating thought process, thereby completing the cycle. On a preventive level, it is vital to recognize the issues involved in breaking this chain and to intervene, whenever possible, in cases where infants and children are experiencing emotional problems and maladjustment.

ENDNOTES

1. Jurg Willi (1975/1982), in *Couples in Collusion: The Unconscious Dimension in Partner Relationships,* explained the meshing of unconscious intrapsychic patterns between two partners that results in increased polarity of traits and behaviors. Thereafter, both partners engage in collusive efforts to maintain the status quo. Willi noted that partner selection often results from the search for repressed or missing elements of self in the partner, which leads to marital conflict.

2. Murray Bowen (1978) found that individuals with a low level of self-differentiation tended to select mates at a similar low level, resulting in a seriously dysfunctional marriage and new family system. It is likely that their choices were attempts to fill a need or void rather than to advance to a higher level of self-differentiation, a movement that would have aroused anxiety.

In *Object Relations Couple Therapy,* David Scharff and Jill Scharff (1991) provided a cogent explanation of partner selection based on the concept of projective identification. From their perspective, marital choices are motivated primarily by attempts to find a person who will complement and reinforce unconscious fantasies. According to Scharff and Scharff, "Projective identification as a concept can now be seen to have the power to offer a conceptual bridge between individual and interpersonal psychology" (p. 53).

3. Books addressing assessment and treatment strategies that deal with the personal growth of each partner are recommended to the reader: *Handbook of Relational Diagnosis and Dysfunctional Family Patterns* (Kaslow, 1996), which includes chapters that focus on treating partners diagnosed with anxiety disorders, borderline disorders, affective disorders, and gender identity disorders; Aaron Beck's (1988) *Love Is Never Enough,* a cognitive therapy perspective on marital relationships; and Guerney, Brock, and Coufal's (1986) description of the Relationship Enhancement (RE) program, which outlines methods for teaching marital partners empathy and listening

skills. The RE program essentially involves educating each partner in a modified form of Rogers's (1951) Client-Centered Therapy techniques.

4. Our preliminary studies of Voice Therapy applied to parenting groups suggest its suitability and value as an effective form of preventive psychotherapy. In "Primary Prevention in Mental Health," Emery Cowen (1983) outlined the essential dimensions of primary prevention programs:

> (a) they must be mass- or group-oriented, not targeted to individuals; (b) directed to essentially "well" people, not to the already affected, though targets can appropriately include those who, by virtue of life circumstances or recent experiences are known (epidemiologically) to be at risk for adverse psychological outcomes; (c) "intentional," that is, rest on a knowledge base which suggests that a program's operations hold promise for strengthening psychological health or reducing psychological maladjustment. (p. 15)

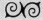

12

Assessment of Suicide Risk

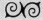

Frank Tobe, a close friend of mine, was on an airplane heading for a business conference in Washington, D.C. He found himself sitting beside Dr. C. Everett Koop, who was at that time the U.S. surgeon general. Excited by my work, Frank found himself enthusiastically talking about my conception of self-destructive behavior and suicide. Koop was interested and spoke about the serious epidemic of suicide in our country. He felt that what was really needed in the mental health field was an accurate predictor of suicide. When Frank told me about his encounter, I was immediately intrigued and decided to develop a predictive instrument based on Voice Therapy theory. I had two goals in mind. First, I felt that a voice scale to determine self-destructive and suicide potential could save lives, and, second, I thought that a scientific study using this type of scale would call attention to the importance of the underlying theory.

My assumption was that a scale of negative voice attacks on the self would parallel self-destructive acting-out behavior, and that if a person scored very

AUTHOR'S NOTE: Portions of this chapter are taken from *The Firestone Voice Scale for Self-Destructive Behavior: Investigating the Scale's Validity and Reliability,* doctoral dissertation, California School of Professional Psychology (Lisa Firestone, 1991); and from the *Firestone Assessment of Self-Destructive Thoughts* manual by R. W. Firestone and Lisa Firestone, copyright © 1996 The Psychological Corporation. Used with permission. All rights reserved.

high on these items, that person would be more likely to injure him- or herself. I began to gather items for the new scale from the negative self-attacks of patients in psychotherapy as well as from participants in my own clinical investigations.

On the one hand, I felt reasonably optimistic that the results would sustain my hypothesis, but on the other, I feared that the phenomena might elude detection because subjects might not reveal themselves honestly in response to the voice statements.

You can imagine my satisfaction when the scale was tested with over 500 subjects and showed very high correlations with suicide attempts and suicide potential. It was both reliable and valid. It provided a mental health professional with a serious measure of each patient's suicide potential, and in addition, the individual items helped the therapist to focus on the specific problem areas of special significance to his or her patient. An outcome of major importance to me was that it supported my contention that voice attacks were closely related to how an individual functions in his or her life. It was apparent that angry, critical voices are at the core of maladaptive behavior in general.

Now, I would like to digress and put these theoretical matters in perspective. I will begin by describing my conception of the relationship between micro-suicide, suicide, and other forms of psychopathology and include a brief review of the literature for the study in question. The technical aspects of our research will be reserved for the "Research Notes" at the end of the chapter.

Psychopathology or "mental illness" can be more accurately conceptualized as a limitation in living, imposed on the individual by inadequate, immature, or hostile parenting, internalized in the form of negative thought processes (voices), and later manifested in self-limiting and/or self-destructive lifestyles. In this sense, varieties of so-called mental illness are subclasses of suicide rather than the reverse (R. Firestone & Seiden, 1987).

All aspects of giving up of self, one's sense of reality, goal-directed activity, and appropriate emotional responses represent a defensive, self-destructive orientation toward life that inevitably leads to neurotic, borderline, or psychotic symptom formation. Emotional deprivation and destructive parenting are the most significant determinants of the degree of psychological maladjustment. Inimical thought patterns and emotional attitudes are introjected or incorporated into the self system and strongly influence or control the relinquishing of one's unique identity and the narrowing of life experiences. Suicide represents the ultimate abrogation of self and the extreme end of the continuum of self-destructiveness. Therefore, it is productive to study this phenomenon as it sheds light on the entire spectrum of "mental illness."

Clearly, suicide, depression, and self-destructive actions are multidetermined, and biological components should be considered in ascertaining their etiology, particularly in bipolar disorders. All mental events have a somatic component, and all somatic events are affected by psychological phenomena.

Human beings are psychosomatic. In our studies, however, we focus primarily on the psychodynamics of emotional disorders and suicide.

This chapter presents research findings (L. Firestone, 1991) that demonstrate the significant correlation between parental introjects or "voices" and self-destructive behavior. The study applied my theoretical construct of the voice to the development of the Firestone Assessment of Self-Destructive Thoughts.

BACKGROUND OF THE STUDY

Self-attacks, "voices," vary along a continuum of intensity from mild self-reproach to strong self-accusations and suicidal ideation. Similarly, self-destructive behavior exists on a continuum ranging from self-denial; self-criticism; self-defeating behaviors, that is, behavior contrary to one's goals, accident-proneness, substance abuse; and eventually to direct actions that cause bodily harm. Clinical evidence supporting the relationship between internal voices and self-destructive living suggested the research potential that would lead to an accurate estimation of an individual's suicide potential.

Data obtained during preliminary studies (R. Firestone, 1988) using Voice Therapy procedures led to the following hypotheses. The source of negative thought processes, and their development within the personality, is related to (a) the projection of negative parental traits onto the child, (b) the child's imitation of one or both parents' maladaptive defenses, and (c) the internalization and incorporation of parental attitudes of overt and covert aggression toward the child. As the degree of trauma experienced in childhood increases, the level of intensity of voice attacks parallels this progression, and there are increasingly angry, vicious attacks on the self. These voices are manifested in an individual's retreat into inwardness, feelings of extreme self-hate, and eventually impulses and directives toward self-destructive action.

In summary, the effects of negative early environmental influences are retained in the form of destructive voices within the adult personality. Thus the voice plays a major role in precipitating and maintaining a wide range of maladaptive behaviors that are mistakenly classified or defined as a disease entity or "mental illness."

BRIEF REVIEW OF THE LITERATURE

The categorization of emotional disturbance as a medical abnormality or illness has been challenged by a number of theorists and clinicians (Feinstein & Krippner, 1988; Laing & Esterson, 1964/1970; Szasz, 1961, 1963, 1978). The suicidologist Edwin Shneidman (1989) emphasized that suicide is *not* an illness; rather, it is

> a human, psychological orientation toward life, not a biological, medical disease.
> . . . Suicide is a human malaise tied to what is "on the mind," including one's
> view of the value of life at that moment. It is essentially hopeless unhappiness
> and psychological hurt—and that is not a medical condition. (p. 9)

In their writing, the suicidologists Kalle Achte (1980) and Norman Farberow (1980) described indirect suicidal manifestations in nonmedical terms, that is, as the methods people use to sabotage their own success, seemingly preferring to live miserable, restricted lives. Clinical and empirical studies tend to confirm our view that "mental illness" represents a narrowing of one's life space, a constriction of experience, and a controlled destruction of the personality.

Psychoanalytic Approaches

Many theorists have identified aspects of a negative internal thought process. In "Group Psychology and the Analysis of the Ego," Sigmund Freud (1921/ 1955) described cases of melancholia in which there is "a cruel self-depreciation of the ego combined with relentless self-criticism and bitter self-reproaches" (p. 109). He went on to state, "But these melancholias also show us something else. . . . They show us the ego divided, fallen apart into two pieces, one of which rages against the second" (p. 109).

In Guntrip's (1969) analysis of Fairbairn's theory of ego psychology, he used the terms *libidinal ego* and *antilibidinal ego* to delineate parts of the split ego. Guntrip linked the punishing ego function of the antilibidinal ego to depression and suicide: "The degree of self-hate and self-persecution going on in the unconscious determines the degree of the illness, and in severe cases the person can become hopeless, panic-stricken, and be driven to suicide as a way out" (p. 190) (Endnote 1).

Cognitive Approaches

Historically, cognitive psychologists, among them Beck (1976), have written extensively about "nonconscious" cognitive processing. Cognitive therapists and researchers (Abramson, Metalsky, & Alloy, 1989; E. Hamilton & Abramson, 1983; Rose & Abramson, 1992; Rose, Abramson, Hodulik, Halberstadt, & Leff, 1994) have investigated the relationship between cognitive patterns, depression, and hopelessness. Studies by Miranda and Persons (1988) also demonstrated that latent dysfunctional schemas can be activated during the asymptomatic period in cases of depression. Deutscher and Cimbolic (1990) noted the relationship between negative attributional styles and different types of depression.

Beck (1976), Ellis (1973), Ellis and Harper (1975), and Kaufman and Raphael (1984) presented similar concepts in their discussions of maladaptive thought processes. Bach and Torbet (1983) described a variety of self-reproaching inner dialogues that indicate attitudes of hostility toward self and anger turned inward upon the self. Beck discovered a discrete group of thoughts, which he termed "automatic thoughts," that precipitate negative feelings and inappropriate or excessive emotional reactions, interfering with the client's ability to cope with life. In a more recent study, Beck, Steer, and Brown (1993) investigated correlations between various dysfunctional attitudes and suicidal ideation in psychiatric outpatients. They concluded that

> the overall severity of dysfunctional attitudes and four sets of specific dysfunction attitudes involving cognitive vulnerability, success-perfectionism, need to impress others and disapproval-dependence were by themselves significantly related to identifying patients who were thinking about committing suicide. (p. 19)

However, they also found that dysfunctional attitudes did not contribute as much to identifying suicidal ideators as did a history of past attempts and degree of hopelessness.

It is apparent that the phenomena described by these clinicians are similar to the self-attacks identified by our subjects through the laboratory procedures of Voice Therapy. However, the concept of the voice and methods of Voice Therapy are more deeply rooted in the psychoanalytic approach than in a cognitive-behavioral model. My theoretical focus is on understanding the psychodynamics of the patient's functional disturbance in the present, and my methods are based on an underlying theory of personality that emphasizes a primary defensive process (R. Firestone, 1988, 1990c).

THE DEVELOPMENT OF THE FIRESTONE ASSESSMENT OF SELF-DESTRUCTIVE THOUGHTS (FAST)

As I noted earlier, my primary purpose in initiating an empirical research project was to predict an individual's suicide potential, because accurate prediction could potentially save lives. I was interested in determining whether the results of the proposed research would be consistent with our theoretical orientation and support our initial findings concerning the continuum of self-destructive behavior. If so, they would be of significant value. Many theorists have noted the continuous nature of self-destructive behavior and restrictive lifestyles, yet this notion or concept had not yet been subject to empirical research. In addition, the research could shed light on the relationship between powerful psychological defenses formed in childhood and later personality malfunctions.

Subsequently, Lisa Firestone elected to conduct the basic research project to fulfill requirements for a doctoral dissertation in clinical psychology. Her study (L. Firestone, 1991) involved the application of Voice Therapy theory to the development of a scale to assess self-destructive behavior. Her goal was to establish the validity and reliability of the scale. It was hypothesized that the scale would reveal valuable information about the content of an individual's negative thought processes. It was expected that one could better assess the seriousness or "dangerousness" of suicide intent by identifying where and with what frequency an individual's thoughts lie along the Continuum of Negative Thought Patterns (Figure 12.1).

Description of the Scale

The "rational" approach (Jackson, 1970) to scale construction was adopted from the onset of the development of the FAST. Items for the FAST were originally chosen on the basis of my theory of the dynamics underlying suicide (R. Firestone, 1986, 1988; R. Firestone & Seiden, 1987). Items were drawn from actual clinical material obtained during my 20-year longitudinal study of the "voice." Items on the scale were made up of self-critical statements or "voices" gathered from patients and subjects over the course of this clinical investigation. It was noted that more extreme "voice" attacks were manifested by individuals who had made past suicide attempts.

Based on a pretest administered to individuals who had made previous suicide attempts and to nonattempters, the scale was shortened and revised. Items found to significantly discriminate between the two groups were retained. The revised scale consisted of 110 items, equally drawn from 11 levels of self-destructiveness that I proposed on the Continuum of Negative Thought Patterns.

Methods

In the main study, the revised questionnaire was administered to 507 subjects currently in psychotherapy. Respondents were tested at sites throughout the United States and western Canada (see the "Research Notes"). They were asked to endorse how frequently they experience negative thoughts or "voices" on a 5-point Likert-type scale. In addition, the subjects were asked to complete a battery of nine other instruments covering diverse areas of self-destructiveness to provide construct validation for the various levels of self-destructiveness I

Levels of Increasing Suicidal Intention	Content of Voice Statements
Thoughts that lead to low self-esteem or inwardness (self-defeating thoughts):	
1. Self-depreciating thoughts of everyday life	*You're incompetent, stupid. You're not very attractive. You're going to make a fool of yourself.*
2. Thoughts rationalizing self-denial; thoughts discouraging the person from engaging in pleasurable activities	*You're too young (old) and inexperienced to apply for this job. You're too shy to make any new friends, or Why go on this trip? It'll be such a hassle. You'll save money by staying home.*
3. Cynical attitudes toward others, leading to alienation and distancing	*Why go out with her (him)? She's cold, unreliable; she'll reject you. She wouldn't go out with you anyway. You can't trust men (women)*
4. Thoughts influencing isolation; rationalizations for time alone, but using time to become more negative toward oneself	*Just be by yourself. You're miserable company anyway; who'd want to be with you? Just stay in the background, out of view.*
5. Self-contempt; vicious self-abusive thoughts and accusations (accompanied by intense angry affect)	*You idiot! You bitch! You creep! You stupid shit! You don't deserve anything; you're worthless.*
Thoughts that support the cycle of addiction (addictions):	
6. Thoughts urging use of substances or food followed by self-criticisms (weakens inhibitions against self-destructive actions, while increasing guilt and self-recrimination following acting out)	*It's okay to do drugs, you'll be more relaxed. Go ahead and have a drink, you deserve it. (Later) You weak-willed jerk! You're nothing but a drugged-out drunken freak.*
Thoughts that lead to suicide (self-annihilating thoughts):	
7. Thoughts contributing to a sense of hopelessness, urging withdrawal or removal of oneself completely from the lives of people closest	*See how bad you make your family (friends) feel. They'd be better off without you. It's the only decent thing to do—just stay away and stop bothering them.*
8. Thoughts influencing a person to give up priorities and favored activities (points of identity)	*What's the use? Your work doesn't matter any more. Why bother even trying? Nothing matters anyway.*
9. Injunctions to inflict self-harm at an action level; intense rage against self	*Why don't you just drive across the center divider? Just shove your hand under that power saw!*
10 Thoughts planning details of suicide (calm, rational, often obsessive, indicating complete loss of feeling for the self)	*You have to get hold of some pills, then go to a hotel, etc.*
11. Injunctions to carry out suicide plans; thoughts baiting the person to commit suicide (extreme thought constriction)	*You've thought about this long enough. Just get it over with. It's the only way out!*

Any combination of the voice attacks listed above can lead to serious suicidal intent. Thoughts leading to isolation, ideation about removing oneself from people's lives, beliefs that one is a bad influence or has a destructive effect on others, voices urging one to give up special activities, vicious self-abusive thoughts accompanied by strong anger, voices urging self-injury and a suicide attempt are all indications of high suicide potential or risk.

Figure 12.1. The Continuum of Negative Thought Patterns

had proposed. The tests included the Beck Hopelessness Scale (Beck, 1978) and the Suicide Probability Scale (Cull & Gill, 1988), among others.

Client participants were administered the battery of tests in a private setting, with the main researcher or a research assistant present to answer questions and communicate with those who might feel disturbed by the testing. Immediately after administering the test, the Beck Hopelessness Scale and the Suicide Probability Scale were scored, and the therapist was informed if any of the scores were in a range of concern.

It was hypothesized that the scale would be able to distinguish between those individuals with a past history of suicide attempts and those without such a history. Both therapists and subjects provided information on the criterion variable (subjects' past suicide attempts). It was found that the sample chosen included 93 persons who had made suicide attempts and 414 who had not.

In addition, we anticipated that the scale would identify a wide range of self-destructive patterns. Combined with my theoretical orientation, the new instrument would provide clinicians with a comprehensive framework for understanding the dynamics of alienation, self-attack, and suicide. The majority of scales previously developed to assess suicide potential focus on descriptive information concerning behaviors known to be correlated with suicide (Endnote 2). In contrast, the FAST is based on accessing and measuring a partially *unconscious* process hypothesized to underlie suicidal behavior. It was expected that this distinction would lend the instrument more discriminatory power in assessing suicide potential.

Results

The results of Lisa Firestone's empirical investigation provided support for the reliability and validity of the Firestone Assessment of Self-Destructive Thoughts (see the "Research Notes"). Perhaps the most promising results were obtained in establishing the criterion-related validity of the scale. It was demonstrated that scores on the scale correlated significantly higher than the Beck Hopelessness Scale or the Suicide Probability Scale with subjects' prior suicide attempts for this particular sample. For example, the Beck Hopelessness Scale showed only 13 of the 93 suicide attempters scoring in the range of severe concern. In contrast, the FAST was found to have 41 individuals of the 93 attempters scoring in the highest ranges of concern, while only 17 individuals scored in either the range of no concern or mild concern. The Suicide Intent Composite, composed of 27 items drawn from Levels 7 through 11, was also found to have a significantly higher correlation with prior suicide attempts than other instruments in the battery of tests.

Discussion

An unexpected but crucial finding of this research involves the reporting of this criterion variable (past suicide attempts). Of the 93 cases where subjects reported a history of suicide attempts, only 38 therapists were aware of this fact.

In other words, for over half the subjects with this serious indication of future suicide potential, the therapist had apparently not asked this important question. Subjects were explicitly aware (having signed releases) that the testing information would be shared with their therapist, which implies that they were willing to tell the therapist about these prior suicide attempts. This finding lends support to the position that clinicians, to some degree, avoid dealing with the difficult topic of suicide. It also strongly supports the idea that clinicians would benefit from making greater use of instruments specifically addressing this topic.

One interesting finding was that subjects reported it was easy to identify with negative thoughts stated in the second person format on the scale. On a number of occasions, clients answering the questionnaire made comments such as these: "I see that my pattern is to be inward and isolated" or "I didn't realize I was talking to myself so much." These comments and others strengthened our informal hypothesis that items on the scale were closely related to internalized thought patterns that were only partially conscious. Answering questions in this format gave respondents a feeling of being understood. Moreover, therapists reported that their clients brought up topics not previously mentioned in their sessions and expressed their emotions more openly and freely in the weeks following testing.

LEVELS OF INTENSITY OF THE VOICE

Clinical Studies

As noted, in laboratory procedures (Voice Therapy) in which subjects verbalized their self-critical thoughts, we were able to identify three levels of the voice in terms of intensity and content: (a) self-critical thoughts and attitudes, (b) self-accusations accompanied by angry affect, and (c) injunctions, often accompanied by murderous rage, to injure or kill oneself.

The levels of intensity correspond to different aspects or functions of the voice that progressively influence maladaptive behaviors along the continuum of self-destructiveness. There are two essential modes of operation. The first refers to thought processes that lead to self-denial—attitudes that are restrictive or limiting of life experience, while the second, self-attack, refers to self-destructive propensities and actions. Some overlap clearly exists between these two aspects of the voice; however, the prohibitive quality appears to be based on the child's imitation of, and adaptation to, the parental defense system, while the malicious aspect of the thought process is more closely related to repressed or overt parental aggression.

The restrictive quality of the voice functions to limit one's experience and stifle one's enthusiasm, spontaneity, spirit, and sense of adventure. These self-attacks restrain or completely block an individual's wants and desires before they can be translated into action. Negative thoughts provide seemingly rational reasons for self-denial, isolation, and alienation from other people.

The malicious aspect of the hostile thought process issues directives to mutilate the self emotionally and/or physically. These thought patterns are accompanied by intense anger against the self. When verbalized out loud, these voices, composed of vicious, degrading self-accusations and injunctions to injure oneself, are very powerful and dramatic. It is important to emphasize that, in almost every case, emotional catharsis appeared to decrease the need for action. Facing up to, and separating from, the enemy within acted to relieve the pressure, and individuals gained a measure of control over self-destructive impulses.

Empirical Findings Related to
Increasing Levels of Self-Destructiveness

The results of an exploratory factor analysis of the FAST (R. Firestone & Firestone, 1996) revealed three factors of increasing self-destructiveness. Composite Factor 1 was labeled the "Self-Defeating Composite" and consisted of Levels 1-5 on the continuum. It includes self-critical thoughts (Level 1), self-denial (Level 2), cynical or hostile attitudes toward others (Level 3), gradual withdrawal into isolation (Level 4), and self-contempt (Level 5). The level of intense anger toward self associated with the thoughts at Level 5 appears to be an important step in the progression toward overt self-destructive acts because it leads to considerable perturbation and psychological pain.

Composite Factor 2, labeled the "Addictions Composite," was made up of all Level 6 items. These items are the types of thoughts that support the cycle of addictions.

Composite Factor 3 is made up of Levels 7-11 and was labeled the "Self-Annihilating Composite." These are thoughts that represent the full spectrum of self-annihilation, from psychological suicide (Level 7, Hopelessness, which urges the removal of oneself from significant others), and thoughts associated with giving up one's priorities and favored activities (Level 8), to self-mutilation (Level 9), to actual physical suicide (Level 10, Suicide Plans, and Level 11, Suicide Injunctions).

For example, Level 8 includes thoughts influencing the individual to give up points of identity and his or her investment in life by indicating that "nothing matters." This type of thought process (the divestment of energy or decathexis) leads to alienation from the self and extinction of the personality (psychological suicide).

Discussion and Interpretation of Findings

Case Study[1]

Composite Factors 1 and 3 are illustrated in statements from an interview with a woman who made a serious suicide attempt and who barely survived through a last minute call for help. At the time of her attempt, she was unaware that a destructive thought process was gradually gaining ascendence over her rational thinking and assuming control of her actions. Later, using the procedures of Voice Therapy, she was able to clearly recall the thoughts she experienced during that period of her life.

In the transcript that follows, one can observe the progression of thoughts and the increasing intensity of her murderous rage toward the self. The interview begins with Sharon describing thoughts associated with feelings of low self-esteem and cynical thoughts toward others, as well as those urging her to isolate herself.

Self-defeating composite.

> I was depressed. I never liked the way I looked. I couldn't look at myself. The way I felt took the form of: "You're so ugly. Who would choose you? You don't really like him—he doesn't matter that much to you. There are other people that he likes—there are other people important in his life."
>
> I was conscious of trying to look okay to my friends, to the people who I was around. I told myself: "Don't let anybody see what's going on. Look okay. Smile if he walks by. Smile. Answer him. Look normal. Don't let anybody know what's going on."
>
> I tried to get alone, because this process occurred when I was alone. I couldn't carry it off if there were other people around. The voice said, "Get alone. You need some time for yourself. Get alone just so you can think."
>
> And once I would get alone, either driving around somewhere or just walking around by myself, then these other voices, the more destructive ones, would start.

Self-annihilating composite. At this point, Sharon's anger toward herself became progressively more intense. As destructive thoughts increasingly dominated her point of view, her self-attacks became more vicious:

> I felt like I was bad, like there was something really bad about me that I couldn't fix. I hated myself. I couldn't stand myself. I don't know why.

---

1 The material in this section is taken primarily from an article titled "The 'Inner Voice' and Suicide," *Psychotherapy, 23* (1986), pp. 439-447. Used with permission.

I thought, "You thought you mattered to him, but you don't any more. You don't matter to anyone! You worm! You don't matter!

"Who would care if you were gone? No one! They might miss you at first, but no one would *really* care!"

During the hours immediately preceding the ingestion of a lethal dose of barbiturates and Valium, Sharon finalized the details of her plan to kill herself. The decision to end her life relieved to some extent the perturbation and psychological pain she had been experiencing during the previous weeks, feelings she expresses in the following sequence:

I had thoughts like "You don't matter to him," and "You don't really like him. You don't like him. He doesn't matter that much to you, either."

Then I thought things like "If you don't matter, what does matter? Nothing matters! What are you waking up for? You know you hate waking up in the morning, why bother? It's so agonizing to wake up in the morning, why bother doing it? End it. Just end it!"

I would think endlessly about the details: "When are you going to do it? Where are you going to do it? How are you going to do it? Come on, when are you going to do it? You've got to find a good time when nobody is going to miss you, when you can get away."

At times the voice would sound rational, like "Look, this is really something you should do. You've thought about it long enough. You decided you're going to do it. Now do it! Quit fooling around and just get it over with."

I know that I took enough pills to kill myself. I remember thinking: "Okay, now do it! Coward! Now do it already. You've got these pills—go ahead, start taking them. Now do it and do it right!"

ORIGINS OF THE VOICE PROCESS

The individuals who participated in our clinical studies traced the origins of their negative or hostile thoughts toward themselves to early family interactions. From these early investigations, we discovered that destructive voices were associated with the core defense the child forms in response to anxiety, pain, and deprivation suffered during the formative years. We concluded that the restrictive, prohibitive aspect of the voice had three major sources: (a) The child takes on, as his or her identity, negative traits that were disowned by the parents, projected onto the child, and subsequently punished. Through the mechanism of projective identification, children adopt their parents' misconceptions of them and maintain this imposed or "induced" identity in the form of the voice and its behavioral consequences throughout their lives. (b) The child imitates and identifies with his or her parent's or parents' personality traits and psychological defenses. (Most often the child is influenced more by the parent of the same sex.) In this manner, children assimilate their parents' defensive modes of coping with the world. (c) Angry self-attacks appear to be more directly related to parental aggression incorporated by the child under conditions of stress or trauma in identifying with his or her attacker. In the interview described above, Sharon was able to identify the roots of the vicious and degrading voices that first caused her pain, then directed her to escape the pain by killing herself.

> This voice was angry toward me: "You'd better do it. It's the only thing you can do. You'd better do it." Like, "I hate you! I hate you!" [*Crying*]
>
> I just had a thought in relation to my mother. I remember feelings directed toward me from her, when she would get angry at me. I knew she wanted to kill me. That's something I remember. I knew she wanted to kill me. I knew it.
>
> I remember being in a bathroom of my house and my eye level was with the sink. So I must have been 5 or something like that. And I remember her getting furious at me for something which I can't remember, and she started hitting me, which was unusual. I don't remember her hitting me often. But she hit me this one time, and she kept hitting me and hitting me until she noticed that I was bleeding, and then she stopped, when she saw that I was bleeding.
>
> I remember that hatred for some reason—her hatred toward me, being directed toward me. "I hate you!" For what? "I hate you." That was like that voice—my own voice. It turned into my own voice hating myself. That's when it was the most vicious.

In an attempt to relieve her distress and fear, Sharon had identified with her powerful, attacking mother. She introjected the hating image of her mother, whom she experienced as wishing her dead. Later, as an adult, she acted out the internalized malevolence in a serious suicide attempt.

Implications

The factor analysis discussed previously suggested that the factor composite "Self-Annihilating" may well contain the primary factors distinguishing suicide attempters from those individuals who represent a lesser threat to self. In other words, individuals who complete suicide and those who attempt it are compulsively acting out the parental death wishes that were directed toward them.

Generally, the most violent actions against the self represent "self-murder" through identification with a covertly hateful or malevolent parent. As discussed in Chapter 5, the child sensing or perceiving unconscious or covert malevolence in his or her parent or parents experiences intense anticipatory fear or terror in relation to survival. The child's tendency is to split off from the identity of the "victim," identify with the aggressor, and later act out his or her parents' murderous rage in the form of self-mutilation or suicide. Thus suicidal behavior represents a self-protective defense mechanism in which there is a sense of triumph over weakness. The helpless child, facing terrifying circumstances with an uncertain outcome, becomes the powerful, omnipotent parent, thereby achieving an illusion of security and mastery.

The research studies described in this chapter tend to validate the connection between negative thought processes (voices) and self-limiting lifestyles, self-destructive behavior, and suicide. There are other important implications. As noted previously, subjects in the early clinical studies (R. Firestone, 1988) identified their voices as parental statements or as representative of the overall attitudes they perceived directed toward them from their parents. Subsequently, the items selected for the scale were obtained directly from data gathered during the earlier studies, that is, from the voice attacks reported by these subjects. The use of this clinical material to construct a scale that was later found to discriminate suicide attempters from nonattempters more accurately than other instruments lends support to the hypothesis that destructive "voices" are associated with self-destructive action and may well represent introjected parental attitudes (R. Firestone, 1986, 1993).

In my opinion, inimical thought processes underlying self-destructive behaviors do *not* originate in an innate aggressive drive or death instinct as postulated by Sigmund Freud (1925/1959) and M. Klein (1948/1964); rather, they are formed in response to a negative or hostile parental environment. I conceive of human aggression as a natural response to frustration and hurt. In the case of suicide, this rage is turned inward against the self.

Every person has suffered some degree of pain in his or her development, has internalized negative voices, and possesses some potential for suicide. Whether or not it is acted out depends on a multitude of factors. However, of utmost importance in predicting suicide is the degree of incorporated parental hostility, particularly parents' covert aggression. I am suggesting that parental death wishes are the primary condition for serious suicidal ideation and action. Other clinicians (Peck, 1983; Rosenbaum & Richman, 1970) have reached similar conclusions, based on data from their clinical studies (Endnote 3). Peck reported the case of a 15-year-old boy whose parents gave him, as a Christmas gift, the gun that his older brother had used to kill himself some months earlier. Commenting on the case, Peck wrote,

Since he [the youngster] already believed himself to be evil and lacked the maturity to see his parents with any clarity, there was but one interpretation open to him: to believe the gun an appropriate message telling him: "Take your brother's suicide weapon and do likewise. You deserve to die."

Rosenbaum and Richman began their controversial article by stating: "We believe that the clinician must ask . . . 'Who wished the patient to die, disappear, or go away?' " (p. 1652).

As noted earlier, there is no single cause of specific symptoms or dysfunctional behavior. All psychological functions are multidetermined. In some cases, somatic aspects clearly outweigh environmental components in the etiology of ego weakness and maladjustment. In most cases, however, it appears that the impact of psychological elements and early family interactions on the child's development exceeds the influence of innate predispositions.

CONCLUSION

Overall, the results of the empirical studies reflect favorably on the concept of the "voice" and the hypothesis that assessing the level and intensity of destructive "voices" would correlate with suicide potential. Further research is suggested, of most importance being a prospective study of 5 or more years' duration, to further evaluate the scale's ability to predict suicide. It would also be of considerable interest to measure the effects or outcome of psychotherapy, testing pre- and posttest responses to the FAST.

Using the concept of the voice and the continuum of self-destructive behaviors to develop the FAST led to a significant correlation with other indices of suicide potential and an even more significant correlation with actual suicide attempts than most suicide theorists have had access to heretofore. As with people's lives in general, all the signs of suicide are guided by these voices. In a sense, one can observe the makings of a suicidal individual in the process. Our data suggest that emotional or psychological malfunction or disturbance is representative of self-limiting and self-destructive lifestyles that can be more usefully conceptualized along a continuum than defined and categorized as disease entities.

RESEARCH NOTES:
SUMMARY OF RESEARCH FINDINGS

Results of Outpatient Study
Developing the FAST

The sample consisted of 93 subjects who had made suicide attempts and 414 who had not. Of the 93 attempters, 76% were women and 24% men. The majority of the sample were white (90%) as were the majority of attempters (87%). Nonwhites made up only 10% of the total sample and 13% of the attempter groups. Unemployed subjects made up only 26% of the overall sample, but they were 43% of the attempted sample. The same was true for income, with subjects in the lower income brackets making up a higher proportion of the suicide attempter group (L. Firestone, 1991).

Internal Reliability:
Consistency of Test Scores

The internal consistencies were evaluated for the sample by estimating Cronbach's (1951) alpha coefficient. Internal consistency estimates for the levels range from .78 for Level 2 to .97 for Level 11. The estimated internal consistency of the total scale was very high (alpha = 0.98).

Validity

A number of procedures were implemented to establish the validity of the FAST: (a) expert reviews, (b) factor analytic studies, (c) correlations with other measures of self-destructive thoughts or behaviors, (d) studies of specificity and sensitivity of the test to discriminate suicidal from nonsuicidal subjects, and (e) incremental validity studies demonstrating the scale's ability to add to our ability to predict suicide.

Content-Related Validity

As noted previously, the original 220-item pool for the FAST consisted of verbatim statements made by clients during Voice Therapy groups. Raters were used to establish the extent to which the items actually represented the 11 levels from the Continuum of Negative Thought Patterns. Those items found to have the highest level correlations were retained.

Hierarchial Construct Validity

A Guttman Scalogram Analysis (the microcomputer program SCALO by Gilpin & Hays, 1990) was conducted to examine the hierarchy of the self-destructive levels represented on the FAST. If dichotomous items are consistent with a Guttman scale, then they are ordered along a single dimension in terms of prevalence of their endorsement. The scalability of responses was determined by comparing observed patterns of data with patterns predicted for a Guttman scale. The level prevalence observed varied somewhat from prediction, with Level 4 (isolation) receiving a higher level of prevalence than any other level. In addition, Level 6 (addictions) and Level 10 (suicide plans) each had slightly lower levels of prevalence than predicted. However, the coefficient of reproducibility (CR) was 0.91, with a standard of 0.90 or higher considered acceptable. The coefficient of scalability (CS) for a slightly modified ordering of the levels (i.e., by difficulty) was 0.66, with a CS of 0.60 as a standard for acceptability.

Construct Validity

Subjects were asked to complete the following battery of questionnaires: the Suicide Probability Scale (Cull & Gill, 1988); the Reasons for Living Inventory (Linehan, Goodstein, Nielsen, & Chiles, 1983); the Beck Hopelessness Scale (Beck, 1978); a 2-question subset of the Survey on Self-Harm (Favazza & Eppright, 1986); the Eating Disorder Inventory (Garner & Olmsted, 1984); the Inventory of Feelings, Problems, and Family Experiences (Cook, 1986), which consisted of three tests, the Internalized Shame Scale, the Problem History Scale, and the Family of Origin Scale; the Monitoring the Future Substance Use Battery (Bachman & Johnston, 1978); an 11-item Socially Desirable Response Set Measure (Hays, Hayashi, & Stewart, 1989); and the CES-D Depression Scale (Radloff, 1977).

The FAST total score was significantly correlated with the Suicide Probability Scale total score, $r = 0.77$ $(p < .05)$, and the Beck Hopelessness Scale, $r = 0.60$ $(p < .05)$. Items from Level 10 (thoughts planning suicide) and Level 11 (injunctions to commit suicide) were correlated with scores on the SPS $r = 0.67$ $(p < .05)$; and $r = 0.80$ $(p < .05)$ with the SPS Suicide Ideation Scale. Items on Level 6 (addictions) were correlated with the Eating Disorder Inventory, $r = 0.40$ $(p < .05)$. Items on Level 9 (injunctions to self-harm) positively correlated with the Survey on Self-Harm Types, $r = 0.52$ $(p < .05)$, and Self-Harm Times, $r = 0.25$ $(p < .05)$. Items on Level 5 (vicious self-abusive thoughts) were correlated with the Internalized Shame Scale total, $r = 0.75$ $(p < .05)$. The FAST total also correlated significantly with therapists' overall evaluation of the self-destructiveness of the clients $r = 0.40$, $(p < .05)$.

However, the FAST total and the Reasons for Living Inventory were not significantly correlated. In fact, the RFL did not correlate significantly with any of the other measures of suicide potential used in the study. Many subjects appeared to find this particular test difficult to grasp.

Criterion Validity Studies

The criterion validity for the FAST was evaluated by comparing scores with the criterion variable (previous suicide attempts). The FAST was found to have higher correlations with the above-mentioned criterion variable (total score, $r = 0.31$ $(p < .05)$ than any of the other measures included in the study $(SPS, r = 0.26,$ and BHS, $r = 0.18)$. Steiger t-ratios were calculated to estimate the significance of the difference between these correlations. The FAST correlation with the criterion variable was significantly higher than all other instruments except the SPS, where the difference was not significant. However, correlations for the FAST Level 10 (thoughts planning suicide) and Level 11 (injunctions to commit suicide) with the SPS total correlation self-reported suicide attempts were significantly larger than with this criterion. These "suicide" levels of the FAST demonstrate a significantly higher correlation with reports of past suicide attempts than any of the other measures administered.

Incremental Validity

A logistic regression analysis was conducted to determine whether or not the FAST could add significantly to our ability to determine suicide potential. A logistic regression coefficient was obtained using the following variables as predictors of past suicide attempts: SPS total score, BHS total score, age, income, gender, race, employment status, and marital status. Subsequently, with the FAST total score added, a logistic regression was run. The difference in resulting logic coefficients was compared χ^2 $(1, N = 383) = 7.268$ $(p < .05)$ and revealed a significant difference. Hence the FAST total score adds significantly to our ability to discriminate those individuals who have made prior suicide attempts and who, by inference, represent a greater potential threat of actual suicide.

Inpatient Study

A second study was conducted with 479 inpatients from various diagnostic categories including schizophrenic patients, patients with major depression, and bipolar disorders. The FAST distinguished suicide ideators from nonideators in each of the diagnostic categories.

Study With Incarcerated Individuals

In a more recent study of 915 incarcerated individuals, participants in domestic violence diversion groups, and individuals with no criminal records, the FAST correctly classified 83% of the suicide ideators.

ENDNOTES

1. According to Fairbairn (Guntrip, 1969), the libidinal ego is the original infant psyche and is "in a rejected state of fear and unsatisfied need . . . [The] newly developing persecuting ego

function [the antilibidinal ego] . . . directs its energies to hating its infantile weakness and striving to subdue it" (p. 188).

Guntrip linked the punishing ego function to depression and suicidal behavior. "In depressed and obsessional persons the central ego [conscious, coping ego] may be all but captured by the antilibidinal ego" (p. 189).

Novey (1955) attributed the unconscious punitive part of the personality to the superego:

> The essential superego is an institution of the unconscious . . . [and] exercises its power through the threat, or the employment, of the special form of anxiety known as guilt or through the anxiety emerging from the threat of withdrawal of its love. (pp. 256-257)

2. Other methods of suicide risk assessment are described in *Suicide Risk: The Formulation of Clinical Judgment* (Maltsberger, 1986) and *Assessment and Prediction of Suicide* edited by Maris, Berman, Maltsberger, and Yufit (1992).

3. Other writers addressing this issue include Arnaldo Rascovsky (1995) in his book, *Filicide,* who stated,

> Primitive myths (Devereux, 1953, 1966, Rascovsky . . . [& Rascovsky], 1968 . . .), rites of initiation, studies of human sacrifice . . . and diverse expressions of the social systems show us that the real or symbolic killing, mutilation, and humiliation of the offspring, in their most varied expressions, constitute practices that have also been universal since the dawn of man (. . . Rheingold, 1964). (pp. 45-46)

and Berliner (1966), who asserted, "The deepest meaning of the Oedipus legend, and parricide and incest, is *infanticide,* not in the simple form of killing a child but also by burdening it with guilt. . . . Suicide is sometimes deferred infanticide" (p. 247).

PART IV

Theoretical Issues

13

The Dual Nature
of Guilt Reactions

The unconscious force which drives people to deny themselves
enjoyment and success, to spoil their chances in life or not to make use
of them, may be more accurately defined as the need for punishment. . . .

The origin and the essential features of moral masochism are strange
indeed, but anyone can perceive a faint echo in himself if he listens to
the melody. We are surprised that the feeling of guilt or the
corresponding wish to be punished can remain completely unconscious.

Theodore Reik (1941, pp. 10-11)

Human beings spend their lives in a restricted range of personal relationships
and experiences. Their freedom and initiative are constricted by a self-
destructive process. Furthermore, their internal conflict is primarily unconscious,
and they are generally unaware of the circle of guilt and shame that limits them.

An important distinction in the literature has been made between guilt
feelings and shame (Endnote 1). In the psychoanalytic literature, shame is
associated with the pre-Oedipal level, and guilt is more associated with the

AUTHOR'S NOTE: The substance of this chapter is taken primarily from an article titled, "The
'Voice': The Dual Nature of Guilt Reactions," *American Journal of Psychoanalysis, 47* (1987),
pp. 210-229. Used with permission.

Oedipal level of development. Kaufman (1980), Morrison (1989), Goldberg (1991, 1996), and H. B. Lewis (1971) identified guilt as self-critical feelings experienced in relation to one's actions, whereas shame is a primary affect related to my concept of negative parental introjects internalized during the pre-Oedipal stage. Voices represent both types of attacks: self-recrimination for behavior, as well as a sense of deep humiliation for perceived inadequacies, of which "exposure means exposure of one's inherent defectiveness as a human being" (Kaufman, 1980, p. 77) (Endnote 2). The range and substance of experience that people permit themselves is regulated by this system of self-accusatory thoughts and injunctions. To whatever degree these self-critical thoughts remain unconscious, they cause considerable damage, and the individual is unable to break the cycle.

I include both concepts when referring to the double bind of moving toward self-activation and moving away from infantile dependency sources, versus retreating from personal goal-directed activity into passivity, symbiosis, and fantasy processes. The concepts of guilt and shame both refer to an insidious process of self-limitation and self-hatred that seriously restricts people's lives. Because of these emotions, people become self-denying, self-defeating, self-destructive, and even suicidal.

NEUROTIC AND EXISTENTIAL GUILT

In the forthcoming discussion, to clarify the distinction between neurotic and existential guilt, I have chosen to omit the distinction between guilt and shame and refer to both processes under the generalized heading of guilt or self-attack. First, I will illustrate how an individual's ongoing motivation is disrupted by harsh judgmental attitudes toward self, incorporated during the early developmental years, causing the individual to back away from life's pursuits. Second, I will emphasize that when an individual does back away, there is a fundamental sense of having violated the self that causes a great deal of additional suffering. I have termed the former *neurotic guilt* and the latter *existential guilt.*

Neurotic guilt may be defined as feelings of remorse, shame, or self-attack for seeking gratification, for moving toward one's goals, and for pursuing one's wants. The person essentially characterizes him- or herself as "bad or selfish." This form of guilt reaction appears to be related to emotional deprivation, parental prohibitions, and faulty training procedures in childhood.

Becker (1964) defined neurotic guilt as "the action-bind that reaches out of the past to limit new experiences, to block the possibility of broader choices" (p. 186). He attributed the cause of this constriction of life to the "early indoctrination" of the child.

In his essay, "The Ego and the Id," Freud (1923/1961) delineated two kinds of neurotic guilt: (a) conscious guilt (conscience) "based on the tension between the ego and the ego ideal . . . the expression of a condemnation of the ego by its critical agency" (p. 51) and (b) an unconscious sense of guilt that Freud believed to be the basis of the patient's "negative therapeutic reaction" to progress or to praise from the therapist. The reappearance of symptoms signified an underlying, unconscious guilt: "As far as the patient is concerned this sense of guilt is dumb; it does not tell him he is guilty; he does not feel guilty, he feels ill" (pp. 49-50).

Freud and Becker perceived neurotic guilt as preventing an individual from achieving satisfaction or fulfillment in life as well as interfering with his or her progress in psychotherapy. My views concerning neurotic guilt are similar both to Becker's and to Freud's formulations. It is my contention that neurotic guilt reactions arise when a person chooses self-actualization. When we choose to go against our inhibitions and spontaneously embrace life, we have to deal with the fear and guilt aroused by our affirmation of individuality and personal power. We experience anxiety from having separated ourselves from dependency bonds with others and are vulnerable to guilt for surpassing our parents and contemporaries.

The second type of guilt, termed *existential* or *ontological guilt,* is triggered by holding back or withholding one's natural inclinations. It is generally experienced by individuals when they turn their backs on their goals, retreat from life, or seek gratification in fantasy. Rollo May (1958) has described this form of guilt as

> rooted in the fact of self-awareness. Ontological guilt does not consist of I-am-guilty-because-I-violate-parental-prohibitions, but arises from the fact that I can see myself as the one who can choose or fail to choose. (p. 55)

> When the person denies these potentialities, fails to fulfill them, his condition is guilt. (p. 52)

Yalom (1980) discusses existential guilt in terms of responsibility and states, "Most simply put: one is guilty not only through transgressions against another or against some moral or social code, but *one may be guilty of transgression against oneself*" (p. 277). According to Yalom, the failure to acknowledge one's existential guilt inevitably leads to confusion, despair, and alienation such as is experienced by Joseph K. in Kafka's (1937/1977) novel, *The Trial.* Constricted by neurotic guilt, leading a banal existence, yet stubbornly unaware of his acts of omission, Joseph K. is imprisoned (symbolically) within the narrow boundaries defined by neurotic guilt and existential guilt.

Abraham Maslow (1968) has also pointed out the sense of loathing experienced when one moves toward security and stasis rather than striving for personal growth or "self-actualization":

> If this essential core of the person is denied or suppressed, he gets sick sometimes in obvious ways, sometimes in subtle ways. . . . Every falling away . . . [from our core], every crime against one's own nature . . . records itself in our unconscious and makes us despise ourselves. (pp. 4-5)

I support Maslow's view of existential guilt. Acting in opposition to one's basic wants has serious consequences; it implies a withdrawal of affect and psychic energy from external objects, a movement toward stillness and psychological death.

Guilt feelings and anxiety reactions are aroused by positive as well as negative circumstances. For example, if people achieve more than their parents did, if they seek gratification of wants denied them in their families, they experience painful feelings of self-recrimination. If, however, they submit to this guilt and regress to an inward posture of passivity and fantasy, they become progressively more demoralized and self-hating. *In a certain sense, each individual is suspended between these polarities of guilt, and they form the boundaries of his or her life experience.*

GUILT AND SEPARATION

> The inordinate force of moral authority derives from the conditions of the first psychological birth, when an infant's physical and psychological survival depended entirely on the protection and approval of her parents. Dread of loss [of the parents] . . . can make cowardly, submissive infants of us all—which is why the human conscience is so largely an instrument of the status quo. It is ruthless in its opposition to change. It preserves the past. (L. Kaplan, 1984, p. 110)

Both guilt feelings and fear arise when there is a threat of separation—separation from the mother, from parents and parental substitutes, and the ultimate separation from self and loved ones in death. There is considerable guilt as an individual moves toward independence and self-realization, thereby separating from imaginary connections with the family. On the other hand, there is existential guilt if one attempts to maintain one's fantasy of connection with his or her family for purposes of security. The failure to differentiate oneself from the mother or other family members inevitably leads to regressive behavior that sets up a pattern of new guilt reactions.

R. D. Laing (1961) portrayed the dualistic nature of guilt relating to destructive bonds in his discussion of collusion:

> The one person does not use the other merely as a hook to hang projections on. He strives to find in the other, or to induce the other to become, the very embodiment of projection. The other person's collusion is required to "complement" the identity self feels impelled to sustain. One can experience a peculiar form of guilt, specific, I think, to this disfunction. If one refuses collusion, one feels guilt for not being or not becoming the embodiment of the complement demanded by the other for his identity. However if one does succumb, if one is seduced, one becomes estranged from one's self and is guilty thereby of self-betrayal. (p. 111)

Laing, in effect, is describing both types of guilt: the guilty feelings aroused when one separates from a fantasy bond and, by contrast, the existential guilt that arises when a person surrenders his or her individuality for the security connection. Being original, nonconforming, separate, and independent fosters anxiety and guilt and may lead to regressive behavior and increased dependency, whereas submitting to the attachment, remaining fused or linked to the family and later to one's mate for imagined safety, also generates feelings of guilt and self-castigation.

Otto Rank was well aware of the contradictory sources of guilt and its dualistic structure. He wrote extensively about guilt reactions in relation to the problem of the "will" and parental prohibitions. However, he perceived that guilt feelings were also reactions to separation experiences. My understanding of the role that neurotic guilt plays in causing a constriction of life-affirming activities is in accord with Rank's thinking. In his essay "Separation and Guilt," Rank (1936/1972) writes,

> The problem of the neurosis itself is a separation problem and as such a blocking of the human life principle, the conscious ability to endure release and separation, first from the biological power represented by parents, and finally from the lived out parts of the self which this power represents, and which obstruct the development of the individual personality. It is at this point that the neurotic comes to grief, where, instead of living, of overcoming the past through the present, he becomes conscious that he dare not, cannot, loose himself because he is bound by guilt. (pp. 73-74)

Rank's reference to the "biological power represented by the parents" calls attention to a special transcendental quality that parents transmit to their children, that is, the possibility of triumphing over death by merging with the parents. However, the illusory merger is costly; the individual is too guilty to "loose himself" from his bonds.

In his synthesis of Rank's work, Becker (1973) writes of children's identification with their parents as being a "special case of the urge for immortality": "The child merges himself with the representatives of the cosmic process. . . . When one merges with the self-transcending parents . . . he is, in some real sense, trying to live in some larger expansiveness of meaning" (p. 152). Both parents and child imagine their merger as somehow imbuing them with immortality. In this sense, the family symbolizes immortality; it is the link in an unending chain of persons passing on unique traits from one generation to the next.

Many parents, in believing that their children "belong" to them, have strong feelings of exclusivity and possessiveness in relation to their offspring. As noted in Chapter 4, this sense of ownership stems partly from parents' deeply held, unconscious belief that through their children, they can achieve immortality. After all, their children are the products of the parents' bodies and extensions of themselves. The more the child is differentiated from the parent in looks, in character traits, in behavior, or in significant career choices, the more guilt he or she feels about breaking the continuous chain symbolically linking the generations. By disrupting this continuity, the developing child becomes acutely aware of his or her vulnerability to death. The child also becomes aware that any movement toward individuality and independence is an assault on the parents' illusion of immortality.[1]

Therefore, in moving away from their families, children experience considerable guilt in relation to the pain and anxiety they believe they are causing their parents. To avoid this guilt, they tend to cling to the bond with their parents by maintaining a sameness with them rather than "living out the parts" of themselves that would cause them to stand out from family patterns and traditions.

Each successive stage of maturity confronts the child and, later, the adult with the basic facts of personal existence—aloneness and separateness as well as vulnerability to death. Each phase is marked by guilt at leaving the parents behind, and by anger and resentment at having to face the world alone. What follows are case examples where people's actions and subsequent guilt feelings led to regression.

Threats of desertion or warnings to the child that he or she will be sent away because of "bad behavior," together with subtle or direct threats of parental illness or an emotional breakdown, occur in families more often than is commonly thought (Bowlby, 1973, 1988). Overprotectiveness toward children is also symptomatic of a strong fantasy bond in the family. I have observed this dynamic operating in "normal" families.

---

1 Kaufman (1980) observed that "the passing on of religious or other cultural practices remains paramount in most families. . . . One must believe as one's parent does and never question their appropriateness for ourselves. Many children are shamed for wanting to consider or follow a religious path or way of life different from their parents." (p. 66)

A 7-year-old boy asked his parents if he could travel with his grandparents to their home in the country. Initially, the youngster was very happy and enjoyed the drive, but later became very agitated and wanted to return home. When questioned about his change of mind, the boy responded with, "Mommy said she would die if something happened to me. I wanted to go back so she won't die, so she can see I'm not hurt." His mother's unintentionally destructive statement about her concern for his safety had aroused the boy's guilt about being away from her for an extended period of time.

Children's guilt about their hostile fantasies of destroying the parental figure has been assumed by some clinicians to be a principal cause of the guilt and depression that they experience during actual separation (M. Klein, 1930/1964). However, other explanations are also relevant and may be more accurate. For example, many parents experience considerable distress at their child's growing freedom and independence, and openly indicate their displeasure. The child senses the parents' pain or grief over the anticipated loss and responds with guilt. If the parents are immature and dependent, these feelings are even more exaggerated, and the child comes to feel that movement toward adulthood and his or her own goals is mean or destructive.

Patients have reported numerous experiences where their parents, mates, or family members responded with episodes of physical illness when they (the patients) moved toward independence.

One young man was successfully manipulated by his mother's illness when he was 18 years old and striking out on his own. On the morning of the young man's departure on a cross-country automobile trip with a friend, his mother developed severe chest pains. She was convinced that she was having a heart attack. The young man's father prevailed upon him not to leave at this time because his departure would make his mother feel worse, and her condition might become critical as a result. Out of a deep sense of guilt, he canceled his trip. Doctors placed his mother under observation, but released her 3 days later without discovering the cause of her symptoms.

This event was indicative of his mother's style of manipulation and significantly affected the young man's approach to life. His guilt generalized to other situations, causing him to be fearful and nonassertive. These types of incidents played a part in the formation of his basic character defenses of self-denial and passivity.

According to Freud (1915/1957), the guilt associated with our illusion of immortality, together with our "daily and hourly" death wishes toward strangers and loved ones alike, engenders a deep sense of guilt about surviving where others die, about enjoying our fortune where others suffer misfortune.

> For strangers and for enemies we do acknowledge death, and consign them to it quite as readily and unhesitatingly as did primeval man. . . . In our unconscious

impulses we daily and hourly get rid of anyone who stands in our way, of anyone who has offended or injured us. (p. 297)

Real and symbolic separation from parents toward whom one has felt ambivalence arouses deep feelings of guilt as though one were leaving them to die while one lives and flourishes.

A 25-year-old woman who was in a lesbian relationship with an insecure and overly dependent partner came to therapy because she wanted to feel more at ease relating to men. As she progressed in psychotherapy, she became freer and more self-assured. Gradually she overcame extreme shyness and began to express an interest in men. Soon afterward, she met a man whom she liked and admired and entered into a sexual relationship.

The relationship progressed, and the couple began to talk seriously about the possibility of marriage. After several months of struggle and internal conflict, she decided to give up the relationship with her girlfriend. After making her decision, she had a terrifying nightmare that left her extremely anxious.

She dreamed that she was walking through a bombed-out city when suddenly she saw her mother, ill and pathetic, beckoning her to come back and get her. Her mother appeared so weak and helpless that the patient could not bear to leave her there among the ruins. Superimposed upon her mother's face were the features of the girlfriend. She returned to her mother's side, lifted her onto her back, and struggled to carry her through the empty city.

She awoke still feeling the weight of this phantom on her shoulders. In the weeks that followed, the patient became disillusioned with her boyfriend, eventually broke off their relationship, and returned to her former lesbian partner.

In reality, the patient's mother had been weak and self-sacrificing while seeking gratification through an overinvolvement with her daughter. The call of the self-denying mother had been too compelling for this young woman to resist. She healed the fracture with her mother symbolically by reconnecting with a woman and renouncing her relationship with a man that had been both happy and satisfying. The nightmare was representative of her guilt and fear of separation.

To summarize, most adults retain strong feelings of being connected to the parent. Independence and individuation disrupt the fantasy bond with one's parents and arouse strong feelings of guilt and separation anxiety.

SELF-HATRED AND GUILT

There is a strong relationship between feelings of guilt and one's feelings of self-hatred. Theodore Rubin (1975) was well aware of the significance of man's propensity for self-hatred and self-destruction, and wrote that "the victim rationalizes . . . guilt as a high sense of responsibility and morality. . . . [But guilt has] a depleting, fatiguing, constricting effect and . . . [is] ultimately destructive to self-esteem and to one's actual person" (p. 73).

In a similar vein, I have emphasized that one of the primary functions of the voice is that of instilling guilt in the individual. Withholding and self-denial are regulated by the destructive thought processes of the voice. The effect of chronic patterns of withholding is an ultimate shutting down, a paralysis, of that part of the individual that strives for emotional health and growth—the part that contributes to feelings of self-esteem.

Clinicians are familiar with the primary guilt reactions experienced by patients when they attempt to overcome inhibitions of the past and actively pursue a more fulfilling life. They understand that this form of guilt is related to early parental training and prohibitions. Similarly, they recognize that many patients feel a sense of guilt when they indulge in self-nourishing habits, for example, masturbating, overeating, drinking to excess, smoking, or drug abuse. Less is understood of the existential guilt aroused by surrendering one's independent point of view and submitting to sameness and conformity. Many therapists are not fully cognizant of the extent to which people feel guilty when they retreat from life and act out this type of self-destructive, self-limiting process. In fact, a person's most stubborn or oppositional behavior centers on this form of guilt.

Individuals go to great lengths to cover up or hide their propensity for self-destruction. Patients in therapy are often the most defensive, disagreeable, and hostile toward the therapist when they are defending the acting out of self-destructive impulses or when they are attempting to deny their self-destructiveness. These urges are perceived by the patient to be humiliating and shameful facets of the personality.

Both patients and psychotherapists fail to appreciate the full significance of the self-destructive process that is set into motion when one adopts an inward lifestyle characterized by self-denial, role-playing, fantasy, and retreat. We recognize the dangers inherent in substituting fantasy gratification for actual satisfactions in the real world when they reach monumental proportions as in the psychoses, yet we remain largely unaware of the extent of microsuicidal behavior manifest by so-called normal individuals as they move through the life process.

SOURCES OF GUILT AND
THE NEGATIVE SELF-CONCEPT

Guilt reactions and shame represent the internalization of parental rejecting attitudes in relation to simple body needs as well as the need for affectionate contact and love. Frustration of infantile urges and primitive hunger caused by emotional deprivation are at the core of guilt feelings and negative feelings toward the self. When parents are unable to sensitively care for and love their children because of their own inadequacies or dependency needs, the child begins to feel guilty for expressing or even having natural wants and needs. As adults, people rationalize their habit of rationing or limiting themselves in an ever-widening range of situations and, as a result, become increasingly alienated from themselves as vital, feeling human beings.

Guilt About Being Alive

If a child was unwanted at birth, or became seriously ill, that child might grow up feeling that he or she was undeserving, had no rights, or, on a deeper level, might feel guilty for even being alive. One subject, an associate, recalled being told by his parents that he had nearly died as an infant during a long illness. After he had grown up, the boy's mother had confided in him that at one point his father had said he would kill himself if the boy died. According to an uncle, his parents were thrilled when the boy lived; however, the weeks of constant fear and concern had evidently taken their toll. The threat of loss had damaged their emotional involvement with their son, and they became more distant from the youngster. His parents' unconscious rejection of him affirmed his sense of being "bad" for being sick and causing his parents concern. As an adult, whenever he became ill or sensed weakness in himself, these feelings were activated. The self-recrimination he felt for inadvertently causing his parents grief was extended and generalized to guilt about enjoying life. It was difficult for this man to maintain a sense of legitimacy, in spite of unusual achievement and dedication.

Guilt About Being
Different From One's Family

Guilt about moving in a direction that is different, or more fulfilling, than experiences in one's family is often expressed in voice terms such as the following: "Who do you think you are?" "You always want your own way!" "You only think of yourself."

In one case, a man verbalized a series of self-attacks representing guilty reactions he experienced about meaningful new friendships he was developing. As he talked, his voice assumed a snide, parental tone, which he later identified as sounding like his father's:

"What are you doing here with these people? What do you need these friends for? You don't need friends! All you need is us, your family. You always were a weird person. When you were a kid, you were so strange. You never wanted to be like us. You always wanted to be different. Who do you think you are?"

The key dynamic in this case concerned the subject's guilt about his movement away from the family and its problems. Achieving more financial success, developing friendships, and choosing to live life more fully than the members of his family gave rise to a considerable amount of anxiety and led to feelings of remorse and self-reproach.

Many people suffer intense guilt about succeeding where those close to them have failed, and in this sense leaving others behind. For this reason, voice attacks are often intensified following a significant success or the realization of a personal goal. For instance, the voice may warn the person that he or she won't be able to sustain or repeat a performance. It often insinuates that an accomplishment was a quirk of fate or that it was the result of deception. This aspect of the voice contributes to the empty feeling that many people notice after they achieve an unusual success.

Many times, contact with a family member will serve to remind the person that he or she has stepped out of line or broken the family tradition. I am pained to be reminded of a patient with a borderline personality disorder who had progressed significantly during 3 years of therapy, changing her hostile, suspicious views of men and integrating fragments of a disorganized ego.

The patient had overcome serious paranoid attitudes, was in the process of forming closer relationships, and in general felt cheerful and well. She was in an optimistic state when her sister, disturbed, called her on the phone.

After the patient told her sister about her progress and her sense of hopefulness, she asked her how she was feeling. Her sister responded bitterly and sarcastically with, "You want to know how I'm feeling? Well, I'll tell you how I'm feeling. I feel like killing myself!"

Tragically, the patient, torn by unbearable guilt feelings about her sister's unhappiness, turned against herself and soon afterward discontinued her sessions. Subsequently, she resumed the isolated lifestyle in which she had existed prior to the psychotherapy.

Although this is a dramatic example of regression following renewed contact with a family member, it is not a singular or isolated phenomenon.

In reviewing the patient's case material, several factors became evident. In her sessions, the patient's feelings of deep remorse and culpability had come to light. For instance, early on she had reported feeling guilty about revealing details of her family life to her therapist. In one session, she had verbalized this voice as follows:

"You don't even know what you're going to say! You have nothing to say! This man doesn't want to hear what you have to say. You'd better keep your mouth shut if you know what's good for you!

"You think you feel good from this session? Well, just wait until morning. You're going to wake up feeling so rotten you won't know what to do. You can't talk to this man and then expect to feel good. You're going to feel terrible if you talk about our family."

In working through the negative transference, the patient developed positive regard for her therapist and had overcome her paranoid expectations of mistreatment and exploitation at the hands of men. Toward the end of therapy, she approached issues that lay at the core of her illness. In one session, she expressed the rage she had internalized early in childhood. She revealed her mother's death wishes toward her as well as her mother's obvious preference for her sister. Her mother's hostile attitudes were incorporated into her antiself system and contributed to the patient's powerful guilt reactions about being different from her sister:

"Why can't you be like your sister? She's beautiful, and look at you! You have the ugliest face. Why don't you just die? Why weren't you one of the ones who died? [The patient's mother had had several miscarriages.] Just get out of here! Just leave me alone!"

Not long after this session, the patient received the significant phone call from her sister. Guilt about her attempt to separate herself symbolically from her sister's wretched outlook on life made it impossible for her to tolerate the difference between her own state of happiness and her sister's depression and misery. Follow-up clearly revealed that the woman's brief phone contact was the key factor in disrupting her adjustment.

THE VOICE AND EXISTENTIAL GUILT

A person may feel consciously guilty for not pleasing authorities, while unconsciously he feels guilty for not living up to his own expectations of himself. (Fromm, 1947, p. 169)

I have consistently found that whenever subjects submitted to neurotic guilt reactions and regressed, they generally "heard" voices telling them that they were no different from their family. For example, one man became deeply concerned that his 5-year-old daughter felt rejected. Whenever he noticed her unhappiness or became aware that he felt distant from her, he tortured himself with thoughts such as these:

"See, you thought you were going to be different. Well, look at your kids. There's the proof! You're no different! What made you think you could be different? You can't change it. You're a failure. You're rotten all the way through."

Rather than acting as a catalyst to improve his relationship with his daughter, this man's guilt, expressed in the form of the voice, only served to demoralize him. It prevented him from feeling compassionate toward himself and his children. Self-critical thoughts, reminding people that they are no different from their parents, have been reported by many individuals as significant factors in their acting against their own interests. Yet, when they act on their conscious guilt, it predisposes existential guilt.

If men and women deprive themselves or their loved ones and act out withholding patterns, their guilt feeds upon itself. They not only castigate themselves for losing the relationship or damaging it—"See, now you have no friends" or "She will never want you back"—but they also feel remorseful and self-hating about hurting others—"You really made him feel terrible," "You have such a bad effect on people." This form of voice attack is characteristic of people who are self-denying and hold back positive emotional responses. Distressed by these guilt feelings, they attempt to compensate for their cutting off genuine feeling by substituting role-determined responses.

In an earlier work (R. Firestone, 1984), I referred to a patient, Joanne, who wrote a letter to her friends in her therapy group describing the guilt and deep-seated feelings of shame that revolved around her self-destructive pattern of living. The following excerpts from her letter demonstrate an unusual understanding of the part played by her voice in preserving her isolated, inward lifestyle:

Self-loathing has become so firmly entrenched in my being, it feels like the very core of me—in some crazy way, self-hatred feels like my "life-force."

I can't hang on to self-hatred around you any more—even with briefest contact of groups and weekly sessions. *No matter how I "insure" the feeling by acts of self-destructiveness during the week—the eating, picking at myself, calling up my mother's voice to ridicule and denounce myself*—you just have to see me, I mean, really see and address the person that's real in me, to strip away the self-hate, even for just a second.

In my case, self-hatred was formed very early, to protect myself from the certain insanity that rejection would have led me into. From there, keeping a layer of fat surrounding me, twisting my face into ugly expressions, kept that basic or primal defense alive in me.

I just remembered that I began being fat at the age of 5, when a friend of the family began showing an interest in me. It was also a time during which I first acted out self-destructiveness, inflicting a concussion on myself, sitting on a live

battery and burning my legs. He was the first to threaten that primary defense
. . . by being nice to me.

This letter was written over 20 years ago, about the same time that my
conceptualization and understanding of the voice process were unfolding. This
patient, who described herself so honestly, showed insight that exceeded my
awareness at that time. For example, Joanne writes of "calling up her mother's
voice" to denounce and ridicule her during the week between sessions. Prior to
therapy, this woman had become progressively demoralized by powerful feelings of self-hatred and a chronic sense of despair and futility. As she improved,
she became more intolerant of her life of guilt and self-loathing and, at the time
she wrote the letter, was making concerted efforts to change behaviors that
caused her to despise herself.

The tragedy is that this woman, who was so painfully intolerant of nice
treatment as a child that she deliberately burned her legs when someone took a
friendly interest in her, could not bring herself to give up her basic defense. She
eventually left therapy and her friends, and today is living the isolated, guilt-rid-
den life she so poignantly wrote about.

MANIFESTATIONS OF
GUILT IN SCHIZOPHRENIA

The end result of a pathological process of regression and self-destructive
behavior, followed by remorse, guilt, and increased self-hatred, can be observed
in the auditory hallucinations of schizophrenic patients in which the patient
actually hears "voices" as distinct from him- or herself. In these cases, the
hallucinated voices continually direct, reprimand, and punish the patient in the
form of parental injunctions. Furthermore, their voices attack them for giving
in to self-destructive impulses, thereby compounding the problem.

Manifestations of guilt and shame in schizophrenic patients often reach
significant proportions whenever there is progress in therapy. Paradoxically,
guilt reactions are also severe when there is regression and acting out of
self-destructive behavior. M. Sechehaye's (1951) classic analysis of Renee, a
regressed schizophrenic girl, clearly illustrates both types of guilt. We are
indebted to Sechehaye for her appreciation of the regressed patient's inability to
accept gratification in reality and her recognition of Renee's need for substitute
or alternative gratification in the form of symbolic realization.

Because of early childhood deprivation, Renee had turned to fantasy for
gratification. The rationale underlying Sechehaye's method of feeding her
patient apples (Renee's personal symbol for the breasts and maternal milk) is
pertinent to our discussion.

While Renee had returned to the oral phase, she would have been angry to receive real milk, and that would have made her more ill. It was necessary for her to receive a symbol and not a reality. Why? Because guilt feelings make it necessary to camouflage the repressed desire. Once the guilt feelings have been calmed (in this case, by having appeased the legitimate desire), one can accept reality. (p. 52)

By offering only symbolic or fantasy gratification, Sechehaye was able to counter the patient's profound feelings of guilt. She was able to "wean" Renee gradually to actual satisfactions and the simple pleasures of reality.

Both M. Sechehaye and Renee herself, in writing about her illness (*Autobiography of a Schizophrenic Girl,* 1951), pointed out that the "flight into madness" was torturous because tremendous feelings of guilt and self-destructive impulses were aroused when regression took place. In the course of treatment, whenever Renee submitted to self-destructive impulses or retreated further into autism, there were strong guilt reactions. The voices instructed Renee over and over again to hurt herself, and it required all her strength to resist. Yet, if and when she gave in to these voices and acted out physical abuse on herself, they became even more intense and derisive.

As she retreated into autism, Renee's guilty reactions focused on three principal themes: (a) the existential guilt of self-betrayal; (b) betrayal of the people who loved her and wished her well, most particularly the therapist who was attempting to help her; and (c) guilt about becoming progressively less functional and thereby presenting a burden to others. Hallucinated voices played an important part in all of her guilt reactions.

The analogy to neurotic behavior and the seemingly perverse actions of normal individuals is clear. People far less disturbed than Renee also feel guilty about actively pursuing their lives. Like Renee, they appear to prefer fantasy gratification to fulfilling their wants in reality. Yet as they choose fantasy, passivity, and self-nourishing lifestyles, they suffer existential guilt. For example, people who give up genuine caring and real interest in their mates for role-playing and a fantasy of love experience considerable torment and remorse.

As individuals retreat from pursuing life fully, they feel ashamed of self-betrayal and the incidental betrayal of their loved ones as well. As is the case in more serious pathology, whenever people become withholding and less adaptive in their overall functioning, they feel guilty about their failures. Any choice of behavior that leads to unnecessary withdrawal and increased dependency intensifies this process. Furthermore, in their attempts to cover up their withdrawal and withholding toward a love object, most people maintain a fantasy bond and act as if they are still pursuing satisfying relationships and personal goals. As a result, their communications become misleading and duplicitous. Their behavior fails to correspond to their stated goals. In other words, they no longer want what they *say* they want. This lack of integrity further intensifies their guilt.

GUILT AND DEATH ANXIETY

In a deep sense, people feel afraid to embrace life in the face of their inevitable fate; they tend to cut off feeling for a life that they know they eventually must lose. They are reluctant to become too attached to other people or to allow others to become close to them because of the pain and grief involved in ultimate separation. They often feel guilty and fearful about enjoying physical pleasure because they wish to remain unaware of being connected to, or trapped in, a body that will die someday. In that sense, their guilt and shame may be an attempt to disown their physical nature because of its obvious impermanence (Vergote, 1978/1988) (Endnote 3).

A form of guilt closely related to separation and death anxiety is "death guilt," described by Robert Lifton and Eric Olson (1976) in their article, "The Human Meaning of Total Disaster." They define death guilt as "the survivor's sense of painful self-condemnation over having lived while others died" (p. 3).

> People who have gone through this kind of experience [a catastrophe involving fatalities] are never quite able to forgive themselves for having survived. Another side of them, however, experiences relief and gratitude that it was they who had the good fortune to survive in contrast to the fate of those [often close relatives] who died—a universal and all-too-human survivor reaction that in turn intensifies their guilt. (p. 5)

Lifton and Olson's concept of "death guilt" coincides with the descriptions of "survival guilt" related by those individuals who were incarcerated in concentration camps and survived the trauma. Bettelheim (1979) emphasized that "these feelings of guilt and of owing a special obligation are irrational, but this does not reduce their power to dominate a life" (p. 27). Elsewhere, Lifton and Olson (1974/1976) relate survivor guilt indirectly to death anxiety and the individual's attempt to cope with the kinds of experiences where this anxiety is aroused. Lifton and Olsen (1976) describe the resultant "psychic numbing—a diminished capacity for feeling of all kinds, . . . [and] apathy, withdrawal, depression, and overall constriction in living" (p. 5) that occurs when these painful feelings of guilt are suppressed. In our terms, the survivor in these situations no doubt possesses a sneering, accusatory voice—"Why did you survive while others died?" or "Did you really deserve to live?"—as part of an unrelenting guilt reaction (Endnote 4).

To feel one's guilt about simply living or valuing one's life can be quite painful. People generally repress these uncomfortable feelings to avoid the pain of positive investment. However, they surface as feelings of self-consciousness, self-attacks, or in apologetic gestures toward others who are less fortunate. On the other hand, when people restrict their lives for any reason, they experience boredom, a sense of emptiness, and feelings of existential guilt. Most people are willing to pay the price of living a defended, self-hating existence (as in the case of Joanne) and choose emotionally deadened, self-limiting lifestyles.

Indeed, a common response to both "survival guilt" and death anxiety is to renounce the very activities and relationships that give life the most value. This process, which is suicidal in nature, diminishes the guilt about choosing life, yet it inevitably leads to the second type of guilt, existential guilt, described by Becker (1973): "Guilt results from unused life, from 'the unlived in us' " (p. 180). This guilt, in turn, is responsible for people's acting out self-destructive impulses in a desperate attempt to atone for acts of omission—in effect, to punish themselves for their withdrawal from life.

DISCUSSION

It is not an accident that the three principal cases described in this chapter had negative outcomes. Guilt reactions can predispose serious consequences and regressions that limit each person's destiny. Indeed, the depth and scope of life open to an individual are defined by the boundaries imposed by neurotic guilt on the one hand and existential guilt on the other—and by the thought process that mediates guilt, the voice. The verbalization of guilt reactions through the procedures of Voice Therapy evokes feelings of compassion and support for the self and for one's personal point of view. In contrast, when the process of voice attacks is *not* interrupted, a person increasingly submits to the injunctions of the voice and progressively abandons his or her real self and unique point of view. By identifying their voices and making them conscious, people can progress and cope more successfully with their self-limiting and self-destructive tendencies.

In our current state of knowledge, my associates and I feel that this technique helps patients isolate and become conscious of the dual nature of their guilt feelings. It is our opinion that Voice Therapy is an effective therapeutic procedure and valuable research tool in understanding the relationship and structure of both neurotic and existential guilt. In challenging the voice in Voice Therapy, one becomes freer to pursue one's life, thereby minimizing regressive trends and the complex of guilt and shame associated with self-betrayal.

ENDNOTES

1. Morrison (1989), in *Shame: The Underside of Narcissism,* provided a clear exposition of the history of theorists' conceptualizations of shame in psychoanalytic, ego psychology, and self psychology systems of thought. He stressed the link between shame and depression, noting that for patients "suffering from narcissistic personality disorders, the relationship of depression to the failure to attain ambitions and ideals may be the most compelling" (p. 81).

2. Kaufman (1980) wrote that, phenomenologically, "to feel shame is to feel seen in a painfully diminished sense" (p. 9). Many individuals feel ashamed of their needs, their need to be touched, to nurture another, the need for affiliation, for love, for sex, and affirmation from others. As the child develops, he or she internalizes shame, which is now "experienced as a deep, abiding sense of being defective, never quite good enough as a person" (p. 75). In *Speaking With the Devil,* Goldberg (1996) described shame as undermining "both the child's sense of well-being and his interpersonal relationships" (p. 38). Goldberg went on to comment,

> If [the child] . . . is unable to express clearly her feelings of hurt and anguish, she develops a disparaging inner "narrative voice" that constantly warns her away from situations in which she might again be hurt or painfully exposed. (p. 38)

3. In *Guilt and Desire,* Vergote (1978/1988) discussed his ideas concerning the origins of sexual guilt: "The danger of religion is that by wanting to triumph over death it can wind up depreciating life" (p. 76). Vergote delineated the harmful effect of religious and cultural patterns on the individual:

> This massive culpabilization of sexuality has some particularly pathogenic effects precisely because it is bound up with and reactivates unconscious representations. If the parents have themselves been mutilated or scarred in the history of their desire, and if their injunctions and prohibitions intensify a religious climate of guilt, the conditions favoring their offspring's development of neurosis converge. (p. 74)

4. Bruno Bettelheim (1979), in *Surviving and Other Essays,* recounted the process of internal self-attack experienced by survivors of the German concentration camps:

> One voice, that of reason, tries to answer the question "Why was I saved?" with "It was pure luck, simple chance; there is no other answer to the question"; while the voice of the conscience replies, "True, but the reason you had the chance to survive was that some other prisoner died in your stead." And behind this in a whisper might be heard an even more severe, critical accusation: "Some of them died because you pushed them out of an easier place of work; others because you did not give them some help, such as food, that you might possibly have been able to do without." And there is always the ultimate accusation to which there is no acceptable answer: "You rejoiced that it was some other who had died rather than you." (p. 27)

14

The Psychodynamics of Fantasy, Addiction, and Addictive Attachments

Fantasy and addiction are co-related aspects of the fantasy bond or self-parenting process. Internal fantasy processes are inextricably involved in the etiology of addictive personality disorders, habit patterns, and attachments. Children deprived of emotional sustenance, threatened by separation anxiety, attempt to form a fusion through fantasy processes. The capacity for imagination can provide partial satisfaction of primitive drives and emotional needs. Therefore, individuals deprived of the necessary ingredients for satisfactory development rely increasingly on fantasy gratification, which partly reduces tension and acts as a painkiller. They develop a defensive self-parenting process in which they are both the parent and the object of parenting.

AUTHOR'S NOTE: The substance of this chapter is taken primarily from an article titled, "The Psychodynamics of Fantasy, Addiction, and Addictive Attachments," *American Journal of Psychoanalysis, 53* (1993), pp. 335-352. Used with permission.

As described earlier, there are two basic aspects to the self-parenting process: self-nourishment and self-punishment. Self-nourishing propensities arise early in life in the form of self-gratifying behavior patterns that become addictive for the rejected child. Reliance on this self-support system is proportional to the degree of deprivation. These patterns manifest themselves in eating disorders or substance abuse. Self-punishing tendencies are also evinced in the form of internal destructive "voices," self-critical attitudes, and behavior that is harmful to self.

As described in Chapter 7, aspects of the self-parenting process can be externalized in the form of addictive interpersonal relationships, that is, a fantasy bond. For example, a man or woman may act out either the grandiose, critical, punitive parent or the helpless, worthless child with their mate, leading to symbiosis, and a fantasy bond is formed. The dynamics of this form of attachment differ from a straightforward relationship. Fantasy processes, acted inward or outward, in conjunction with primitive self-nurturing feeding patterns, can become a survival mechanism for those who suffer deprivation in childhood.

Reliance on this mechanism tends to be progressively incapacitating, as dependence on fantasy interferes with goal-directed activity in the real world. A negative spiral of frustration, fantasy, and addiction, followed by increased frustration, is set into operation. When addictive patterns are acted out in couples and families, they jeopardize personal relationships. For example, a style of sexual relating characterized by a lack of real feeling can take on a mechanical quality that leaves each partner feeling empty and emotionally hungry.

The important issue here is that addictive patterns can come to be preferred over satisfaction in the interpersonal environment. People fearful of taking a chance again develop an inward lifestyle in which risks are limited and achievements are curtailed. *Thus all human beings exist in conflict between an active pursuit of goals in the real world and a reliance on fantasy gratification.* In the course of the developmental sequence, psychological equilibrium is achieved when a person arrives at a particular solution to the basic conflict. This equilibrium is often attained at the expense of satisfying object relations and is threatened by warm or constructive events that contradict earlier painful or traumatic experiences.

The defensive process eventually becomes addictive. It persists for long periods after deprivation has ceased and predisposes negative behavioral responses. For example, we have shown that individuals who exist primarily in an inward state of fantasy drastically reduce their emotional transactions with others. A withholding style of relating is manifested and both giving and taking are restricted. Once the fantasy process and associated behaviors are established, they must be defended against intrusions at all costs. It is important to note that the process of gratifying oneself in fantasy and that of seeking satisfaction in the external world are mutually exclusive. Thus real satisfaction represents a threat to the fantasy process.

APPROACHES TO ADDICTION

A number of theoretical models related to the etiology of addiction have been delineated (Bell & Khantzian, 1991; Hopson, 1993; Morgenstern & Leeds, 1993). A recurring theme emphasized by these models is that seemingly diverse forms of addictions are actually interrelated. Hall, Havassy, and Wasserman (1990), for example, based their studies of alcoholism on the premise that "commonalities exist across the addictions on important psychological dimensions" (p. 180).

Factors cited as predisposing causes of addiction are the inability to manage or regulate intense affects such as aggression, primitive forms of shame and guilt, and inadequate ego development (Adams, 1978). The formulations of Khantzian, Mack, and Schatzberg (1974) are closely related to my view of the defensive function served by the self-parenting process. They conceptualized heroin addiction as a compensatory "self-caring" mechanism. They concluded that the drug becomes the only means for achieving the security and satisfaction that should have been experienced in the early relationship with the mother.

> We have been impressed with a rather specific ego impairment having to do with self-care and self-regulation that characterizes many addicted individuals. (p. 163)

> Their response has been to revert repeatedly to the use of opiates as an all-powerful device, thereby precluding other solutions that would normally develop and that might better sustain them. (p. 164)

Blatt, McDonald, Sugarman, and Wilber (1984) pointed out another motive underlying opiate addiction, that of the "need to find support and assistance in the modulation and regulation of intense and painful depressive affects such as feelings of inadequacy, guilt, worthlessness, and hopelessness" (p. 163).

Other theorists have commented on the addict's internalization of harshly judgmental parental figures. Thomas Szasz (1975) suggested the importance of a superego in addiction whose function is to persecute the drug user. Wurmser and Zients (1982) observed that addicted adolescent patients often feel " 'split' into the compliant, kind, yet false self, and the nasty, cruel, vengeful, spiteful self" (p. 547). Studies of affect regulation and self-soothing mechanisms in infants and reconstructive studies of adult patients (Gaddini, 1978; Krystal,

1990; Tolpin, 1971) indicate that both aspects of self-parenting, that is, compensatory self-nourishing and self-punishing behaviors, are closely associated with a wide range of addictive disorders in adult individuals who suffered deprivation during infancy or early childhood (Endnote 1).

A DEVELOPMENTAL
PERSPECTIVE ON ADDICTION

The ability of human beings to create in fantasy an image of themselves and the fulfillment of their goals can set the stage for psychological disturbances, especially those of an addictive nature (Endnote 2). Often new parents find that the infant's cries arouse painful emotions in them, bringing to the surface suppressed feelings from their own childhood (Demos, 1986). Mothers and fathers will do almost anything to shut off these anxiety-provoking cries. The attempts of parents to allay painful emotions in their offspring can deprive the children of even the minimal frustration experiences necessary for normal development, and teach them self-nurturing habit patterns that eventually limit them as fully functioning human beings. In many cases, techniques employed by parents to soothe the child actually serve to addict him or her to specific tension-reducing routines (Levy, 1943; Mahler et al., 1975; Sroufe & Ward, 1980). We are particularly interested in cases where parents employ the excessive use of (a) drugs for children suffering from colic, (b) Ritalin for "hyperactive" children (Endnote 3), and (c) pacifiers and other means of quieting the child that predispose addiction, as was the case with E. reported in Chapter 6.

Parents use the same psychological techniques for numbing pain in their children that *they* developed as a part of their own defenses. Infants can sense parents' discomfort, anxiety, and unwillingness to make real contact. They learn early on to adjust their responses accordingly (Kumin, 1996; Stolorow, Brandchaft, & Atwood, 1987) (Endnote 4). As they grow older, they become refractive to warm affectionate contact, connect to others without feeling, tend to be overly dependent, and eventually turn to substances and/or compulsive routines to eliminate pain and reduce tension.

The intergenerational cycle of addictive propensities has also been well documented in the literature, as discussed in Chapter 3. Parents transmit their addictive disposition to their children through role modeling. In spite of their parents' attempts to influence their offspring otherwise, children imitate these habit patterns beginning at an early age. The transmission of parental defenses, behaviors, and attitudes through the process of imitation, particularly during the preverbal phase, has a powerful impact on later personality development (Bandura, 1971).

HEALTHY FUNCTIONING
VERSUS ADDICTIVE LIFESTYLES

One can develop a comparative model of mental health versus psychopathology in terms of the self-parenting process. The degree to which a person depends on self-nurturing mechanisms and internal fantasy processes can be conceptualized as a smooth progression ranging from external object gratification to complete autistic involvement in self-gratification. In general, the differences between healthy functioning and serious psychological disturbance are quantitative, rather than qualitative, as depicted in Figure 8.2. However, as one progresses through the continuum and there is extensive damage and more serious regression, there are qualitative changes, such as delusions, hallucinations, and thought disturbances.

Three States of Fantasy Involvement

For purposes of edification, the functions conceptualized as ranging along this continuum can be arbitrarily divided into three categories that describe an individual's resolution of the central conflict: Category 1, the person with extreme propensities for fantasy and isolation, that is, the psychotic individual; Category 2, the person who uses elements of reality primarily to reinforce and support an ongoing implicit, partly conscious, or unconscious fantasy process rather than really investing in relationships and career; and Category 3, the person who lives a realistic committed life whose actions match aspirations and capabilities (Endnote 5).

Self-actualizing individuals (Category 3) have a good deal of personal integrity, that is, their words are consistent with their actions. In contrast, people who are self-denying (Categories 1 and 2) lack integrity in relation to their desires or motives and cannot communicate honestly.

Individuals in Categories 1 and 2 often respond with anger or rage to real love, recognition, and success. These reactions are generally suppressed or repressed because they are irrational or inappropriate. They are redirected and internalized in the form of self-criticism and self-attack or elaborated into paranoid attitudes toward the source of approbation or gratification, that is, the person or persons responsible for the positive experience. Acting out may take various forms such as unresponsiveness, bitterness or coldness, misinterpretation of kindness or approval, suspicion as to others' motives, withholding of positive traits, poor performance, manifestation of signs of inadequacy, and other inappropriate responses. These acting-out behaviors are an important factor influencing the deterioration and breakdown in career and personal relationships over the course of time.

Individuals in Category 2 merely give the impression or illusion of seeking satisfaction in reality. They use real events as a means of reinforcing or "feeding" their most prized fantasies, and value form over substance in interpersonal relationships. In a destructive, addictive attachment, fantasy-bonded individuals place a strong emphasis on ritual or role-determined responses. Concurrently, they often treat each other indifferently or disrespectfully. Indeed, a fantasy bond is a destructive type of relationship in which elements of self-parenting are projected and reciprocated to the detriment of both participants. There is a desperate holding on to the other person, with a corresponding lack of genuine relatedness.

In considering the dynamics of couple relationships from this perspective, one can determine where each partner is on the continuum by observing his or her reactions to genuine affection or a satisfying sexual encounter. For example, following a close sexual experience, an inward person may withdraw almost immediately, whereas an individual pursuing *real* gratification would more than likely remain close and seek a repetition of the experience. In the first case, the sexual experience is often used as a means for maintaining an illusion of closeness and relatedness. On a deeper level, the withdrawal indicates the person's discomfort or anger at the disturbance to his or her psychological equilibrium, that is, defensive process.

Unusual support, personal accomplishment, or recognition upset the defensive balance. People shy away from gratification of their most precious fantasies because real successes challenge fantasy processes and there is a heightened sense of loss of control and strong feelings of increased personal vulnerability. As noted, many people mistake an internal image or feeling of love for the behavior or outward expressions of affection, respect, and concern for another person. For example, a man, recently married, complained to his wife that she had been distant from him for several days and he had begun to feel rejected and fear a loss of her interest in him. She responded, "How can you say that? I haven't been distant; I've been thinking about you a lot. In fact, all week I have been having sexual fantasies about you and feeling very excited."

It is difficult to convince people who are trying desperately to preserve a fantasy of love that they are not in a loving relationship. They know that they *feel* love and attraction, they spend considerable time *thinking about* it, yet their outward expressions of affection may be limited or even contradicted by hostile or rejecting behavior toward their mates or families.

Again, for purposes of delineation, there is a good deal of difference in the feelings, responses to favorable events, and behaviors of individuals in Category 2 as compared with Category 3. In the former, people's emotional responses or variations in mood are related to experiences that affect fantasy images rather than to real events in their everyday lives.

SELF-NOURISHING HABITS
AND ADDICTIVE PAINKILLERS

Self-nourishing habits can be categorized as "ego-syntonic" in that they are originally perceived as positive and arouse minimal conflict with normal ego functioning. Until their use becomes clearly self-destructive or potentially dangerous, they are in consonance with the person's ego (S. Freud, 1916/1963). However, well-established self-nurturing habits become progressively self-limiting and self-destructive because they interfere with a person's capacity to cope with day-to-day life. When these behaviors are associated with a more generalized retreat from the world, they no longer feel acceptable to the self and arouse considerable guilt (R. Firestone, 1985). People are extremely defensive about their addictive patterns, fantasy involvement, inwardness, and depersonalization.

Addictions

As children grow older, they develop increasingly sophisticated habits and techniques with which to parent or symbolically feed themselves. Nail-biting, smoking, excessive drinking, masturbation, addictive sex, or drug abuse are some of the activities that are relied upon for self-gratification, relief of tension, and partial fulfillment of needs. Addictive reactions associated with a self-nourishing lifestyle can be divided into four groups: (a) addiction to physical substances, (b) addiction to ritualistic behavior and routines, (c) self-gratifying modes of sexual relating, and (d) addictive attachments.

Addiction to physical substances. Food often becomes a primary focus for children who are starved for emotional sustenance in the family situation. In these cases, food takes on a special meaning other than simple enjoyment and gratification of a physical need. When food is consistently used as a drug or painkiller to minimize or defend against painful emotions and experiences, it becomes part of an addictive pattern. The addiction to food is manifested in repetitive cycles of overeating and dieting as well as in binges and subsequent purges. These self-feeding patterns are inward, self-centered, and functionally maladaptive as they interfere with other areas of a person's existence.

Anorexia nervosa, a condition that can reach life-threatening proportions, is also associated with self-parenting in that the patient is exercising total control over food intake. These patients, the large majority of whom are young women, are generally cut off from affect and lack a clear awareness of the sensation of hunger. The anorexic patient's symptomatology of refusing food reflects a desperate attempt to ward off the extreme anxiety or panic associated with maternal feeding experiences. Noting the prevalence of inadequate or inconsistent maternal care in the childhood of women with eating disorders, Kim Chernin (1985) points out that

> this sense of the mother's actual or impending breakdown has burdened the childhood and adolescence of women with eating disorders. Again and again we find a vision, carefully hidden, of the mother's inner collapse and emotional crisis. (p. 77)

> Virtually every woman who has come to talk to me about a serious problem with eating believes that her mother experienced stress so severe in mothering her that . . . we are forced to wonder whether it was a breakdown. (p. 72)

The use of substances to satisfy oneself is closely correlated with oral deprivation and maladaptive parenting. When children suffer unusual frustration, they resort to compensatory self-nourishing habit patterns. Later, there is an attempt on the part of these individuals to comfort themselves and relieve their own tension. In every case, the addiction supports a pseudoindependent posture and an illusion of self-sufficiency.

As noted earlier, the dynamics in eating disorders revolve around the central issue of control and self-parenting. The same issues are central in drug abuse and alcoholism. The negative thought process or voice plays an important role in addictive self-feeding patterns. First, it induces the person to indulge the habit, and later punishes the person for acting out. Voices that seduce the alcoholic to indulge his or her habit, with such thoughts as "Take one more drink, you need to relax," are then followed by voices of self-recrimination, "You're so weak, you drunken bum!" In attempting to alleviate the pain of these self-recriminations, an individual invariably resorts to more painkillers, and the cycle continues.

It is very difficult to break these patterns, because the anxiety allayed by the use of substances comes to the surface during withdrawal, leaving the patient in a state of disorientation and helplessness. There are painful emotions of sadness or rage that are complicated by childlike or regressive behavior when patients attempt to abstain from the use of these substances.

Addiction to routines and habitual responses. Repetitive behaviors and rituals come to have addictive properties; they tend to dull one's sensitivity to painful feelings and lend an air of certainty and seeming permanence to a real life of uncertainty and impermanence. Obsessive or compulsive patterns that temporarily reduce anxiety become habitual and later foster anxiety. When these habits intensify, they can become seriously maladaptive. In the "normal" range of functioning, many people become addicted to routines and personal habits such as TV watching, the necessary morning cup of coffee, video games and computer games, compulsive reading, shopping, and many others.

Often, routines and compulsive behaviors are perceived as acceptable, or even desirable. Despite the fact that physical-fitness programs are beneficial to one's health, jogging, running, and compulsive exercising are potentially addictive because they are primarily inward, self-involved, and narcissistic activities. The dynamics of compulsive workers reflect similar needs. So-called normal individuals use what might otherwise be considered constructive work activities to isolate themselves, cut off feelings, and soothe their pain. Basically, people with compulsive work habits effectively retreat from relationships and essentially ruin their lives while using defensive rationalizations that justify hard work. Bookkeepers, accountants, computer programmers, and others who work at repetitive, mechanical tasks have unique opportunities to cut off feelings and depersonalize, whether they intend to or not. When these activities take on an addictive element characterized by long hours and great difficulty pulling oneself away from the task, they have a destructive effect.

Routine or excessive masturbation to reduce tension is generally a symptom of emotional deprivation. The child discovers early on that touching his or her genitals not only leads to pleasant sensations but tends to neutralize emotional distress. This activity can develop into a self-soothing, isolated method of taking care of oneself. When habitual masturbation persists into adulthood and is preferable to sexual activity with another, it is representative of a self-feeding process.

Disturbed children often masturbate compulsively. In a residential treatment facility, one youngster with a pervasive developmental disorder masturbated excessively before falling asleep each night. As part of an experimental treatment plan, the nurses offered him a glass of milk each night. They also left a glass of milk on the night table next to his bed. Within a few days, there was a dramatic reduction in masturbatory activity. Evidently, the boy's willingness to accept *real* nourishment from the nurses freed him from the compulsive need to satisfy himself.

ADDICTIVE ATTACHMENTS

The gradual decline in personal relating, sexual attraction, and desire that occurs in many relationships and marriages has its basis in the self-parenting process. Early in a relationship, the new love object begins to threaten the defensive psychological equilibrium firmly established in each individual. As noted earlier, insecurity and lack of tolerance of intimacy are the principal causes of marital failures. People try to preserve their original feelings of attraction and love while, at the same time, they hold on to habitual methods of self-gratification and a pseudoindependent posture. The dilemma created by the attempt to achieve these two mutually exclusive orientations is obscured by a fantasy of love and closeness, and real love, friendship, and concern are gradually replaced by an intrusive, possessive style of relating.

Later, when either partner moves away from the addictive attachment toward independence or autonomy, symptoms similar to those manifested in withdrawal from chemical dependency are aroused in the other. These symptoms include feelings of desperation, emotional hunger, disorientation, and debilitating anxiety states. The intensity of these emotional reactions indicates the powerful nature of the imagined connection or fantasy bond existing between the partners.

One woman, in describing her reasons for marrying, inadvertently defined the essence of addictive attachment:

> I knew I was afraid of being in a *real* feeling relationship with any person, man, or woman, and I knew, too, that I was terrified of being alone. Forming a fantasy bond with my husband was a solution. I could stay somewhat distant from him yet I would always have somebody *there for me.*

Incidentally, this couple slept wrapped in each other's arms, while acting out hostility and abuse toward each other during waking hours. The relationship ended in a bitter divorce.

The child born to a couple involved in a fantasy of love while acting out behavior that is emotionally distant, rejecting, or outright hostile to one another will be provided with little emotional sustenance. Children growing up in this atmosphere learn to "take care" of themselves through fantasy and self-nourishing behaviors, thereby completing the intergenerational cycle.

THERAPEUTIC INTERVENTIONS

A necessary objective in treating addicted patients is to provide them with an authentic relationship during the transition from relying on addictive substances to seeking and finding satisfaction in genuine relationships outside the office setting (R. Firestone, 1990c). Therapists actively confront the patient's self-nourishing habit patterns without being judgmental or parental, while, at the same time, the transitional relationship with the therapist makes reality more rewarding. The approach is twofold in its focus: (a) it challenges and disrupts the addictive patterns, and (b) it encourages movement toward real gratification and autonomy in the external environment.

Therapy With Schizophrenic Patients

In my early work with schizophrenic patients, I came to understand the important role that fantasy played in the psychotic regression. Deprivation of love and care in interpersonal relations results in anxiety states that disturb the psychological equilibrium, and this tension is relieved by fantasies of fusion. The primary fantasy therefore is the "self-mothering" process or the incorporation of the maternal image within the self as a nourishing and controlling agent (R. Firestone, 1957).

Two kinds of activities are required in the treatment of schizophrenic patients: The therapist must counteract the psychotic dream solution, thereby disturbing the psychological equilibrium and creating anxiety. Concomitantly, he or she needs to encourage the patient to "take a chance again" and learn to reinvest in personal relationships. This is accomplished by the consistent provision of love and sensitive care by the therapist over an extensive time period.

An important aspect of the therapy involves restriction or control over the patient's life, actively limiting the acting out of psychotic propensities. Both control and affection (love-food) are necessary to counteract the effects of an inadequate emotional environment. My methodology challenged patients' idealization of the mother and provided the emotional support that enabled them to progress through the early stages of development where they had previously been fixated.

Therapy With Addicted Patients

The ultimate goal of therapy is to help patients move away from compulsive, addictive lifestyles so that they can expand their lives and tolerate more gratification in reality. As described in Chapter 10, manifestations of the self-parenting process are challenged at every level—affectively, cognitively, and behaviorally—through (a) intense feeling release, (b) verbalization and identification of negative thought patterns (Voice Therapy), and (c) corrective suggestions for behavioral change.

Patients' lack of self-control and compulsive involvement in self-nourishing behavior patterns point up an important prerequisite for therapy: It is necessary for the patient to give up addictions before any real therapy takes place. This creates an incredible paradox. The alcoholic or drug addict must give up these substances to get well, yet this is the presenting problem. Nevertheless, no real therapy will take place as long as these patterns are acted out.

In spite of this dilemma, a therapist of strong character, concerned and sensitive, can establish a preliminary contract with the patient on this issue. Early on, the therapist points out, in nonevaluative terms, the serious consequences of the patient's addiction. It is important that patients *not* relate to their behavior as a moral issue, but that they become aware, on a feeling level, of the harm they are inflicting on themselves through the continued use of substances. The therapist's warmth, independence, and maturity are essential in gaining and holding patients' respect and trust so that they will continue to be motivated to give up the addiction. If the patient refuses to enter into such an agreement at this time, prognosis is poor.

This approach is not limited to working with patients where addiction and drug abuse are primary. Contracts with respect to abstinence as a prerequisite for therapy have been shown to be effective in all types of therapeutic endeavor. The prohibition against commonly used self-nourishing habits such as smoking, drinking of alcoholic beverages, excessive use of medication, or acting out, as a precondition for therapy, is a powerful treatment method in and of itself. Interference with these addictive patterns fosters a state of deprivation, which, in turn, arouses anxiety and renders repressed feelings more accessible. In my work with an intense feeling release therapy, I found that, as a result of these preconditions, patients felt close to their underlying pain, which led to deep catharsis and the development of their own crucial intellectual insights. Patients who continued to control the acting out of habitual addictive patterns progressed rapidly and made important behavioral changes, whereas those who reverted to addictions and acting out were limited in their therapeutic gains.

Case Study

Mrs. R., 25, was referred for therapy immediately after her second serious suicide attempt. In the initial interview, she disclosed pertinent details of her personal history, revealing a life characterized by emotional turmoil, intense self-hatred, drug abuse, patterns of binge eating, and a progression of casual sexual relationships devoid of feeling. In addition, she was the mother of an unwanted, unplanned-for young child.

Mrs. R.'s erratic mood swings—exuberant states alternating with severe depression—suggested a diagnosis of cyclothymic disorder overlaid with psychoactive substance dependence. The patient's distrust and suspicions were evident at the outset (she felt disillusioned and had failed at previous attempts at therapy). Nevertheless, she responded well to my directness and insistence that she abstain from heavy drug use while undergoing treatment. She gradually developed trust and excitement in the therapeutic process.

An entry from Mrs. R.'s journal, in which she recorded her thoughts and feelings early in therapy, reveals dimensions of the patient's addictive lifestyle and her intolerance of real feeling and intimacy in interpersonal relationships.

I grew up not wanting much out of life, living in the short term from day to day, always having suicide as the final out when things would get rough. Early in childhood I learned to satisfy myself—not to count on anyone else to be sensitive enough—to only count on me. That has had a profound effect on my life.

I found the closeness and feeling I felt on rare occasions to be followed by fear and self-gratification. If I make love and feel really close, I feel a compulsion to masturbate and satisfy myself. If I am excited, I tone it down with Valium. At a party, feeling somewhat happy and content, a drink turns everything into a fantasy—takes the edge off—makes the lights brighter, jokes funnier, but the contentment disappears.

The first phase of treatment dealt directly with uncovering the patient's voice attacks. Mrs. R. learned to identify and verbalize the malicious, self-accusatory thoughts that dominated her thinking. In analyzing her suicide attempt, she expressed the feelings of hopelessness she felt at the time, in terms of voices:

"You thought things were going to be different this time, but you were wrong! You can't change the way you are with a man.

"You're just a bad person. Who cares about you? Nobody! They don't give a shit! Nobody would even notice if something happened to you."

Mrs. R.'s drug use prior to her suicide attempt acted to diminish her inhibitions, making it easier for her to carry out her destructive plans. In one session, she articulated the voices that had urged her to escape the unbearable psychological pain she was in by taking a lethal dose of sleeping pills:

"Look, things are closing in on you. They'll never get any better. You can't eat, you can't sleep, you can't get any peace of mind.

"Don't be such a coward. This is something you have to do. It's the only way out! You've got to get together enough pills to really do it!"

The patient experienced intense feelings of anger and sadness as she identified the strong self-attacks that had gained complete control over her behavior. In bringing these hostile voice attacks to consciousness and recognizing their relationship to actual parental attitudes toward her, she was able to separate the internalized patterns of destructive thinking from her own point of view, a process that led to an overall improvement in her emotional state.

In the second phase of therapy, Mrs. R. began to uncover painful memories of incidents from her childhood that she had partially or completely repressed. In feeling-release sessions, she relived key traumatic events in growing up. Reexperiencing the longing and desperation of that period of her life provided her with important insights into her pattern of compulsive overeating.

> During the session, I felt very small. It seemed as though I was sitting in a high-chair in a kitchen. I could see my mother standing in front of the refrigerator, grabbing any food she could get her hands on, and shoving it into her mouth— very fast. She didn't look at me; she didn't even see me. I asked her to look at me, to feed me. I cried for a long time, feeling that she would never feed me, because she didn't even see I was there.

The material in this session touched on painful themes at a primitive, preverbal stage of development, relevant to frustration and fixation on an oral level. Mrs. R. recognized her mother's hostility and abject neglect of her as a child. More painful was the realization that her mother's own life had centered on compulsive, self-feeding patterns.

In another deeply moving session, the patient disclosed how she came to be inward and secretive about her eating disorder.

> As a child, my mother didn't want me to get fat, so she put me on a very restricted diet. She didn't let me eat much and often I was starving.
>
> I would smuggle food to my closet and hide it. I spent a lot of time planning what to take—it had to be something that wouldn't get old, smell, or rot. I finally took cookies, but I couldn't take just one or two because she might notice, so I took the whole package, so she might not remember she bought them.
>
> I would sit in my closet and eat the whole bag. I would feel sick, unsatisfied. I was afraid to get caught or leave evidence, so I would tear up the package and hide the pieces in the toes of my shoes. When she wasn't home, I would take the pieces of the package outside to the trash.

In other deep feeling sessions, she remembered her father's sexualized involvement with her as an adolescent and reexperienced her anger at his intrusiveness. She came to understand his rage and beatings as a manifestation of his disturbed sexual feelings toward her. Integrating the material from these sessions provided the patient with a more realistic view of her parents and reawakened a sense of compassion for herself in relation to the damage she had sustained in her early life.

Later, in Voice Therapy sessions, Mrs. R. identified a soothing, seductive voice that urged her to indulge in eating binges, followed by vicious thoughts of self-recrimination. In collaboration with me, she formulated plans for breaking her addictive use of Valium, diuretics, and food, and translated her plans into action. For a short time, she underwent symptoms of withdrawal, including feelings of disorientation, near-panic states, and increased voice attacks. These reactions gradually diminished in intensity as she refrained from these self-destructive patterns.

As she gave up her dependency on physical substances, Mrs. R. focused on improving her personal relationships, particularly with men. She became seriously involved with a man, whom she married within the year. It started as a relatively positive union, but soon manifested many of the addictive qualities that characterized the patient's previous lifestyle. Mrs. R. used the relationship as a self-nourishing process in that, in her addictive orientation, she attempted to exert absolute control over the sources of external gratification from the interpersonal environment. This process of substituting addictive attachments to objects for an addiction to substances is not uncommon, and difficult to work through in psychotherapy.

Symptoms of deterioration in the relationship included Mrs. R.'s extreme dependency and her erratic fluctuations between angry, provoking manipulations that caused her considerable guilt, and apologetic gestures. Anticipating rejection, she continually sought reassurances of love and demanded proof that she was special, thereby "feeding" strong narcissistic needs. In attempting to control and dominate her husband, Mrs. R. lost much of the sexual attraction she originally felt toward him, and there were serious problems in the couple's sexual relationship. The rare occasions on which Mrs. R. was able to respond sexually and personally were often followed by periods of retribution and abuse, indicating the patient's intolerance for being less defended and vulnerable.

Another crisis arose when Mrs. R. had a brief episode in which she ran away. It appeared that the responsibilities of motherhood (she had recently given birth to another child) had aroused strong dependency needs and fears of being depleted, and there was a regressive pattern. During the postpartum period, Mrs. R. experienced strong self-attacks about her perceived inadequacies as a mother. In a session following her return home, she verbalized the specific voice attacks that had strongly influenced her to run away:

"You don't know how to take care of a baby! You just make him feel bad. What have you got to offer a baby? You don't care for anybody. You've never cared for anybody in your whole life!"

As she continued, her voice became louder and increasingly angry and malicious.

"Can't you see what a bad effect you have on your husband? He's always worrying about you. He'd be better off if he didn't have you to worry about. Your baby would be better off without you, too. Why don't you just leave? Everybody would be better off without you!" [*Cries*]

It was clear to the patient that the self-destructive action of temporarily deserting her family had corresponded to the voice attacks she verbalized in the session.

Outcome. The process of consistently identifying her self-attacks and working on corrective suggestions over an extended time period eventually freed the patient from the addictions and self-destructive habit patterns she had maintained for most of her life. It is interesting to note that the patient's symptoms progressed from actual suicidal behavior to running away (a partial suicidal pattern), to microsuicidal thoughts and actions, and eventually were reduced to a subclinical level.

Mrs. R. became more cheerful, experienced considerably less misery and depression, modified her debilitating feelings of self-hatred and self-deprecation, and, at termination, was functioning at a good level. Follow-up 2 years later indicated that the patient's fluctuations in mood were well within the normal range; there was stability in her personal relationships, and she continued to develop in other areas of her life.

CONCLUSION

Based on our clinical experience and therapeutic position, we have come to the conclusion that all patients, indeed all people, suffer from some degree of addiction that interferes with their living fully. Our primary goal is to help people come to terms with the painful feelings and frustrations that caused them to retreat into fantasy and self-nurturance. Most patients believe on a deep level that they cannot survive if they have to face the primitive wants and the rejection they experienced early in life. Indeed, they are terrified of being in a wanting state and experiencing frustration. People will be self-denying, restrict their personal goals, and otherwise limit themselves, as this is under their control. They are comfortable to express a need when they feel that they are guaranteed it will be met. However, they are terrified of indicating their wants honestly and having them refused or rejected. They react to this situation as though it were life-threatening. They respond as though they were still as vulnerable as they once were when they were young children, utterly dependent on their parents to keep them alive.

Regardless of the specific techniques, interventions, or therapeutic approach, patients must become aware of their ongoing needs and desires and use the therapeutic situation to ask directly for what they want. The inevitable limits to personal gratification inherent in the structure and discipline of the therapeutic encounter lead to frustration of the patient's infantile needs. Patients learn that they can survive without the therapist's "parental support" and come to terms with their anger at being frustrated.

This is the crux of positive or lasting therapeutic progress with addicted individuals, for in the course of facing their anger at the inevitable frustration, they strengthen their independence and relinquish the fantasy bond with their parents as well as dependency on internal sources of fantasy gratification. Insight and growing awareness of the fact that they can never obtain the gratification they needed so desperately as children, that, in fact, these needs are no longer vital to adult survival or happiness, can help addicted individuals to expand their boundaries, get more enjoyment out of life, and remain free of self-parenting addictions.

ENDNOTES

1. Tolpin (1971), in her discussion of the internalization of the transitional object (blanket) as a self-soothing device, noted that

> the infants who suffer maternal deprivation cannot re-create "good enough" mothering experiences because they have never experienced them. . . . A fixation on the need for the functions of the idealized parent imago occurs, and the personality is "addicted" to the functions of an external regulator. (p. 331)

2. Research has shown that fantasy can be rewarding under conditions of physical deprivation. In one study (Keys, Brozek, Henschel, Mickelsen, & Taylor, 1950), volunteer subjects deprived of food and kept on a minimum sustenance diet reported that they spent hours daydreaming about food, which partly alleviated their tension and hunger drive.

3. LynNell Hancock (1996) reported that 1.3 million children in the United States between the ages of 5 and 14 take Ritalin regularly. The rate of Ritalin use in this country is at least five times higher than in the rest of the world.

4. Recent studies in infant development have yielded information about the precursors of both normal and inadequate affect regulation in the young infant. Ivri Kumin (1996) synthesized new data from infant studies with attachment theory, psychoanalytic concepts such as projective identification, and the concept of affect attunement from self psychology.

5. Freud (1914/1957) portrayed the characteristic behaviors of individuals in "Categories 1 and 2" as follows:

> [The patient has] substituted for real objects imaginary ones from his memory, or has mixed the latter with the former; and on the other hand, he has renounced the initiation of motor activities for the attainment of his aims in connection with those objects. (p. 74)

15

The Essential Paradox
of Psychotherapy

> It is all right to say, with Adler, that mental illness is due to "problems in
> living,"—but we must remember that life itself is the insurmountable
> problem.
>
> *Ernest Becker (1973, p. 270)*

The tragedy of the human condition is that man's awareness and true self-consciousness concerning existential issues contribute to an ultimate irony: Man is both brilliant and aberrant, sensitive and savage, exquisitely caring and painfully indifferent, remarkably creative and incredibly destructive to self and others. The capacity to conceptualize and imagine has negative as well as positive consequences because it predisposes anxiety states that culminate in a defensive form of denial.

Therapeutic progress inevitably leads to a heightened sense of awareness and new levels of vulnerability. We are reminded of Freud's commentary that we

AUTHOR'S NOTE: The material in this chapter is taken primarily from "The Dilemma of Psychotherapy," in *Voice Therapy: A Psychotherapeutic Approach to Self-Destructive Behavior,* Human Sciences Press (1988). Used with permission.

cure the miseries of the neurotic only to open him up to the normal misery of everyday life. Prior to therapy, people's defensive patterns served the function of numbing them to the pain inherent in everyday living. A breakdown of these defenses and the associated misery were most frequently the driving force behind the individual's motivation to seek psychotherapy. Abandoning habitual defenses, while opening patients up to life, also causes them to be more sensitive to reality and increases their exposure to a world that is abrasive and destructive to the undefended person. In addition, the conventions and mores of society are generally opposed to the state of honesty, openness, and vulnerability brought about by the process of dismantling major defenses.

Moving away from the imagined safety of familiar support systems, individuals experience their aloneness. They feel considerable guilt and fear in separating from dependency bonds. Although more capable of sustaining genuine and close relationships, they find themselves in a high-risk situation. In their personal interactions, they may now feel deeply wounded by retaliation from others who are defended and cannot accept their liveliness, generosity, warmth, and acknowledgment. On a societal level, there is a great deal of unavoidable suffering and anguish inherent in living an undefended life. One is constantly aware of such external issues as crime, poverty, economic recession, financial setbacks, illness, and the potential threat of deadly viruses or a nuclear holocaust. Finally, all people are confronted with an insurmountable problem in life—the fact that they are trapped in a body that will certainly die. Recovering aspects of their child selves and emotional vitality makes them more poignantly aware of the inevitable loss of self through death.

Who wants to live with this new awareness, this heightened vulnerability to rejection, loss, and death? Therein lies the dilemma, for how can the therapist symbolically influence the patient to embrace life fully in the face of a predictable future with a negative outcome?

The patient's dilemma is evident from the beginning of the therapeutic process. The basic conflict centers on the choice between avoidance or contention with the realities of life. Individuals in crisis enter therapy desperately searching for relief from painful symptoms, failures, phobias, anxiety reactions, or depression. In the majority of cases, motivation to seek help reflects a desire to escape from this pain. At the same time, patients want to hold on to basic character defenses and stubbornly refuse to give up self-nourishing habits or dependency bonds that, if maintained, would continually lead to symptom formation. Thus a person's motives in seeking professional help may seriously conflict with the goals of a conscientious approach to the psychotherapeutic endeavor. In this condition, patient and therapist find themselves at odds.

DEFINITIONS OF PSYCHOTHERAPEUTIC
"CURE": SOME PERSPECTIVES

All definitions of therapeutic "cure" or improvement point toward an integrated, feeling self and a positive adaptation to life that allows the individual
more flexibility and exposure to real experience. However, a nondefensive
approach to life obviously has its disadvantages as well as its advantages. The
problems involved in retaining an open and vulnerable orientation have been
described by a number of clinicians. Wolberg (1954), in writing about the
dilemma of psychotherapy, stated, "Society itself imposes insuperable embar-
goes on certain aspects of functioning. It supports many neurotic values which
necessitate the maintenance of sundry defenses for survival reasons" (p. 554).

Consider also Rank's, and Becker's (1973), cogent descriptions of the paradox faced by the "cured" patient: "It is not so much a question as to whether we
are able to cure a patient, whether we can or not, but whether we should or not"
(Rank, quoted by Taft, 1958, p. 139).

On the other hand, people do not necessarily remain successfully defended.
As Rollo May (1983) indicated in the following statement, the "adjusted," yet
self-protective, patient may feel less anxious and be symptom-free; nevertheless,
his or her adaptation to society has its own negative consequences in a loss of
freedom:

> The kind of cure that consists of adjustment, becoming able to fit the culture, can
> be obtained by technical emphases in therapy. . . . Then the patient accepts a
> confined world without conflict, for now his world is identical with the culture.
> And since anxiety comes only with freedom, the patient naturally gets over his
> anxiety; he is relieved from his symptoms because he surrenders the possibilities
> which caused his anxiety. (pp. 164-165)

Clinicians face a difficult task in evaluating the effects of psychotherapy.
Many researchers "argued that traditional assessment methods are too global,
imprecise, and rooted in a 'medical model' conceptualization of psychological
problems" (Stiles, Shapiro, & Elliott, 1986, p. 170). In addition, psychoanalysts
tend to feel that the "subtleties of dynamic change could not be captured by
symptom scores or personality inventories" (p. 171). In terms of actual attempts
to measure therapeutic success precisely or scientifically, there is conflicting
evidence to support the hypothesis that patients really improve over the course
of treatment (Endnote 1). Whereas a number of studies indicate a point of view
that there is no apparent change associated with therapy sessions, many others
demonstrate favorable outcomes. The problem is that these measurable changes
occur in circumscribed areas referring to specific, operationally defined, discrete

aspects of the patient's personality and may fail to register other equally important, but more subtle, developments.

Although there is still considerable disagreement about the issue of evaluation, a vast accumulation of clinical and personal data from both therapists and patients exists indicating that the psychotherapy experience is valuable and has considerable impact. Seligman (1995), citing the substantial benefits of psychotherapy reported by patients in a recent survey conducted by *Consumer Reports,* concluded that effectiveness studies, in combination with efficacy studies, could "provide empirical validation of psychotherapy" (p. 965). It is a matter of unusual complexity. For example, in estimating positive change, the extent to which therapy may have prevented further deterioration cannot be scientifically assessed. In some instances, patients may have been significantly helped in the sense that the sessions prevented more serious regression or eventual institutionalization.

The key issue in evaluating outcome in psychotherapy lies in determining how one defines the "healthy, well-adjusted" individual. Psychotherapeutic "cure" is defined by various clinicians in terms of the patient's increased ability to function and respond appropriately to his or her interpersonal world. For example, Freud (1930/1961) described the healthy or nonneurotic individual simply as one who is able to derive satisfaction from love and work (Endnote 2). Carl Rogers (1951), in his investigations, defined positive change in terms of patients' perceptions of self: "The result of therapy would appear to be a greater congruence between self and ideal" (p. 141). Rogers interpreted these findings as demonstrating that the therapeutic relationship allows the patient to experience "himself as a more real person, a more unified person" (p. 142). The *Firestone Assessment of Self-Destructive Thoughts* (R. Firestone & L. Firestone, 1996), which relates to the continuum of self-destructive behavior, could potentially serve as an outcome measure, in that change over the course of therapy could be measured in a relatively objective manner, similar to Rogers's assessment techniques. One would expect the improved patient to endorse items in the lower range of the continuum rather than in the higher ranges representing more serious forms of self-destructive behavior, including suicide. Mowrer (1953) emphasizes that a mentally healthy patient takes a "realistic problem-solving approach," which, in turn, allows his or her "emotions, now in proper context . . . [to be] both proportionate and appropriate" (pp. 148-149). Arthur Janov (1970) describes the "well patient" as a "real adult" who no longer needs the destructive, limiting defenses that, prior to therapy, had kept the patient alienated from his or her genuine feelings.

My concept of "cure" is similar in many respects to Janov's conclusion. I perceive the healthy, adjusted individual as moving *toward* the pursuit of gratification in the interpersonal environment, and *away* from defenses and addictive behaviors and lifestyles. The patient is now free of the compulsive repetition of familiar, destructive patterns, opening the possibility for continuous change and development.

As can be seen from the above statements, the road to mental health is paradoxical in many respects. In the following pages, I explore the dimensions of the patient's dilemma and the fundamental issue of choice: whether to reinstate or strengthen defenses, destructive fantasy bonds, and deadening habit patterns in a renewed attempt to avoid pain, or to live fully, with appropriate emotions, meaningful activity, and compassion for oneself and others.

PARADOX OF FEELING

A psychologically healthy person has a strong emotional investment in living and will respond with appropriate affect to both good and bad experiences in life. Basing one's emotional reactions on real events and circumstances, rather than a self-protective posture, leaves one open to painful feelings.

For example, on Wednesday, July 26, 1995, a man turns on the evening news and within 3 minutes is bombarded with the following stories:

- five people killed and many injured in a terrorist bombing on a Paris subway train
- a survey showing over 2.4 million children physically abused in the United States last year
- the embargo lifted on arms supplied unilaterally to warring factions in Bosnia
- contaminated supply of aspirin detected in several states
- trial of mother indicted for murdering her two small sons ends with guilty verdict—jury to decide between the death penalty and life imprisonment

What quality of experience affects the feeling person alive to the realities of life?

Defenses are almost mandatory when one is faced with man's inhumanity to man. Yet cruelty and injustice are an outgrowth of dishonest and defended patterns of thinking and living that preclude the human's compassion for him- or herself and fellow human beings.

Many patients mistakenly believe that improvement in therapy will make them *less* sensitive to the pain of everyday living and more impervious to distress arising from failure, rejection, or loss. In general, our findings indicate an opposite trend. Emotionally healthy individuals are acutely sensitive to events in their lives that impinge on their sense of well-being or that adversely affect the people closest to them. Indeed, they appear to be *more* responsive, not less, to emotionally painful situations that are real than prior to therapy. However, more important, by fully experiencing their emotional reactions, they are better able to cope with anxiety and stress and are far less susceptible to infantile regression and neurotic symptom formation.

Those individuals who are inward and cut off from feeling often have melodramatic overreactions to minor personal slights or imagined rejections, yet they may display a curious lack of feeling or affect in response to real adversity. Role-determined emotions and conventional reactions tend to dominate their responses, and at times they appear to be one step removed from directly experiencing the world around them. Their defenses act to suppress feelings; consequently, their reactions are more automatic and cerebral. In an important sense, defended persons have disengaged from themselves as hurting children and now, as adults, lack feelings of compassion for themselves and others.

In contrast, psychologically healthy individuals are more open to their emotions and can tolerate irrational, angry, competitive, or other "unacceptable feelings." Therefore, they are not compelled to act out these feelings on friends and family members. This manifestation of mental health has broad psychological implications. For example, in cases of both emotional and physical child abuse, we found that the inability to accept feelings of anger, hostility, and resentment caused many parents to extend these feelings to their offspring. Later, when the parents were able to recognize and accept destructive feelings in themselves toward their children, tension was reduced and damaging responses were minimized.

A prevailing view of emotional suffering has been that it is unacceptable and that people who are in psychological pain are sick or abnormal. To the contrary, only by experiencing the painful emotions that arise in life can people feel joy or experience genuine happiness. Furthermore, when painful feelings are accepted or allowed full expression, there is a corresponding reduction in compulsive reliving and attempts to manipulate or control others in the interpersonal environment.

Many individuals are reluctant to experience or express deep feelings of sadness. The anticipation of these feelings appears to arouse primal fears and considerable tension, whereas the actual experience of sadness frequently brings relief. After expressing emotional pain or deep feelings of sadness, people usually feel more unified or integrated and report a stronger sense of identity. For example, in therapy groups with young adolescents, we observed that when the youngsters expressed previously suppressed feelings of sadness, their outlook on their problems shifted considerably to a more positive perspective. Prior to these group discussions, many of the youngsters had been involved in acting out negative, hostile behaviors. It appeared that they engaged in these actions in an attempt to avoid underlying feelings of sadness that they perceived as being embarrassing or unacceptable.

GUILT AND FEAR REACTIONS
ARISING FROM BREAKING BONDS

In Chapter 13, I emphasized that movement toward emotional health and independence creates both guilt and fear. These reactions often have their basis in the family's interpretation of separation. For example, Joseph Richman (1986) cited what he believes to be an important factor contributing to suicide attempts in adolescents. His studies stressed the fact that the suicidal patient's family frequently perceives the adolescent's moves toward independence, particularly the establishment of peer relationships outside the family circle, as being extremely threatening to family cohesiveness or even family survival. Writing about the "myth of exclusiveness" symptomatic of these disturbed families, Richman (1986) stated, "The formation of outside friendships and relationships is labeled as disloyalty" (p. 32). Richman defined the relationships that exist between these family members as "symbiotic bonds" wherein "the development of uniqueness or individuality in a key member opens up the threat of separation and must therefore be opposed or 'corrected' " (p. 19).

The guilt reactions documented by Richman are typical for individuals striving to separate from destructive bonds with parents and parental substitutes. Parents and mates who are immature and dependent are capable of manipulating the guilt feelings of improved patients, causing considerable damage and often precipitating serious setbacks. They are intimidating and controlling of one another by acts of direct intimidation and hostility, by judgmental and condemning attitudes that support the voice, and by "falling apart" or other self-destructive actions. Indeed, anything that reinforces one's inner sense of "badness" can be damaging.

Initially, a patient's progress or improvement leads to intensified internal voice attacks about the new developments. However, as described, when people refuse to submit or alter their behavior based on these attacks, they can eventually adapt successfully to their new circumstances. It is almost as though the "voice," when ignored, like the parents themselves, gets tired of nagging and cautioning and is finally quieted. Paradoxically, people are afraid of losing the constant companionship of their destructive voices. Just as self-assertion and movement toward independence from the family bond disrupt a vital support system, separation from introjected parental voices severs an important symbolic tie.

Living without imaginary bonds or connections, with the relative absence of voice attacks, leaves one in a state of uncertainty and ambiguity. James McCarthy (1980) in *Death Anxiety: The Loss of the Self* describes Erich Fromm's interpretation of man's basic existential dilemma in terms of his choice between health and mental illness:

Fromm elegantly dichotomized the two simple possibilities of adult emotional response into autonomy and health versus regression and despondency. (p. 97)

In Fromm's view, an adult who remains overly attached to his parents avoids the anxiety inherent in the awareness of living as a distinct, separate entity. (p. 96)

To some extent, all people cling to internal and external security mechanisms because they are frightened of their aloneness. The experience of being separate and alone can be terrifying when it is related to primal feelings of helplessness, dependency, and repressed infantile feelings. On the other hand, the feeling inherent in being a separate adult person can be exhilarating.

PROBLEMS IN PERSONAL RELATIONSHIPS

Paradoxically, a sensitive, compassionate human being evokes negative as well as positive reactions in other people. Many people lash out with hostility when they are loved, befriended, or treated with unusual kindness. In protecting themselves, they unintentionally cause damage to the individuals closest to them. In this sense, people cannot be innocently defended. To defend against anxiety, pain, and sadness—emotions that are inherent in personal relationships—they must push away or punish other individuals who care for them. For example, the man who perceives himself as cold or unattractive will be suspicious of a woman who shows an interest in him; a woman who has an image of herself as unlovable will punish the man who offers her love. Generally speaking, punitive responses will be set into motion whenever a defended person is treated with unusual consideration, respect, or affection. Therefore, a person who has developed increased empathy and understanding as a result of therapy will often be retaliated against whenever he or she is the most giving and understanding.

A number of writers are sensitive to this issue and have described the paradox in significant works. Notably, Carson McCullers (1940), in *The Heart Is a Lonely Hunter,* depicts the philosophy that the beloved always resents and hates the lover. This phenomenon is so common that almost every person at some time has had the experience of being rejected following intervals of special closeness. A patient related an incident from his early adolescence that bears on this subject.

As a young child, he had experienced physical abuse at the hands of a brutal, cruel father. His mother, suffering from a chronic illness that necessitated repeated hospitalizations, was unable to intercede or protect the youngster. When he was 12 years old, the patient's family moved to a new neighborhood. Although the boy was stronger physically, his father's beatings continued unabated. However, there was some respite in this new setting. A neighbor, a married man with no children of his own, took an interest in the youth and treated him with kindness. For several months, the patient enjoyed his friendship with this man and the activities that they shared, especially fly-fishing.

Early one morning, after undergoing a particularly severe beating from his father, the boy, humiliated and angry, gathered several piles of dog feces and deposited them on the neighbor's doorstep. He then smeared some across the front door, rang the doorbell, and hid in the nearby bushes. He thought it would be funny, but instead, when the man answered the door, the boy felt sickened by what he had done. He never told anyone about this reprehensible act. The event effectively ended the association with the neighbor as the patient's shame was so intense that he was unable to respond to the man's overtures of friendship.

Years later in a therapy group, he recounted the event and experienced the grief and remorse for lashing out at the only person who had ever treated him with tenderness and consideration during his youth.

This story points out an important truth—that we are prejudiced against those who tempt us to lower our barriers and expose us once again to pain and rejection. Most people have considerable anger, albeit unconscious, toward a person whom they feel is responsible for "luring" them into a less defended position.

There are many other painful issues that psychologically healthy individuals face in everyday interactions. Their strength and self-confidence frequently arouse dependency feelings in others who then turn to them for support and leadership. This increased responsibility or emotional load puts more pressure on the improved individual at the same time that he or she is moving away from his or her own dependency relationships. Self-assurance and a positive outlook are often misinterpreted as vanity or greeted with jealousy and suspicion. If a person develops leadership potential and becomes powerful and effective in his or her field of endeavor, his or her motives are often misunderstood or interpreted as exploitive. People who have a neurotic, victimized orientation to life mistakenly perceive assertiveness as meanness.

In general, these distrustful attitudes are supported by a distorted interpretation of the Judeo-Christian ethic that condemns actions based on self-interest. The social order reinforces the voice process and, later, the self-limiting, self-destructive individuals it has helped produce create a form of social pressure, thereby completing the cycle. In this sense, society represents an amalgamation of the defense systems of its members, leading to a kind of Orwellian perspective wherein love is feared, hated, or distrusted; selflessness and self-denial are admired; honest striving is condemned; and strength is suspect.

Moreover, our society is permeated with mixed messages concerning these issues. Competitiveness and entrepreneurship are highly valued and encouraged while, at the same time, success and power are given negative connotations or condemned. Examples of negative power, passive-aggressive manipulations, and rejection of honest competition prevail. A humanitarian concern with the rights of the "underdog" has led to an unfortunate and incorrect assumption: that those who are successful achieved their advantages at the expense or disadvantage of others. The reason that this view persists is that many people have never developed psychologically beyond the conception of themselves as victims (which they often *were* as children) and are geared for failure rather than success. Thus the tyranny of the helpless and powerless can become a form of blackmail to the individual who is pursuing his or her needs.

People who are alive to their experiences may unconsciously hold back their enthusiasm, sensing that their vitality might threaten a person who is more self-denying. Worse, they may even lose their sense of excitement altogether in the presence of others who are limiting themselves and are not pursuing their goals or priorities. For example, a person delighted with the purchase of a new car would not rush over to show it to a friend who just lost his job. A woman in a happy love relationship feels self-conscious describing her life to a friend who is a wallflower and has no dates. In my clinical experience, I have observed that people are vulnerable to negative social pressure from unhappy or self-sacrificing family members. As noted previously, they find it difficult to surpass the parent of the same sex, personally or vocationally, without experiencing considerable guilt.

Emotionally healthy people are acutely aware of duplicity and dishonesty in others. In addition, their open style of communication may threaten or disturb more inward, defended people who are uncomfortable with directness and who are afraid to hear the truth. An honest person is susceptible to blackmail and manipulation by mates or family members who may break down emotionally or become self-attacking when confronted. Attempts to communicate often bring out angry, punitive reactions in people who are defensive.

Close scrutiny will reveal that most marriages and family constellations are characterized by intimidating, controlling, self-hating, or self-denying behavior on the part of one member or another. In addition, the martyred position assumed by many individuals produces a sense of guilt in their close friends, associates, and family members. Similarly, the tyranny of illness and weakness exerted by disturbed individuals clearly has manipulative effects. Consider, for example, the man whose doctor orders him to strictly control his diet because of a diabetic condition, yet who continues to eat improperly and develops increasingly serious symptoms. Obviously, his wife is alarmed and deeply concerned. Many people unconsciously use self-destructive behaviors as threats to gain leverage over others and strengthen dependency ties. These destructive manipulations and a variety of other adverse personal reactions impinge on the world of the "cured" individual with a potential for causing considerable distress.

INCREASED DEATH ANXIETY

Most people have little awareness of how much they are afraid, even terrified, of freely pursuing their goals, achieving personal power, and finding satisfaction in loving interactions. Prior to therapy, the patient may have underestimated the pain and anxiety involved in establishing a new identity and in developing long-lasting relationships that are free from a fantasy bond. The essential dilemma of "cure" may be stated as follows: The patient who progresses in therapy faces an increased awareness of death and intensified feelings of death anxiety. As he or she reaches out to life, there is a greater realization of a finite existence.

In his book *Death Anxiety,* James B. McCarthy (1980) cites three components of the fear of death as delineated by the philosopher Jacques Choron: "The fear of dying, the fear of what happens after death, and the fear of ceasing to be" (p. 10).

I believe that our existential anxiety centers on our dread of cessation of consciousness and loss of self. The fantasy bond is a basic survival mechanism because it is connected in an individual's mind with immortality. There are myriad manifestations of the fantasy bond that are used in one's efforts to deny and transcend death (see Chapter 16). However, each attempt to gain control over death ultimately ends in despair because no project or belief can guarantee an individual the survival of his or her corporeal body. The discontinuity of one's personality, identity, body, consciousness, and awareness is a truth that one cannot escape.

When a fantasy bond is threatened, people are defensive and angry at those who challenge it. Indeed, the intensity of their reaction to these "enemies" is in many ways similar to medieval crusaders who attempted to impose their religious beliefs on "heretics" in the fanaticism of the bloody holy wars—that is, to protect their conception of eternity.

Book burning, control of political thought, propaganda, and rewriting history are barbaric examples of this type of paranoia. Altering or denying the truth of experience disturbs an individual's basic sense of reality and is a primary causative factor in mental illness. In a sense, all defenses represent a dishonest choice of magical safety over real and appropriate insecurity.

No death—a car accident or a plane crash, an extended illness, a slow and painful deterioration, senility, or even a quiet death in one's sleep—is acceptable to a fully alive, feeling person who has invested meaning and affect in his or her life experience. Simone de Beauvoir (1966/1976) wrote the following about her mother's death:

> The knowledge that because of her age my mother's life must soon come to an end did not lessen the horrible surprise. . . . There is no such thing as a natural

death: nothing that happens to a man is ever natural, since his presence calls the world into question. All men must die: but for every man his death is an accident and, even if he knows it and consents to it, an unjustifiable violation. (p. 526)

PROGRESSIVE SELF-DENIAL AS AN ACCOMMODATION TO DEATH ANXIETY

Living with the poignant awareness that we share an unavoidable fate with all human beings appears to be too agonizing for many of us to endure. Consequently, we slowly commit suicide, causing anguish to those who care about us. The voice plays a central role in the process of progressive self-denial, predicting and rehearsing negative outcomes; advising the individual to reject positive experiences over which he or she has no control; and guiding the person toward negative consequences that are more under his or her control. Just as people tend to protect themselves against potential rejection in personal relationships by withdrawing interest and affect, they are able to gain an illusory sense of control over death by withholding their emotional involvement in life itself.

The voice's predictions and injunctions to avoid excitement and spontaneity support people's desperate efforts to accommodate this fear by persuading them to give up meaningful activities and close association with others. Ironically, in deadening themselves in advance, people barely notice the transition from living to dying.

Despite a person's strong tendency to adopt a lifestyle that would ease the dread surrounding death, I feel it is possible to adopt a positive philosophical outlook. Margaret Mead (1956/1960) eloquently depicted the dimensions of this choice in *The Age of Anxiety:*

Acceptance of the inevitability of death, which, when faced can give dignity to life . . . ennobles the whole face rather than furrowing the forehead with the little anxious wrinkles of worry. Worry in an empty context means that men die daily little deaths. (p. 177)

My sentiments are similar, as I feel that one's awareness of a finite existence makes life and living all the more precious. My position suggests that we embrace life fully and cherish every aspect of real experience, however temporal.

CONCLUSION

The dilemma faced by patients who have progressed and developed in psychotherapy is essentially no different from that faced by every human being.

The alternatives are clear: Without challenging destructive aspects of ourselves as represented by the voice, we will gradually submit to an alien, inimical point of view and shut down on our authentic self and unique outlook; on the other hand, disrupting powerful, self-protective defenses intensifies our awareness of life's tragic aspects and threatens at times to overwhelm us with feelings of helplessness and dread.

The patient's fear of change is related to each dimension described earlier: an increased potential for feeling and experiencing both happiness and distress; the problematic nature of one's closest relationships; the circumstances of a troubled world; and, finally, the fear of losing through death everything one has gained through expanding boundaries. Juxtaposed against this fear is the patient's knowledge that only by relinquishing defenses and fantasy bonds can one avoid inflicting incidental damage on other individuals, most painfully one's children. In addition to expanding opportunities for personal gratification, remaining vulnerable and undefended becomes an ethical or moral choice, given the alternatives.

Ideally, an effective psychotherapy would enable the patient to discover an implicit moral approach toward him- or herself and other human beings. In recognizing and gradually giving up the authority of the voice as an antifeeling, antilife, regulatory mechanism, a person feels far less victimized or blaming and far more an investigator, as it were, uncritically accepting and examining one's most irrational thoughts and feelings, while at the same time viewing others and the world with a very real curiosity and concern. As Thomas Malone (1981) said, "The task of psychotherapy is to make the ordinary a full experience . . . to uncover, or reactivate . . . the experiential dimensions of the ordinary experience" (p. 91).

I have concluded that there is no hidden significance to life that may be uncovered; rather, it is only each individual's investment of him- or herself, feelings, creativity, interests, and personal choice of people and activities that is special. Indeed, we imbue experience with meaning through our own spirit rather than the opposite, and our priorities and personal meaning express our true identity. The dilemma of psychotherapy has an important positive aspect in that the awareness of death itself could serve to enhance life's value for each of us.

ENDNOTES

1. A number of studies address the problem of measuring change in psychotherapy, including "The Germ Theory Myth and the Myth of Outcome Homogeneity" (Beutler, 1995), which cited evidence challenging the "Psychotherapy Outcome Equivalence" myth, that is, that all psychotherapies are the same in terms of effectiveness and/or outcome. Another critique by Gottman and

Rushe (1993), "The Analysis of Change: Issues, Fallacies, and New Ideas," pointed out several fallacies regarding research studies.

Hollon, Shelton, and Davis (1993), in "Cognitive Therapy for Depression: Conceptual Issues and Clinical Efficacy," reviewed findings from outcome studies of cognitive therapy used for depressed patients. Horvath and Luborsky (1993) provided a comprehensive examination of research on the relation between a positive alliance and success in therapy, and variables affecting the alliance, in their article, "The Role of the Therapeutic Alliance in Psychotherapy."

For a review of outcome studies in couples therapy, see N. S. Jacobson (1993), Halford, Sanders, and Behrens (1993), and N. S. Jacobson and Addis (1993). For single-case research, see the Special Section (Jones, 1993) in the *Journal of Consulting and Clinical Psychology,* which includes six outcome studies of single-case research. Orlinsky, Geller, Tarragona, and Farber (1993) introduced two measures for investigating patients' internal representations of their therapist, the Therapist Representation Inventory and the Intersession Experience Questionnaire, in their article, "Patients' Representations of Psychotherapy: A New Focus for Psychodynamic Research."

A more recent analysis of change in psychotherapy can be found in Seligman's (1995) article, "The Effectiveness of Psychotherapy: The *Consumer Reports* Study," which compares efficacy studies with "effectiveness studies," specifically the 1995 *Consumer Reports* study of 4,100 patients surveyed, showing that patients benefited substantially from psychotherapy, long term better than short term, with no specific modality doing better than any other modality for any disorder. Four meta-analyses of over 200 controlled outcome studies with children and adolescents can be found in Weisz, Weiss, and Donenberg's (1992) article, "The Lab Versus the Clinic: Effects of Child and Adolescent Psychotherapy."

2. Freud (1930/1961) in "Civilization and Its Discontents" discussed the "purpose of human life" in terms of the pleasure or satisfaction man is able to derive from his work: "No other technique for the conduct of life attaches the individual so firmly to reality as laying emphasis on work; for his work at least gives him a secure place in a portion of reality, in the human community" (p. 80).

PART V

Social Concerns
and Existential Issues

16

Psychological Defenses Against Death Anxiety

When I was 16 years old, I saw the world as turned upside down. I saw people trivializing their lives by bickering, struggling, and dramatizing their experiences while failing to focus on issues of personal identity and ignoring existential reality. I had a strong realization that they were living their lives as though death did not exist and that powerful defenses operated to deny this information. I sensed that this denial played a part in people's insensitivity and inhumanity to other people; their conformity and lack of a definitive point of view; their passive, dulled, victimized, paranoid orientation toward life experiences; and their disregard of themselves as unique feeling entities.

At that time, I was aware of only the most rudimentary defenses against death anxiety, that is, the identification with causes, religious ideologies, the imagined

AUTHOR'S NOTE: The substance of this chapter is taken primarily from "Psychological Defenses Against Death Anxiety," in *Death Anxiety Handbook: Research, Instrumentation, and Application* (1994), pp. 217-241 (R. A. Neimeyer, Ed.), Taylor & Francis, Inc., Washington, D.C. Reproduced with permission. All rights reserved.

continuity of life through one's progeny, and attempts to live on through creative works and contributions that would have everlasting value. Although I was not cognizant of the combined impact and influence of psychological defenses on society and culture, I did recognize that there was collusion among parents and family members to deny death and maintain the defensive process at the expense of children who expressed a natural curiosity and fear. There was a conspiracy of silence and avoidance about the subject of death.

After many years of clinical experience, I have come to understand that human beings adapt to death anxiety by giving up their lives in the face of death. As mentioned in the previous chapter, this defense contributes to a withdrawal of feeling from personal relationships, which in turn transforms genuine relating into a fantasy bond of security. The formation of this destructive tie eliminates and destroys the true bond that could exist between people who love one another.

My purpose in this chapter is to describe specific defenses against death anxiety in the context of the cultural framework that supports them. I have shown how early trauma leads to defense formation and how these defenses are reinforced as the developing child gradually becomes aware of his or her mortality. Thereafter, people adapt to death anxiety through a process of self-denial and withdrawal of interest in life-affirming activities. The denial of death through progressive self-denial leads to premature physical or psychological death, reinforces an antifeeling, antisexual existence, supports the choice of addictive attachment over genuine involvement, love, and concern, and predisposes alienation from others and from personal goals.

By moving out of the familiar safety of this adaptation and expanding their lives, people begin to experience their aloneness, separateness, and existential anxiety; the more invested they are in life, the more they have to lose. Generally, they respond to this anxiety on a preconscious or unconscious level by forming defenses without being aware of them. Paradoxically, patients who progress in psychotherapy place greater value on their lives yet are more apprehensive of death. Without recognition of this underlying pressure, some degree of regression may follow significant improvement. On the basis of extensive clinical data, I have concluded that there is a correlation between the degree of individuation, self-actualization, and life satisfaction of an individual and painful feelings of deep sadness and concern about the finitude of life.

RECENT TRENDS IN EXISTENTIAL THOUGHT

Existential philosophers and psychotherapists have written extensively of people's attempts to transcend their dualistic nature and the fact of mortality. Until the last two decades, however, fear of death (the complete transformation or termination of one's existence as one knows it) has been almost completely excluded from psychoanalytic theory or has been equated in a reductionistic way with castration fears and other anxieties. Regarding this omission, M. M. Stern (1972) wrote,

> It is surprising that psychoanalytic psychology, despite its characteristic tendency to uncover the hidden truth behind all denials and repressions, nevertheless, in its studies up to this day has rather neglected the fear of death, our steady companion. (p. 901; translated by J. E. Meyer, 1975, p. 84)

With few exceptions (Endnote 1), most classical psychoanalytic themes of the human response to death have been derived from Freud's (1915/1957) well-known dictum: "Our unconscious . . . does not know its own death" (p. 296).

In contrast, Becker (1973), J. E. Meyer (1975), and M. M. Stern (1968, 1972) contended that reactions to the realistic fear of death are of the utmost importance in the development and continuation of neurosis. Meyer (1975) emphasized that the part played by death and dying in neurosis had "until now barely been considered" (p. xi). Stern argued that working through the fear of death is an indispensable part of every treatment, and the failure of adaptation to this fear is an important cause of neurosis.

Frankl (1946/1959) asserted that individuals have the capacity to transcend tragic aspects of the human condition. He stated,

> I speak of a tragic optimism, that is, an optimism in the face of tragedy and in view of the human potential which at its best always allows for: (1) turning suffering into a human achievement and accomplishment; (2) deriving from guilt the opportunity to change oneself for the better; and (3) deriving from life's transitoriness an incentive to take responsible action. (p. 162)

"HEALTHY" VERSUS "MORBID" VIEW OF DEATH

There are two views concerning the impact of death anxiety on human affairs. Proponents of the "healthy" view of death assert that the fear of death is not natural and the child who receives good maternal care will develop a sense of basic security and will not be subject to morbid fears of losing support, being annihilated, or dying. A corollary from this approach, the "life satisfaction" point of view proposed by Searles (1961), Hinton (1975), Yalom (1980), and others, states that death anxiety is a manifestation of unfulfilled strivings in life and is "*inversely proportional to life satisfaction*" (Yalom, 1980, p. 207). They postulate that the fear of living leads to, or is transformed into, the fear of death;

however, I believe that it is more logical to consider that the fear of death transforms or alters the life experience.

According to Becker (1973), proponents of the "morbid" view (so named by proponents of the "healthy" view) claim that although "early . . . experiences may heighten natural anxieties and later fears, . . . nevertheless the fear of death is natural and is present in everyone" (p. 15). Becker, one of the major supporters of this proposition, argued persuasively that the dread of death leads to denial on many levels:

> Everything that man does in his symbolic world is an attempt to deny and overcome his grotesque fate. He literally drives himself into a blind obliviousness with social games, psychological tricks, personal preoccupations so far removed from the reality of his situation that they are forms of madness—agreed madness, shared madness, disguised and dignified madness, but madness all the same. (p. 27)

Becker did not fail to take into account emotional pain and frustration during childhood that intensify and are equated with death anxiety. He believed that psychological defenses were essential for survival during the formative years, given a child's "precocious or premature" nature and his or her involvement in

> the most unequal struggle any animal has to go through; a struggle that the child can never really understand because he doesn't know what is happening to him, why he is responding as he does, or what is really at stake in the battle. (p. 29)

The child, facing such a battle, eventually gives up the struggle in despair, building "character" defenses to conceal inner defeat. In another work (R. Firestone, 1985), I described the crucial point at which the child gives up: "Soon . . . they [children] learn that they too must die and discover that they cannot sustain their own lives. . . . At this critical 'point of futility,' their sense of omnipotence is deeply wounded. People rarely recover from this final blow" (p. 242).

Despite the fact that death is inevitable for all human beings, thoughts of dying rarely intrude into the average person's consciousness. By denying death or displacing the fear of death onto other concerns, most people are able to function in their everyday lives without being overwhelmed by anxiety and dread of their anticipated end. Zilboorg (1943) observed this obliviousness to death:

> Therefore, in normal times we move about actually without ever believing in our own death, as if we fully believed in our own corporeal immortality. . . . We marshal all the forces which still the voice reminding us that our end must come

some day, and we are suffused with the awareness that our lives will go on forever. (p. 468)

CULTURAL PATTERNS OF DENIAL

Zilboorg (1943), Becker (1973), Choron (1964), and others have pointed out the vital function that cultural norms, rituals, and institutions serve in anesthetizing people to existential realities. Human beings created a social order to help them avoid the fact of their mortality. However, Levin (1951) also emphasized that the fear of death has been used "by societies primitive and civilized as a mechanism of control and repression" (p. 264) (Endnote 2).

I perceive all societies and complex social structures as generally restrictive of individuality and personal expression in the face of existential anxiety. To some extent, all cultural patterns or practices represent a form of adaptation to people's fear of death. Much of people's destructiveness toward themselves and others can be attributed to the fact that they conspire with one another to create cultural imperatives and institutions that deny the fact of mortality. Becker's (1973) views concerning the incidental destructiveness of defenses and their projection into society are closely aligned with my own thinking. Becker (1973) stated,

> If we had to offer the briefest explanation of all the evil that men have wreaked upon themselves and upon their world since the beginnings of time right up until tomorrow, it would be not in terms of man's animal heredity, his instincts and his evolution: it would be simply in *the toll that his pretense of sanity takes,* as he tries to deny his true condition. (pp. 29-30)

DEATH ANXIETY AND INDIVIDUATION

A number of theorists subscribe to the view that the process of individuation intensifies the fear of death. Rank (1941) conceptualized neurotic persons as having transformed the fear of death into a fear of living. He wrote extensively about anxiety states aroused by individuation.

> In this sense, the individual is not just striving for survival but is reaching for some kind of "beyond," be it in terms of another person, a group, a cause, a faith to which he can submit, because he thereby expands his Self. (pp. 194-195)

Maslow (1971) agreed with Rank's formulations concerning the close relationship between the fear of death and the fear of standing alone, as an individual, out of the crowd. Maslow believed that this fear manifests itself during a person's most fulfilling or peak experiences, when he or she has a profound sense of being separate from the group:

> We fear our highest possibilities (as well as our lowest ones). We are generally afraid to become that which we can glimpse in our most perfect moments. . . . We enjoy and even thrill to the godlike possibilities we see in ourselves in such peak moments. And yet we simultaneously shiver with weakness, awe, and fear before these very same possibilities. (p. 34)

My clinical experience has shown that most individuals live out their lives enmeshed in the kind of "other power" described by Fromm (1941), Maslow, and Rank—in couples, groups, or nationalistic causes—so that they never (or rarely) experience the shiver of weakness to which Maslow alluded. The majority are terrified of differentiating themselves from their original families and of not conforming to accepted cultural norms.

ORIGINS OF THE CORE DEFENSE

As discussed in Chapter 6, psychological defenses originate before the child develops a concept of death, that is, prior to the experience of death anxiety. However, the way a child is treated within a culture that denies death and the manner in which parents defend themselves against their children play a significant part in the child's development. In attempting to protect themselves against feelings of helplessness and vulnerability in the face of death, many parents unknowingly distance themselves from their offspring.

The unwillingness of defended parents to allow repressed emotions to reemerge during tender moments with their children is a major reason those parents find it difficult to sustain loving, affectionate relationships with them.

In the early developmental years, frustration and emotional deprivation lead to the formation of a fantasy bond—an imagined connection with the mother— that becomes the core defense. Later, children's discovery of mortality, first their parents' and later their own, destroys their illusion of self-sufficiency and omnipotence, and is therefore the proverbial last straw. This new awareness causes a general tendency to withdraw libido, or genuine feeling for themselves and others, in favor of defenses and self-parenting behaviors that shield them from the consciousness of being alone and exposed to death.

Secondary defenses, including the prediction of rejection, the anticipation of negative outcomes, self-critical thoughts, and cynical views of the self and others function to protect the fantasy bond. These views are maintained by the voice process in its support of every defense against death anxiety. The voice process is at the core of microsuicidal behavior, self-denial, and self-limitation, instigating and rationalizing methods of accommodation to death.

Children's Reactions to Death

Clinician studies (Anthony, 1971; Lester, 1970; Nagy, 1948/1959; Rochlin, 1967) have shown that a child's denial of the knowledge of death may be almost immediate or may develop gradually. Nagy conceptualized three stages in children's understanding of death. Rochlin (1967), on the basis of play therapy sessions with children ages 3-5, came to the following conclusion:

> Very young children seem to learn that life ends. They apply this information to themselves. . . . The clinical facts show that the child's views of dying and death are inseparable from the psychological defenses against the reality of death. They form a hard matrix of beliefs which is shaped early and deep in emotional life. It appears not to alter throughout life. (p. 63)

Anthony (1971) reported cases of immediate denial of mortality followed by adverse reactions to the denial: "Clifford [3 years, 10 months] in his happiest mood . . . suddenly exclaimed: 'I shall never die!' . . . [However,] both he and Ruth [another child who stoutly denied death] showed anxiety during the months following their assertion of immortality" (p. 156).

Research studies (Kastenbaum, 1974, 1995) have contributed empirical findings regarding children's reactions to death. Kastenbaum (1974) reported that more than three fourths of the respondents to a questionnaire expressed the opinion that children "are better off not thinking of death and should be protected from death-relevant situations by their parents" (p. 12). In more recent research, including interviews with mothers of schoolchildren, Kastenbaum (1995) found that

> *experiences, attitudes, and ways of coping with death are part of the intimate flow of life between children and their parents* . . . [and that] *parents who are not able to cope with a child's death-related curiosity on a simple, naturalistic level because of their own discomfort may be perpetuating the anxieties for still another generation.* (pp. 200-201)

I have observed numerous children cutting off feeling, becoming inward and distant from others, and manifesting hostility as they went through the process of realization. Their questions indicated a significant increase in anxiety and concern about death. One child (age 4 years, 6 months), after learning about death, became increasingly preoccupied with fairy tales about princes and princesses who live forever. She was often disturbed by nightmares; however, she was unable to recall the contents of her dreams. In general, the frequency of nightmares about death decreases during later childhood and early adolescence, a fact that may indicate preadolescents' increased ability to repress thoughts about death and dying. This notion is supported by several empirical studies (I. Alexander & Adlerstein, 1958/1965; McIntire, Angle, & Struempler, 1972) (Endnote 3).

The apparent tranquility of the latency period may be related more to the repression of death anxiety than to the repression of sexual impulses. Many child developmentalists have commented on the obvious defended attitude of children during this period. For example, Anthony (1971) asserted, "Denial of personal mortality is only one among several ways in which the child gradually becomes able to assimilate emotionally and intellectually the realities of his physical and social environment" (p. 163).

J. E. Meyer (1975) drew attention to the fact that life and death are central themes in adolescence, "as is clearly shown by the frequency with which young people attempt to commit suicide." Meyer suggested that the loss of a love relationship "may easily cause the adolescent to step across the boundary of the will to survive" (p. 27).

Relationship Between
Separation Anxiety and Fear of Death

There are a number of affects common to separation anxiety and the fear of death, as well as certain differences between the two. One affect inherent in both reactions is the fear of being cut off from others, alone and isolated from fellow humans. This fear of object loss recapitulates the infant's anxiety at being separated from the mother.

An individual's profound terror, however, is caused by contemplation of the obliteration of the ego. This dread goes beyond separation anxiety. The cessation of the ego's existence in any knowable or recognizable form is horrifying. Any promise of an afterlife, reincarnation, or union with a universal consciousness is, at the deepest level, not convincing. The anticipation of the death of the ego is particularly agonizing to a person who lives a happy, fulfilling life, possesses a strong sense of personal identity, and is involved in a mutually rewarding love relationship. These people report that thoughts about dying also lead to a painful sense of their loss to significant others.

INDIVIDUAL DEFENSES
AGAINST DEATH ANXIETY

Clinicians may find it difficult to identify defenses specifically related to death anxiety because defenses are instituted before the patient becomes aware of the anxiety on a conscious level. Regressive trends are activated as an individual suppresses death anxiety. There is a retreat to an earlier stage of development, a level at which the individual was not fully aware of death (R. Firestone, 1990a). These regressive trends may persist throughout a person's life.

The arousal of death anxiety generally leads to an increased reliance on defensive behaviors and self-protective lifestyles. Any negative event or reminder of death, such as illness, rejection, accident, or tragedy, can precipitate feelings of death anxiety, which in turn may lead to a retreat to specific, idiosyncratic defenses typically used in times of stress. For example, I treated one young man who witnessed his father's sudden collapse from an apparent heart attack. Even though the "attack" was diagnosed as food poisoning and the father recovered quickly, the young man pulled sharply away from his wife and children, as well as from his father, for whom he had a great deal of affection. In the months that followed, he gained considerable weight and became progressively less efficient at work. These symptoms persisted for well over a year, despite the fact that his father had recovered his health almost immediately after his brief illness.

Basic defenses against death anxiety and their projection into the social structure can be delineated. These defenses are not discrete entities, but they may be categorized for the purpose of clarity as follows.

Self-Nourishing Habits

Self-parenting behaviors are closely tied to children's earliest feelings of omnipotence and self-sufficiency and in adulthood support people's illusions of mastery over their world, their lives, and their death. Just as the infant and young child partially relieve primitive feelings of hunger by fantasies of connection, thumb-sucking, and masturbation, adults come to use increasingly more sophisticated versions of self-nourishing habits to relieve emotional pain and existential anxiety. Indeed, we are currently in the throes of a drug problem of epidemic proportions in our society, as adolescents and adults strive to obliterate the pain of their existence with every means at their disposal. The United States has become an addictive society, perhaps partly as a response to the anxiety surrounding the possibility of nuclear destruction. The family—the agent of socialization—while encouraging children to find ways to suppress feelings and events, cannot later discourage them from adopting painkillers that shelter them from reality. The majority of parents exist in an unfeeling, albeit comfortable, state in which they are removed from genuine emotional contact with their spouses and children. Denying themselves satisfaction in personal interactions, they come to rely on self-nourishing habits and routines as a substitute and, by example, teach their offspring a lifestyle of addiction.

Interesting studies indicating the relationship between death anxiety and addiction can be found in the work of Rado (1933, 1958) and J. E. Meyer (1975). They stressed the obvious indifference to the future in addictive personalities.

Death appears to be completely foreign to the conscious thought process of these individuals who, according to Rado (1933), firmly believe in their personal invulnerability and immortality.

Preoccupation With Pseudoproblems

It is my contention that death anxiety and the fact of death give rise to a basic paranoia that is then projected onto real-life situations. In other words, paranoia is a suitable response to existential truths, inasmuch as powerful forces that are beyond their control *are* affecting human beings, are alien to their physical and mental health, and eradicate any possibility of ultimate survival. Many individuals project this paranoia onto encounters in life that do not justify an intense reaction of helplessness and powerlessness. People often overreact to these events with rage, fear, and panic. J. E. Meyer (1975) pointed out that the displacement of problems connected with death is apparent in agoraphobia, fear of cardiac arrest, animal phobias, and, most particularly, claustrophobia. Meyer cited von Gebsattel's (1951) reasoning in relation to the agoraphobic person's defense against annihilation anxiety: "Where anxiety cannot take on its true meaning, it assumes the form of fear and shifts its true meaning into an apprehensive attitude of fear, in which the threats of daily life play an exaggerated, even an immoderate role" (Meyer, 1975, pp. 37-38).

Most people seem intolerant of a simple, satisfying life and prefer to occupy their minds with melodrama and pseudoproblems while shutting off feeling for real issues in their lives. When preoccupied with these concerns, they are tortured by the dramatization of real-life situations but seem to be immune to death anxiety.

Vanity: Specialness

Vanity may be defined as a fantasized positive image of the self that an individual uses to compensate for deep-seated feelings of inadequacy and inferiority. It represents remnants of the child's imagined invincibility, omnipotence, and invulnerability that live on in the psyche, always available as a survival mechanism at times of great stress or when the person becomes too conscious of the fallibility of his or her physical nature and the impermanence of life. It expresses itself in the universal belief that death happens to someone else, never to oneself.

Zilboorg (1943) described this defense, "specialness," that sets one apart from one's neighbors and gives one a feeling of immunity from death: "We must maintain within us the conviction that . . . we, each one of us who speaks of himself in the first person singular, are exceptions whom death will not strike at all" (p. 468).

A soldier going into battle is well acquainted with this deep-seated belief that the bullet will not hit him—his comrades may fall to the left and right, yet his life is charmed. The popular novel *The Right Stuff* (Wolfe, 1983) accurately described this defense as superstition accepted as fact: The test pilots who crashed obviously don't have "the right stuff."

Voices build up an individual's self-importance and support an inflated self-image. Many patients report thoughts about being exceptional, special, and capable of performing at unrealistically high levels. When performance falls short of perfection, severe self-castigation and demoralization can result. However, individuals are willing to live with the tension associated with vanity in a desperate attempt to avoid feeling subject to death, as "ordinary" people are.

A compensatory image of exaggerated self-importance often extends to beliefs about marriage and the family. By being specially chosen, preferred over all others, people convince themselves that this preference guarantees them immortality through specialness. Society's conventions, mores, and institutions support a myth of exclusive and enduring love in couples. Married couples vow to "forsake all others," renounce old friends, and systematically exclude new ones (potential rivals) from their small kingdom to preserve the illusion that they are forever preferred. When this illusion is destroyed, there are dire consequences. Many times this fantasy is interrupted by the discovery of the partner's unfaithfulness, leading to catastrophic anxiety.

Male vanity and its corresponding buildup by women are fairly commonplace in our society, perhaps because they are so closely linked to the denial of death. As part of the socialization process, men learn implicitly that they are to be the head of a household, always preferred by their wives, and therefore better than other men. Women are able to control men by manipulating their vanity, by deferring, or by making "their man's" life and interests the center of their universe, and themselves the center of his existence. Both roles are damaging to the real feelings that once existed in the relationship. Again, on a societal level, stereotypical views of male superiority and strength and female inferiority and weakness support these unrealistic images.

Addictive Couple Bonds

The impact that defenses against death anxiety have on relationships by perpetuating the formation of destructive bonds has not been fully recognized. As a clinician, I am invariably impressed by the extent to which people appear to want debilitating, conventional forms of safety, security, and "togetherness," yet reject genuine closeness with their loved ones. They tend to relive early, painful experiences from childhood in their present relationships and, at the same time, maintain a fantasy that they somehow can escape death by merging with another person.

One reason that people avoid intimacy and closeness is their fear of losing the partner through rejection or death. One of my clients was delayed by an accident on the freeway while driving home from work one day. As he slowly approached the scene of the accident, he saw an overturned car that looked like his wife's. The man felt his heart pounding: What if his wife had been involved in the accident? As he drove nearer, he realized it wasn't his wife's car. He shuddered as he saw an ambulance attendant covering the face of a person lying on a stretcher. He could not get the image of the body on the stretcher out of his mind. When he reached home, he was still shaken and tearfully told his wife about the accident and his fears for her safety. Two weeks later, the client suddenly realized that he had not made love to his wife since the night of the accident. In a session, he revealed, "I numbed my feelings of attraction for my wife, trying to somehow erase the image of her in that accident from my mind."

Gene Survival

As described in Chapter 4, most parents believe that their children "belong" to them, and they experience intense feelings of exclusivity and possessiveness in relation to their offspring. To the extent that children resemble their parents in appearance, characteristics, and behavior, they are their parents' legacy, providing evidence to the world after the parents die that their lives had been meaningful (R. Firestone, 1988). Both parents and children imagine that this ownership or union somehow imbues them with eternal life. The promise that parents hold out to their offspring, that of the possibility of triumphing over death by merging with them, is costly because the individual feels too guilty to individuate and live his or her own life. Society strongly supports parents' assumption that they have proprietary rights over their children. Despite all facts about children's misery and teenage troubles, most courts of law hold sacred and inviolable parents' rights over their children's lives and destinies, except in cases of blatant child abuse or neglect.

INSTITUTIONALIZED DEFENSES
AGAINST DEATH ANXIETY

Nationalism, Totalitarianism, and the "Ultimate Rescuer"

The fear of death drives people to embrace various causes, groups, and totalitarian regimes in an unending search for immortality and security. It has been my experience that behaviors such as desperate dependence on a group, idolization of a leader, and mindless allegiance to a cause are all defenses against death fears. Individuals tend to transfer the primitive feelings that initially characterized the bond with their parents onto new figures and ideologies. In discussing transference, Rank (1936/1972) described the dynamics of forming a bond with persons and groups for the purpose of preserving one's life:

> With human beings this whole biological problem of individuation depends psychically on another person, whom we then value and perceive psychologically as parents, child, beloved friend. These several persons represent then for the individual the great biological forces of nature, to which the ego binds itself emotionally and which then form the essence of the human and his fate. (p. 82)

According to Kaiser (Fierman, 1965), people's compelling need to surrender or completely submit their will to another person or group through a "delusion of fusion" represents the universal neurosis. In this form of denial, the leader of the group becomes the "ultimate rescuer," and the cause a bid for immortality. The illusion of fusion and connection provided by being part of a patriotic or nationalistic movement is addictive and exhilarating because of the false sense of power it gives the individual.

The fear of leaving the security of the family for a world of decision and responsibility (the fear of individuation) can be avoided by conforming to the standards and values of the "kinship circle," "group," "nation," or "fatherland." Allegiance and identification with the group feeds narcissistic, omnipotent feelings and inflates a sense of self-importance. On the other hand, as Fromm (1964) pointed out, submission and conformity keep the individual "in the prison of the motherly racial-national-religious fixation" (p. 107).

Fromm extended Freud's (1921/1955) formulations about group behavior to include couple relationships that have elements of a symbiotic, dependent tie. My own analysis of marital relationships has shown that most people act out dominant/submissive (parent/child) modes in their coupling. In these cases, one partner becomes the ultimate rescuer, responsible for the other's decisions, happiness, and life. Both partners collude to preserve this polarization because, on an unconscious level at least, it offers an illusion of safety and strengthens a sense of immortality.

Religious Doctrine

> In both recent and ancient times certain Christian milieus have been so obsessed with sinfulness, particularly of a sexual nature, that one is led to posit an analogy between this exacerbated sense of sin and obsessional neurosis. (Vergote, 1978/1988, p. 72)

Traditional religious ideologies of both Western and Eastern cultures have contributed to a collective neurosis by unwittingly reinforcing people's tendencies to deny the body or obliterate the self (destroy the ego). Misinterpretations of teachings originally meant to enhance spiritual and humane qualities have led to a self-denying, self-sacrificing, passive orientation to life in many individuals. For example, in the fifth century, St. Augustine's interpretation of the story of creation led to his adopting a view of nature that was "utterly antithetical to scientific naturalism" (Pagels, 1988, p. 130). Ever since, theologians have postulated that the punishment for Adam's act of disobedience was death and have held out the promise that if individuals deny sexual desire and bodily pleasures, their soul will triumph over the body and survive death.

In a similar manner, many people have misunderstood the teachings of Taoism and Buddhism, assuming that all desire, striving, and will (the ego) must be given up to attain enlightenment. Suzuki, Fromm, and DeMartino (1960) and Watts (1961) have attempted to overcome this misinterpretation of Eastern philosophers in their discourses on Zen Buddhism.

The question arises as to why millions of people blindly follow religious dogma based on distortions or misinterpretations of the original teachings. Dostoyevsky (1880/1958) partly answered this question in *The Brothers Karamazov,* listing, among other reasons, transcendence over the body that must die, a guarantee of perpetual care from the institutionalized church, and the union with a powerful being.

> But we [the church] shall keep the secret and for their own happiness will entice them with the reward of heaven and eternity. (pp. 304-305)

> The most tormenting secret of their conscience—everything, everything they will bring to us, and we shall give them our decision for it all, and they will be glad to believe in our decision, because it will relieve them of their great anxiety. (p. 304)

As is true of relationships and sexuality, to use a spiritual teaching, whether of a god or a Buddha, to procure an absolute, unqualified security in the face of a realistically uncertain future often destroys the inherent value and meaning of that teaching. Moreover, religious ideologies based on distortions of the basic teachings tend to support a collective self-destructive process. Philosophies of self-sacrifice and self-denial of the personality or body that equate thought with action are in essence a form of thought control. Traditional religion's dogma of selflessness represents an externalization of the individual's destructive voices that underlie feelings of shame about basic wants and needs. These judgmental values have a devastating effect on people's lives because they support the internal voice's negative injunctions.

An Antisexuality, Antifeeling Existence

Secular attitudes toward sex and the human body derived from traditional religious beliefs could be construed to be institutionalized sexual abuse because they cause so much damage to people in their sexual lives. In my clinical experience, I have found that virtually every patient has developed a negative point of view about his or her body, especially the sexual region. In socializing their children, parents are under tremendous pressure from society to teach restrictive values and narrow, distorted views of sexuality. For example, parents typically perceive sex as dirty, or as a function that should be hidden or compartmentalized (Berke, 1988; Calderone, 1974/1977). Children internalize this distorted view of sex as a negative thought process, and their adult sexuality and closest relationships are profoundly influenced by it.

Perhaps because feelings arise in the body, society has also created strong prohibitions against feelings, especially anger and sadness. People are taught to feel only in a socially prescribed manner. Children are socialized to suppress their genuine feelings, particularly those that would indicate that they are in pain. Parents who protect themselves against feelings of sadness and vulnerability related to death cannot help but stifle these same emotional responses in their children. Admonitions such as "Don't wear your heart on your sleeve!" "Why get so upset?" and "You're too thin-skinned, too sensitive" effectively suppress the child's expression of feelings. Efforts to restrict or suppress people's natural expressions (of both sexuality and "unacceptable" emotions) lead to an increase in human aggression and immoral, acting-out behavior.

Progressive Self-Denial

The circumstance faced by all human beings is analogous to the situation faced by the convict on death row. Just as prisoners faced with the knowledge of the exact hour of their execution often attempt suicide to escape the unbearable anticipatory anxiety, "normal" individuals commit emotional or subclinical suicide in an attempt to accommodate death anxiety. In both cases, the suicide is a desperate act to avoid the dread surrounding the awareness of death (R. Firestone & Seiden, 1987).

It is noteworthy that the indications or signs of suicidal intention delineated by the suicidologists Shaffer and Shneidman (MacNeil-Lehrer Productions, 1987) parallel the basic defenses against death anxiety. The symptoms and behaviors in patients that alert therapists to the possibility of suicide are similar to those that "normal" people use to keep themselves dulled to an awareness of death. These symptoms include isolation, substance abuse, an unconcern with physical surroundings, misery and guilt reactions, and a progressive withdrawal from relationships and favored activities.

Psychosis and depersonalization are exaggerated forms of defensive accommodation to the fact of death. The less serious version of reconciliation to this existential reality in "normal" people includes feelings of estrangement from loved ones and from the world, an impairment of the feeling of being alive, a sense of not being connected to one's body (disembodiment), and the sense of no longer being touched by events, that is, isolation from affect (J. Meyer, 1975). These symptoms can be found, albeit on a subclinical level, in a large majority of individuals in our society.

The negative thought process, or voice, diminishes one's motivation for purposeful goal-directed behavior. It controls suicidal tendencies and mediates a systematic decathexis process. People withdraw investment and interest from their most meaningful associations and increasingly trivialize their experiences. Most individuals are unaware that they are acting against their own best interests and fail to question their loss of vitality and enthusiasm. The voice supports their diminished investment in life with familiar rationalizations: "This vacation is too expensive, too much trouble to arrange. Why not stay home?" or "Why begin this project at this stage in your life? You probably won't be around to see it finished" or "You're too old for sex."

Nowhere is the evidence supporting this hypothesis more clear-cut than in Voice Therapy sessions. For example, one of my clients, approaching his fiftieth birthday, decided to give up his avocation of flying and sell his private plane. He told himself that flying was too dangerous for someone his age. He reported thoughts such as "You're not as alert as you once were. You should just stay on the ground." Subsequently he became deeply depressed. His friends, concerned about his loss of vitality, urged him to take up flying again. Their encouragement sparked his interest and he decided to continue flying and work toward his instrument rating. The renewed activity acted to dispel his depressed mood and his voice attacks.

As people move into middle age, many become fearful and apprehensive, and the defense of withdrawing libido from favored activities and relationships is accelerated. The voice becomes more dominant, exerting increasing influence by dictating and rationalizing self-denying behavior. Society reinforces the defense of self-denial by maintaining certain standards regarding "age-appropriate" behavior. Consensually validated attitudes on the part of most members of our society support disengagement from life in every area of human endeavor: early retirement, segregated retirement communities, a giving up of participation in athletics and other physical activities, a diminished interest in sex, a reduction in sexual activity, and a decline in social life. Remaining involved and energetic often elicits disparaging remarks from one's friends, relatives, and children, comments that reinforce the voice: "Still playing baseball at your age? You must be crazy!" Similarly, signs of romance in the elderly bring on ridicule: "You're a fool to be in love at your age."

Thus conventional attitudes about so-called mature behavior disguise a process of self-denial that appears to be almost universal, and people are able to gradually ease themselves out of the mainstream of life. They become emotionally deadened to life, yet maintain their physical existence.

DISCUSSION

As noted earlier, a number of theorists subscribe to the view that death anxiety masks unfulfillment and dissatisfaction with one's life. However, my clinical experience supports the converse proposition: Death anxiety is related to degree of individuation and self-actualization. As I have shown, most people, beginning in early childhood, try to deny death on an immediate, personal level and gradually adapt to the fear of death by giving up, or at least seriously restricting, their lives. Most individuals never reach an optimal level of differentiation or individuation because they stubbornly refuse to step outside their customary defenses (Kerr & Bowen, 1988). They fear that they will experience a recurrence of the full intensity of terror and dread that tormented them as children when they first learned about death. However, people who live defended, constricted, and unfulfilled lives in an attempt to minimize death anxiety are often tortured by ontological guilt about a life not fully lived.

My clinical data support the hypothesis that death anxiety increases as people relinquish defenses, refuse to conform to familial and societal standards, reach new levels of differentiation of the self, or expand their lives. Many of my clients have reported having death dreams immediately after a particularly happy or fulfilling experience. In addition, serious, long-term regression often follows an atypical success or achievement in high-functioning adults.

Finally, a negative therapeutic reaction or intensified resistance to the therapy process often indicates that clients have reached a certain stage in their therapy in which death anxiety is intensified. In becoming aware of the damage they sustained in their early development, they often react with anger and outrage. As described in Chapter 10, experiencing this murderous rage in sessions is symbolically equivalent to expressing death wishes toward the parents. Intense guilt and separation anxiety arise during the symbolic destruction of parental figures. At the same time, the client is moving away from, or completely severing, the fantasy bond with the family and the sense of "belonging" that previously functioned as a powerful defense. Reactions to expressing anger over childhood abuses, combined with the anxiety involved in breaking with the family bond, may well be a key factor underlying therapeutic failure.

Viewing death anxiety as natural, that is, taking the "morbid" view of death, and as proportionally related to degree of individuation, facilitates an understanding of the full range of clients' resistance: their fear of change, the stubbornness with which they cling to a negative concept learned in the family, episodic regressions related to significant improvement or progress, and the anxiety involved in termination. It clarifies why patients persist in holding on to feelings of vanity and omnipotence and explains their fear of nonconformity and personal power, their overriding need for illusions of fusion, and the impact of destructive bonds on interpersonal relationships. In contrast, the life-satisfaction/ healthy view of death may itself be a defense against death anxiety, because it denies the reality that people can conceptualize their own death. This view in all probability confuses death anxiety with the existential guilt inherent in withholding from life's satisfactions.

CONCLUSION

In this chapter, I have attempted to elucidate the manner in which people defend themselves against the fear of death. My approach has not been philosophical in the sense of expressing either optimism or pessimism about the dilemma humans face. My interest has been in the impact that defenses against death anxiety have on individuals and on society. I have outlined a theoretical framework that integrates psychoanalytic and existential thought concerning defense formation and its effect on the developing personality.

The data supporting this approach to death anxiety are primarily observational and longitudinal; thus there is a compelling need for experimental studies. Two types of research that might be fruitful are (a) clinical and empirical studies in which children's thoughts, feelings, and attitudes toward death are elicited and assessed at various stages in their development and (b) research studies in which increased reliance on defense mechanisms known to be associated with the arousal of death anxiety is measured in experimental and control groups. Recent studies (Greenberg et al., 1990; Rosenblatt, Greenberg, Solomon, Pyszczynski, & Lyon, 1989; S. Solomon, Greenberg, & Pyszczynski, 1991) have demonstrated the feasibility of such empirical investigations.

The formulations set forth in this chapter have crucial implications for psychotherapy. First, the state of vulnerability to death anxiety brought about by the process of dismantling major defenses needs to be taken into account by clinicians. McCarthy (1980) has addressed this concern:

> If the goal of the psychoanalytic work is the patient's freedom and autonomy, and the patient retains the unconscious fears that autonomy equals death or the loss of the self, then the positive outcome of the analysis may be as anxiety-provoking as the original inner conflicts. (p. 193)

Indeed, the intensity of death anxiety appears to be in proportion to clients' freedom from neurotic propensities. I have found that many clients concerned with the trivialities of life and obsessed with worries about personal conflicts and pseudoissues have viewed death with a kind of friendly acceptance. Unless therapists recognize the implications of therapeutic progress related to the arousal of death anxiety, they run the risk of misinterpreting many of their clients' reactions, symptoms, and communications.

Second, let me repeat that it is more pragmatic to conceptualize mental illness as a form of suicide (related to the attempt to achieve control over death) than to consider suicide and microsuicide as a subclass of mental illness. This formulation provides a clearer perspective on the underlying meaning of clients' symptoms and distress.

Finally, therapeutic progress may be disappointing to the client, because it does not lead to a state of prolonged happiness. In fact, by opening us up to genuine feeling about our lives, improvement gives us a sense of personal freedom that makes us more aware of potential losses. Appropriate affect as contrasted with melodramatic reactions deepens our sadness about the poignancy of life, death, illness, and aging as well as permitting us to enjoy the excitement and thrill of genuine positive experiences. The inevitability of future loss is a real problem for human beings, yet when we face this issue without defending ourselves, our lives become rich, powerful, and sweet, and we are capable of true intimacy, friendship, and love. Indeed, the choice to invest in a life we must certainly lose leads to tenderness and compassion for ourselves and others.

ENDNOTES

1. Otto Kernberg (1980) is one exception. He focused on existential issues in his analysis of narcissistic patients. Kernberg cited Jaques (1970), *Work, Creativity, and Social Justice.* What is now needed, Jaques suggested, is to "begin to mourn our own eventual death. . . . Such a working-through is possible if the primal object is sufficiently well established in its own right and neither excessively idealized nor devalued" (p. 61).

2. Levin (1951) quoted Freud's statements regarding the origins of culture, as follows:

[It was] because of the very *dangers* with which *nature threatens us* that we united together and created culture, which, amongst other things, is supposed to make our communal existence possible. Indeed, it is the principal task of culture, its *raison d'etre,* to defend us against nature. (p. 261)

Freud included among these dangers the "painful riddle of death, for which no remedy at all has yet been found, nor probably ever will be" (Levin, 1951, p. 262).

3. In a large-scale study involving 598 children conducted by McIntire et al. (1972), the 7- and 9-year-olds were the most willing to accept the irreversibility of death, and older children showed increasing interest in reincarnation (approaching 20%). I. Alexander and A. Adlerstein

(1958/1965) used a word association test combined with psychogalvanic skin reflex to test children's reactions to death-related words. They found that "two subgroups, 5 through 8 and 13 through 16, show significant decrease in skin resistance. No reliable differences on this measure are found in the 9 through 12 group" (p. 122). In other words, latency age (9-12 years) children appeared to have less response to death-related words. J. E. Meyer (1975) confirmed these findings:

> The fact that death quite early plays a role in the child's life has obviously gone largely unnoticed, as has the fact that death . . . between the eighth year and puberty becomes step by step subject to a process of repression that in many respects runs parallel to the development of sexual taboos. (p. 82)

17

Origins of Ethnic Strife

You've got to be taught to hate and fear.
You've got to be taught from year to year. . . .
You've got to be taught before it's too late,
Before you are six or seven or eight,
To hate all the people your relatives hate,
You've got be carefully taught!

Lyric excerpts from "You've Got to Be Carefully Taught"
by Richard Rodgers and Oscar Hammerstein II

The words of this song from the musical *South Pacific* pertain to one aspect of a powerful defense mechanism that reifies the family, shrouding it and other forms of group identification in a fantasy bond that assures immortality in the face of death anxiety. The fantasy bond, an illusory connection with another or others, offers security at the expense of self-realization, autonomy, and individuation. The fantasy solution arises to counter interpersonal trauma and separation anxiety, and it must be protected from all intrusion. This protection predisposes aggressiveness, hostility, and malice toward those who challenge its function.

The combined projection of individual defense mechanisms into a social framework makes up a significant aspect of culture. These consensually vali-

AUTHOR'S NOTE: A version of this chapter has been accepted for publication in *Mind and Human Interaction.*

dated social mores and rituals in turn influence individual personality development. Members of a given social group or society have a considerable stake in how they perceive reality, and their emotional security is fractured when individuals or groups express alternative perceptions. Cultural patterns, religious beliefs, and mores that are different from our own threaten the core defense that acts as a buffer against terrifying emotions. People will fight to the death to defend their customs and traditions against others who perceive and interpret reality in different terms.

The distinctive elements that support cultural integrity and loyalty in a specific group or society are at once a source of beauty and of human destructiveness. Paradoxically, the myriad cultural patterns and racial, religious, and ethnic differences make for creative individuation and fascinating variations in the world scene yet at the same time arouse insidious hostilities that could eventually threaten life on the planet. Indeed, racism and ethnic strife are the major problems facing us at the turn of this century (Hacker, 1992; Moynihan, 1993; Schlesinger, 1991) (Endnote 1). Although issues of economics and territoriality are also stimuli for intergroup hostility, I support the position that ethnic hatred constitutes the more significant threat at this point in history. The rapid advance of technology and destructive potential is far outracing our rationality (Mumford, 1966). Unless we understand the nature of the psychological defense mechanisms that play a major part in people's intolerance and savagery, the human race will be threatened by extinction.

This chapter examines the dynamics of what I consider to be the most important underlying cause of controversy and violence in the world today: an individual's need to maintain powerful defenses of repression and denial when faced with the terrifying awareness of his or her aloneness and mortality. As noted in the previous chapter, to develop a complete dynamic picture of how people construct self-protective defenses and their subsequent aggression, one must recognize that the fantasy bond, formed in response to inadequate or destructive parenting in early childhood, is later reinforced as the youngster experiences a growing awareness of death. Thereafter, a person's most profound terror centers on contemplation of the obliteration of the ego, the total loss of the self. People employ both idiosyncratic, individual defense mechanisms and social defenses to protect themselves against death anxiety.

Much of human aggression can be attributed to the fact that the individual conspires with others to create cultural imperatives, institutions, and beliefs that are designed to deny his or her true condition. These socially constructed defenses never "work" completely as a solution to the problem of our mortality; if they did, there would be no need for controversy and no reason to go to war over differences in religion, race, or customs. On some level, people remain unsure despite strong and rigid belief systems (Berger & Luckmann, 1967). The fear of death still intrudes into their consciousness, particularly when they are confronted by others with alternative resolutions that challenge their own. Unfortunately, people are willing to sacrifice themselves in war to preserve their nation's or religion's particular symbols of immortality in a desperate attempt to achieve a sense of mastery over death. In this situation, actual death is often preferable to the anticipatory anxiety and uncertainty surrounding the imagination of a death beyond our control.

VIEWS OF ETHNIC STRIFE

There are a number of perspectives related to the causes of racial conflict, terrorism, and war. These may be roughly divided into the following areas of inquiry: (a) theories and research concerning the origins of human aggression, (b) theories that specifically link group identification to aggressive warlike behavior, (c) research of social psychologists in relation to prejudice and racism, and (d) Ernest Becker's existential/psychological synthesis on the origins of social evil. Space does not permit more than a cursory review of these approaches.

Theories of Human Aggression

Many scholars view human aggression as the key issue in ethnic strife and war. Research studies conducted by primatologists and social scientists have been based for the most part on the assumptions that human beings are naturally aggressive because of their close kinship with the primates who are aggressively competitive for mates and territory (Ardrey, 1966; Goodall, 1986; Lorenz, 1963/1966; Maccoby & Jacklin, 1974). Freud contended that the aggressive drives (id), based on a death instinct, are so powerful that they must inevitably prevail over reason (ego) or conscience (superego). In recent years, this point of view has come under severe attack (Berkowitz, 1989; Eron, 1987; Fromm, 1986). A number of theorists contend that prevailing theories on aggression (the instinct theory, the aggression-frustration model, and social learning theories) are contradictory and confusing and should be reexamined to clarify the specific environmental conditions that arouse aggressive impulses and violent acts in individuals. Lore and Schultz (1993) have argued that "there is now sufficient information to demonstrate that popular views on the nature of aggression in both humans and animals need major revision" (p. 17).

I agree with those who challenge the Freudian contention that aggression is a derivative of the death instinct. I subscribe to N. Miller and J. Dollard's (1941) view that aggression is primarily frustration-derived and that human beings are not inherently destructive, aggressive, or self-destructive (Endnote 2). They become hostile, violent, or suicidal because of the pain or frustration they experience in relation to deprivation of basic needs and desires and later in response to death anxiety. My understanding of human aggression also takes into account social learning theory (Bandura & Walters, 1963), that is, children learn through example (role modeling) to imitate a parent's aggressive behavior. Those theorists who believe in the death instinct as the most powerful driving force in the id are naturally pessimistic about humankind's future, whereas the belief that aggression is based on frustration and other environmental factors offers a more hopeful outlook and implies constructive action.

Approaches to Group Identification

A number of theorists assert that group identification is a major causative factor in religious, racial, and international conflict. Freud's (1921/1955) work on the subject, which stressed the "mindlessness of the group mind," supports my own thesis that group membership offers a false sense of superiority, specialness, and omnipotence to individuals who feel helpless and powerless in an uncertain world. Erich Fromm (1941, 1950) traced the social and psychological elements of the Nazi movement to their sources in the Age of Reformation. He explained that existential fears of aloneness and the "terrifying responsibility of freedom" compel people to take actions as a group that would be unthinkable to them as individuals:

> There is nothing inhuman, evil, or irrational which does not give some comfort provided it is shared by a group. . . . Once a doctrine, however irrational, has gained power in a society, millions of people will believe in it rather than feel ostracized and isolated. (Fromm, 1950, p. 33)

Extending these concepts to religious groups, Freud (1921/1955) argued that believers naturally experience malice and animosity toward nonbelievers:

> Those people who do not belong to the community of believers . . . stand outside this tie. Therefore a religion, even if it calls itself the religion of love, must be hard and unloving to those who do not belong to it. (p. 98)

Lasch (1985), in his introduction to Chasseguet-Smirgel's (1975/1985) book *The Ego Ideal: A Psychoanalytic Essay on the Malady of the Ideal*, notes that Freud's notion of group dynamics, that is, the group as a "revival of the primal horde, with the leader as a father-figure," may not be as comprehensive as the version proposed by Chasseguet-Smirgel. Lasch (1985) writes,

> Especially in the modern world, groups seem to find their dominant fantasy not in submission to the father but in collective reunion with the mother. 'The group is auto-gendered. It is itself an all-powerful mother. Group life organizes itself

not around a central admonitory figure but around the group itself.' The group thus represents the 'hope of a fusion between the ego and the ego ideal by the most regressive means.' (p. xv) (Endnote 3)

It is my hypothesis that identification with a particular ethnic or religious group is at once a powerful defense against death anxiety and a system of thought and belief that can set the stage for hatred and bloodshed. Conformity to the belief system of the group, that is, to its collective symbols of immortality, protects one against the horror of facing the objective loss of self. In merging his or her identity with that of a group, each person feels that although he or she may not survive as an individual entity, he or she will live on as part of something larger that *will* continue to exist after he or she is gone (Endnote 4).

Prejudice and Racism

Researchers have asserted that affective factors and mechanisms of social influence, including those of conformity and childhood socialization (Lambert & Klineberg, 1967), need to be included in studies of racism (Byrne, 1971; Cialdini & Richardson, 1980; Duckitt, 1992; Goldstein & Davis, 1972; Meindl & Lerner, 1984; Moe, Nacoste, & Insko, 1981; Tesser, 1988). Hamilton (1981) has called attention to the fact that cognitive approaches to prejudice have serious limitations; one is their neglect of affect (Endnote 5). He suggested that people attach more emotion to their distorted views of "different" groups than to their most significant interpersonal relationships: "If there is any domain of human interaction that history tells us is laden with strong, even passionate, feelings, it is in the area of intergroup relations" (p. 347).

Studies concerning people's need to maintain self-esteem or feelings of self-importance are relevant to our discussion of prejudice. Becker (1962) and S. Solomon, Greenberg, and Pyszczynski (1991) have proposed that self-esteem functions as an anxiety buffer against death anxiety: "A substantial portion of our social behavior is directed toward sustaining faith in a shared cultural world view (which provides the basis for self-esteem) and maintaining a sense of value within that cultural context" (S. Solomon et al., 1991, p. 118).

In my work, I have described a number of defensive maneuvers that people use to bolster their sense of self-importance. The defenses of disowning one's own negative or despised characteristics and projecting these traits onto others help one maintain self-esteem, albeit falsely, and provide the basis for prejudice and racism. People of one ethnic group tend to dispose of their self-hatred by projecting it onto their enemies, perceiving them as subhuman, dirty, impure, and inherently evil (Holt & Silverstein, 1989; Keen, 1986; Niebuhr, 1944; Silverstein, 1989) (Endnote 6). Subsequently, they behave as though they can achieve perfection and immortality only through the removal of this imperfection, impurity, and evil from the world.

Becker's Approach to
Ethnic Wars and Death Anxiety

In his analysis of the phenomena of religious wars and ethnic "cleansing," Ernest Becker (1975) also discussed the use of displacement and projection described above:

> Men try to qualify for eternalization by being clean and by cleansing the world around them of the evil, the dirty. . . . The striving for perfection reflects man's effort to get some human grip on his eligibility for immortality. (pp. 115-116)

In his book *Escape From Evil,* Ernest Becker (1975) explored the relationship between the fear of death and the social evil that finds its primary expression in warfare. I am aligned with Becker in hypothesizing that existential dread is the foremost predisposing influence at the core of man's inhumanity to man. Becker and other theorists (Lifton, 1973; Toynbee, 1968b) viewed cultural patterns and social mores as constructions by human beings to alleviate death fears, and understood that they generally resulted in aggressive acts against others. Since antiquity, people have believed that they were immortal to the extent that they had power over others and that victory, particularly in a religious war, was an indication of God's favor. Becker (1975) wrote,

> No wonder the divine kings repeatedly staged their compulsive campaigns and inscribed the mountainous toll of their butchery for all time. . . . Their pride was holy; they had offered the gods an immense sacrifice and a direct challenge, and the gods had confirmed that their destiny was indeed divinely favored, since the victories went to them. (p. 106)

It is important to stress that the defense mechanisms of displacement and projection also play a significant role in maintaining feelings of divine sanction and specialness within religious groups and nations. As noted previously, they are the dynamic forces underlying racism and genocide. Allegiance and identification with the group, while at the same time devaluing others ("outsiders," "aliens," "immigrants," those who do not belong), feeds narcissistic, omnipotent feelings and inflates a sense of self-importance.

In summary, I propose that the terror of death, the feeling of utter helplessness in contemplating the cessation of existence as one knows it, provides the impetus driving members of a group or citizens of a nation to build up grandiose images of power at the expense of other groups or nations, to act on their projections and distortions, and to attempt to eliminate impure and despised enemies from the face of the earth.

INTERPERSONAL DYNAMICS
UNDERLYING GROUP IDENTIFICATION

To develop a better understanding of ethnic strife, it is necessary to examine the parallels between the psychodynamics in extended groups and societies and those operating in couples and families. This explanation of group dynamics must begin with a knowledge of the individual patterns of psychological defense that arise in response to stressful conditions. Interpersonal tension in the family system leads to hostile, guarded, and defensive behaviors that are acted out on family members and later extended to outsiders. When groups or societies emerge, the individual patterns of defense of the members are pooled and combine to form cultural attitudes and stereotypes.

A Developmental Perspective

The most powerful and effective denial of death is to be found in the fantasy bond (Chapter 6). Once the fantasy bond is formed, there is a marked tendency to withhold one's feelings in interpersonal relationships and a strong resistance to intrusion. This resistance is inevitable because if the core defense were to break down, the person would be faced once again with the pain of the original trauma. When the fantasy bond is threatened, it gives rise to a powerful fear reaction as the defended person anticipates being subject to anguish beyond his or her tolerance level.

In the context of defending the fantasy bond, negative thought processes, "voices," foster distrust and hostility toward others. Critical thoughts and abusive attitudes toward oneself are always projected to some extent onto other people. Stereotypes, prejudicial attitudes, and racial biases are extensions of these fundamentally hostile and distorted views of others that provide a pseudorational basis for aggressive acts against people who are perceived as different (Endnote 7).

As described earlier, the idealization of parents and family is part of the core defense or fantasy bond. This defense is difficult to refute as one moves out in life and attempts to expand one's boundaries because, to a large extent, it is supported by society's belief in the sanctity of the family. Only in the most blatant instances of child abuse and neglect does the collective idealization of the family break down. For example, people were outraged at the parents who allowed their children to live and eventually die in the insane and oppressive cults of Jonestown and Waco, Texas. However, they were reluctant to extend their vision to comprehend the fact that these incidents were an extreme manifestation of the complete power, proprietary interest, disrespect, and possessiveness "normal" parents righteously impose on their children's lives.

In preserving an idealized image of their parents, children must dispose of their parents' actual negative qualities. They block from awareness those parental characteristics that are especially threatening and displace them onto other people at the expense of the out-group. By judging their parents as right or superior, and others as wrong or inferior, children, and later adults, preserve their illusions about the family. Stereotypes, prejudice, and racist views represent extensions of these distortions into a cultural framework (Berke, 1988; Lasch, 1984) (Endnote 8). Because they are based on a core psychological defense, they stubbornly persist in the face of logic and contrary evidence. Moreover, in idealizing the family, an individual adopts his or her parents' distortions and biases and imitates their negative responses to people who are seen as different. In this manner, prejudicial attitudes toward specific groups of people and individuals are transmitted intergenerationally.

Feelings of vanity and specialness are also part of the defense system that protects an individual against death anxiety. These defenses manifest themselves in the idealization of the group and leader just as they do in the idealization of the family. *Vanity* refers to omnipotent attitudes, an aggrandized image of self that compensates for deep-seated feelings of inferiority and that provides the individual with a special exemption from death on a fantasy level. It is important to note that the extension of vanity as a defensive mechanism to a cultural pattern that exists on a regional or national level has led to virulent racism and genocide throughout history. As noted by Sheldon Solomon (1986), "All isms potentially lead to schisms."

As adults, most individuals tend to form relationships with significant others in a way that duplicates the imagined connection with the parents. This transference of emotional reactions from early interactions with parents to one's mate and to groups and institutions in a society is largely responsible for the submissive behavior observed in members of a group. In extending the parent/child aspect of the self-parenting process to their couple relationships, individuals intermittently act out dominant/submissive modes in their interactions. Both partners find it difficult to disengage because the polarized patterns provide an illusion of safety and wholeness and eventually foster a sense of immortality on an unconscious level.

Once an addictive attachment is formed within the couple, it must be defended at all costs against being disrupted. Anything that threatens to disturb an individual's method of defending him- or herself arouses considerable fear; this rise in anxiety results in both aggressive and regressive reactions. In much the same way, people who form a fantasy bond in a group context to cope with death anxiety also react to threats with hostility and angry retaliation. In both cases, the hostility is based on the perceived threat of breaking the illusory connection.

As discussed in Chapter 4, most parents imagine that their children are extensions of themselves and that they will somehow live on forever through their offspring. In using the child in this way, parents feel the obligation to impose their standards, beliefs, and value systems on their children, no matter how distorted or maladaptive they are. Having been "properly socialized," most children relinquish their autonomy early in life, and guilt prohibits them from breaking away from the dependency bond with their parents. They find it difficult or virtually impossible to live their own lives with integrity, independent of destructive group and societal influences (Milgram, 1974). Thus the process of socialization sets the pattern for the adult's conformity to the group.

When the parental atmosphere is immature, frightened, hostile, or overly defended, the family takes on the quality of a dictatorship or cult, wherein powerful forces operate to control other family members, fit them into a mold, "brainwash" them with a particular philosophy of life, and manipulate them through guilt and a sense of obligation. Children brought up in this manner become mindless, authoritarian personality types that are easily exploited by power-struck leaders and manipulated into a destructive mass (Adorno, Frenkel-Brunswik, Levinson, & Sanford, 1950; Fromm, 1941; Shirer, 1960).

The Development of Rigid Belief Systems in Individuals and Groups

The degree of hostility and intolerance people express toward those of different group identification, religious persuasion, or race is influenced by the extent to which they rely on the fantasy bond as a source of security. People who have been damaged to a significant extent in their early family interactions are more defensive and rigid with respect to their beliefs than their less damaged counterparts and tend to react with fear and hostility to racial and cultural differences (Ehrlich, 1973).

Most individuals, though defended, are not usually emotionally disturbed to the extent that the existence of a group with different views causes them to strike out with aggressive or violent acts. However, the majority can be induced into an intense state of hatred or rage by a leader who has pathological needs and who manipulates their fear and insecurity to achieve power (Fromm, 1941; Shirer, 1960).

If the personality makeup of people in a society or nation is rigid and intolerant, their social mores and conventions tend to reinforce a general movement toward a prejudicial view of others. Entire societies are capable of becoming progressively more hostile, paranoid, or psychologically disturbed in much the same manner that the defended individual becomes mentally ill

(Endnote 9). Indeed, the more a society is built on insecurity and inflexible belief systems, the more "sick" it becomes, and the more dangerous to world peace.

This phenomenon was most clearly exemplified in the evolution of a particular authoritarian Germanic personality type that tyrannized Europe and was responsible for the Holocaust. The superior, destructive attitudes toward minorities and the sadism manifested to the extreme in the concentration camps represented an acting-out by many Germans of internalized aggression toward their child selves. Abused and mistreated as children under the guise of order and discipline, they had come to consider themselves as inferior, unworthy, and unclean. In an attempt to absolve themselves of their self-hatred, they then projected these characteristics onto anyone they saw as different and less powerful, such as the Jews and gypsies. They were compelled to mistreat these minority groups in a manner similar to the way they had been mistreated as children. This acting-out helped to compensate for deep-seated feelings of inadequacy and powerlessness (Endnote 10). Many individuals in post-World War I Germany denied their feelings of inferiority by conceptualizing themselves as a "superrace"—a tragic form of social madness (Endnote 11).

SOCIETAL DEFENSES AGAINST DEATH ANXIETY

The progressive suppression of feeling in our society has led to an increase in aggression, violence, and criminality, accompanied by a heightened indifference to the suffering of human beings. A multitude of conventional defenses and cultural patterns militate against facing the fact of mortality and are used by people in an effort to deny and transcend existential finality. As delineated in the previous chapter, there are two major forms of defense that have evolved into unique cultural systems: (a) religious dogma, including belief in an afterlife, reincarnation, or union with a universal unconscious (Toynbee, 1968a), and (b) group identification and nationalism, idolization of the leadership, and mindless allegiance to the group cause.

Religious Doctrine

For the most part, religious doctrine consists of consensually validated concepts of existential truth. In a mistaken cause, people strive for selflessness, whereas, perversely enough, only by being themselves and accepting their true nature can they contribute to mankind through positive, life-affirming action.

Transcendence over the body that must die, the postulation of a soul or spirit, and the union with a powerful being have been the principal motivations for people's allegiance to religious beliefs. Religious dogmatism generally supports a self-destructive process of self-limitation and self-abrogation, yet restricting or suppressing people's natural desires (i.e., sexual and aggressive thoughts and feelings) unwittingly contributes to an increase in the incidence of violence and immoral acting-out behavior (Vergote, 1978/1988).

There are variations in the warlike tenor of religious groups; some have an aggressive desperation attached to their beliefs, while others are peace loving and generate far less animosity toward people of different persuasions. Religious dogma that is rigid, restrictive, and inflexible functions to instill strong hatred and malice in believers toward nonbelievers. In fact, some religious factions endorse or demand individual sacrifice in war as a basic tenet of their doctrine; a heroic death in a religious war guarantees entry into the afterlife. A primary commitment of these extremist groups is to war and to suicidal terrorist acts.

The current Middle Eastern and Balkan conflicts are based largely on religious motives. According to political analysts, the "ethnic cleansing" taking place in Yugoslavia represents yet another stage in a 600-year-old conflict that began with a religious war during the 14th century.

In the 6 intervening centuries between the original religious war and the present-day bloodshed, with the exception of a brief interlude (Endnote 12), the people involved in the fighting have maintained a hatred based on old forms of logic and reasoning that no longer have any application to their everyday lives (Moynihan, 1993; Owen, 1993; Puhar, 1993; Schmemann, 1992) (Endnote 13).

Nationalism and Other "Isms"

> Wherever there is the jealous urge to exclude there is the menace of extinction. I see no nation on earth at present which has an all-inclusive view of things. I say it is impossible for a nation, as such, to hold such a view. . . . [Eventually] nations will disappear. The human family does not need these water-tight compartments in which to breathe. There is nothing any longer which warrants the survival of the nations, since to be Russian, French, English, or American means to be less than what one really is.
>
> *Henry Miller (1947, p. xxii)*

> Nationalism is an infantile disease, the Measles of Mankind.
>
> *Albert Einstein*
> *(quoted in Dukas & Hoffmann, 1979, p. 38)*

Nationalism, communism, capitalism, and other "isms" function as a narcotic, a psychic painkiller that fosters a deep dependency in people who are searching for comfort, security, and relief from ontological anxiety. Totalitarian regimes are generally associated with the outcome of the vacillations of socioeconomic forces, but their roots lie in the psychological makeup of the individual. In any system other than a functioning democracy, the individual subordinates the self in relation to an idea or a principle and experiences a false sense of power. The illusion of fusion and connection that comes from being a part of a patriotic or nationalistic movement is exhilarating and addictive. Any cause, whether potentially good or evil, is capable of fostering a corresponding addiction in the individual.

RECENT EMPIRICAL RESEARCH

Empirical studies that noted an increased reliance on defense mechanisms to maintain self-esteem as a result of the experimentally manipulated arousal of death anxiety provide support for our hypotheses (Rosenblatt et al., 1989; S. Solomon et al., 1991). In discussing the implications of this research in terms of "terror management theory," Greenberg et al. (1990) noted that

> people's beliefs about reality [and their cultural expressions of such beliefs] provide a buffer against the anxiety that results from living in a largely uncontrollable, perilous universe, where the only certainty is death. (p. 308)

> Enthusiasm for such conflicts [religious wars and ethnic conflict] among those who actually end up doing the killing and the dying is largely fueled by the threat implied to each group's cultural anxiety-buffer by the existence of the other group. (pp. 309-310)

CONCLUSION

In "Thoughts for the Times on War and Death," Freud (1915/1957) articulated his views of the inevitability of war: "So long as the conditions of existence among nations are so different and their mutual repulsion so violent, there are bound to be wars" (p. 299).

Freud's pessimism concerning the future of humankind was due largely to his deterministic view of human aggression based on his notion of the death instinct, yet it also reflected the stress and turmoil of the times he lived in. I have shown that human hostility and violence are responses to painful issues of emotional frustration in growing up, compounded by death anxiety. Psychological defenses that minimize or shut out psychological pain are collectively expressed in restrictive, dehumanizing cultural patterns that people feel must be protected at all costs. My conception that aggression stems from frustration and fear rather than from instinct is congenial with Becker's (1975) view: "It is one thing to say that man is not human because he is a vicious animal, and another to say that it is because he is a frightened creature who tries to secure a victory over his limitations" (p. 169).

The explanation set forth here not only provides a clear perspective concerning the underlying meaning of prejudice, racism, and war but this outlook is also more positive, pragmatic, and action oriented. It offers hope for the future, whereas the deterministic conception of humankind's essential savagery may well provide a self-fulfilling prophecy. Indeed, pessimistic forecasting generally precludes constructive action, and people feel progressively more demoralized and helpless.

In this chapter, I do not attempt to offer a simple solution to the struggle for peace nor do I feel there can be one. However, the lack of an immediate, obvious course of action or definitive pragmatic program should not be interpreted as cause for pessimism, and the hope for peace should not be abandoned on those grounds. I offer guidelines explaining human aggression that, if properly understood, could lead to an effective program of education. This program would enable individuals to come to know themselves in a manner that could effectively alter destructive child-rearing practices and social processes that foster aggression. People must retain feeling for themselves in spite of psychological suffering. Only by piercing our character armor of denial and challenging the use of painkilling addictive substances and habit patterns can we manage to halt the slaughter.

Freud (1915/1957) shaded his own pessimistic view when he declared that people might benefit from an awareness rather than a denial of their mortality: "Would it not be better to give death the place in reality and in our thoughts which is its due, and to give a little more prominence to the unconscious attitude towards death which we have hitherto so carefully suppressed?" (p. 299).

To find peace, we must face up to existential issues, overcome our personal upbringing, and learn to live without soothing psychological defenses. In a sense, we must mourn our own end to fully accept and value our lives. There is no way to banish painful memories and feelings from consciousness without losing our sense of humanity and feeling of compassion for others. An individual *can* overcome personal limitations and embrace life in the face of death anxiety. Such a person would find no need for ethnic hatred or insidious warfare.

ENDNOTES

1. In *Two Nations: Black and White, Separate, Hostile, Unequal,* Hacker (1992) points out that African Americans are outside the mainstream in America's economy and that their civil rights are not safeguarded. Moynihan (1993) in *Pandaemonium: Ethnicity in International Politics* urges a discipline or study of ethnicity—an understanding of the forces of nationalism, class, and race that contribute to ethnic conflict.

2. My understanding of human aggression also takes into account social learning theory (Bandura & Walters, 1963; Berkowitz, 1989). Okey (1992) reviewed diverse theoretical ap-

proaches to aggressive behavior in his article "Human Aggression: The Etiology of Individual Differences."

3. Janine Chasseguet-Smirgel's (1975/1985) formulations seek to explicate the development of the ego ideal during the pre-Oedipal phases. Her chapter "The Ego Ideal and the Group" sets forth a conceptualization of group dynamics that differs from Freud's. She argues that group phenomena can be explained as an acting-out of regressive fantasies of merger with the mother figure: "As far as Nazism is concerned, the return to nature, to ancient Germanic mythology represents an aspiration to fusion with the omnipotent mother" (p. 83).

4. See Bettelheim's account (1943/1979) of this phenomenon, where prisoners in a German concentration camp imagined they could survive as a group on one occasion where they were required to stand all night in subfreezing temperatures. More than 80 perished, but survivors reported that during the event they "felt free from fear and therefore were actually happier than at most other times during their camp experiences" (p. 65).

5. Studies conducted by Tajfel, Flament, Billig, and Bundy (cited by Turner, 1978) also showed that "the variable of social categorization per se is sufficient as well as necessary to induce forms of ingroup favouritism and discrimination against the outgroup" (p. 101). Turner expanded Tajfel's work by including social competition as an important factor influencing group discrimination.

6. Rheinhold Niebuhr (1944) in *The Children of Light and the Children of Darkness* addressed the theme of ethnic pride, prejudice, and defenses against death anxiety. He stated,

> Racial prejudice, the contempt of the other group, is an inevitable concomitant of racial pride; and racial pride is an inevitable concomitant of the ethnic will to live. . . . Human life is never content with mere physical survival. There are spiritual elements in every human survival impulse; and the corruption of these elements is pride and the will-to-power. (p. 139)

7. A special subcase of group bias can be observed in "identity politics," prevalent on American campuses and in the workplace. Gitlin (1993), noting this separatist movement, declared, "The long overdue opening of political initiative to minorities, women, gays, and others of the traditionally voiceless has developed its own methods of silencing" (p. 172).

8. In *The Tyranny of Malice,* Berke (1988) related psychodynamics to social psychology in showing how envy, greed, and jealousy extend to cultural imperatives operating between nations. See Chapter 11, "National Pride," in which Berke stated, "Nationalism is to the State what narcissism is to the individual. It is a form of national narcissism, the expression of a perverted or pathological self-absorption and pride" (p. 258).

9. Kerr and Bowen (1988) noted that societies can become regressive as the force for togetherness and lower differentiation of self of its members become more prominent during times of stress and chronic anxiety.

10. This pattern persists today in reunited Germany, where angry hordes have been conducting demonstrations against foreigners in the same aggressive style (Grass, 1993; Joffe, 1993; Kahn, 1993).

11. Fromm's (1941) *Escape From Freedom* and Shirer's (1960) *The Rise and Fall of the Third Reich* document the impact of various social forces and historical events on the German people. A particularly cogent description of these phenomena can be found in Shirer's "The Mind of Hitler and the Roots of the Third Reich" (pp. 80-113), in which he traces the psychological underpinnings of a "German personality type" to the Thirty Years' War and the Peace of Westphalia in 1648. Shirer states that "Germany never recovered from this setback. Acceptance of autocracy, of blind obedience to the petty tyrants who ruled as princes, became ingrained in the German mind" (p. 92). In Fromm's book, see Chapter 4, "Freedom in the Age of Reformation," as well as Chapter 6, "The Psychology of Nazism," which traces the roots of the willingness on the part of many people to submit to totalitarian rule, resulting in Germany's policies of aggression and "ethnic cleansing."

12. Until 1991, under the influence of a powerful leader and united against a common enemy since World War II, these warring groups in Yugoslavia lived together in peace.

13. David Owen (1993) traced one factor in the Balkan conflict to the massacre of the Serbians by the Germans and some Croatians and Muslims in the 1940s: "Now the Serbian political leaders are reminding every Serb of all those past misdeeds to justify new ones" (p. 7). Puhar (1993) documented child-rearing practices in southern Yugoslavia: "The two countries [in Europe] with the highest infant mortality rates have so far (in 1990) been unable to produce successful democratic movements: Yugoslavia (28.8) and Albania (44.8) [per 1,000 live births]" (p. 375).

18

The "Good Life"

M y concept of the "good life" is not founded on moral precepts or philosophical systems; rather, it is based on sound principles of mental hygiene deduced from clinical practice and empirical research. An understanding of the internal and external forces that are confining, toxic, or demoralizing to human beings has led me and my associates to speculate about the type and quality of experience that would be conducive to people's well-being and therefore growth enhancing. Although this chapter represents a broadening of my perspective, the generalizations still apply on a clinical level. Indeed, people who have adopted the tenets of the "good life" to varying degrees have progressed in every aspect of their personality functioning.

Human beings exist in a state of conflict between the active pursuit of their goals in the real world and an inward, self-protective defense system characterized by reliance on fantasy gratification and manifestations of self-nurturance. The more an individual is damaged in early life experiences, the less willing he or she is to undertake the risks necessary for self-actualization. The resolution of the core conflict in the direction of a defended lifestyle has a profound negative effect on an individual's overall functioning. The defended person's life is significantly distorted by a desperate clinging to addictive attachments, a dependence on self-nourishing habit patterns, strong guilt reactions, low self-esteem, and a distrust of others, whereas, ideally, an undefended or mentally healthy individual exists in a state of continual change, moving toward increased autonomy and enjoying more satisfying relationships.

The autonomous individual generally feels more integrated, has a stronger sense of self and a greater potential for intimacy, and is more humane toward others. However, the mentally healthy person, who is relatively free of symptoms and the compulsion to repeat familiar destructive patterns, must live with a heightened sense of vulnerability and a more acute sensitivity to emotionally painful situations and ontological anxiety.

Individuals who are open and less defended appear to be responsibly reactive to events in their lives that impinge on their well-being. There is a poignant and painful reaction to life's tragic aspects, and there tends to be an increase in an awareness of death anxiety, that is, these people are investing in a life they know they must certainly lose. I perceive that positive movement toward health and adjustment implies moving *away* from defenses, support systems, and painkillers in the direction of openness, feeling, and emotional responsiveness, while changing from an inward, self-parenting posture to an active pursuit of gratification in the external world.

The feeling inherent in being a separate adult person can be exhilarating. It can be compared to sailing on uncharted seas, where one always faces the unexpected—without guidelines, without established regimens, but with complete responsibility for one's destiny. One needs courage for the voyage, but one's reward is an adventurous life—the "good life."

The process of identifying the dictates of the voice and regaining feeling for oneself leads to the development of countermeasures—ways of living and being that challenge the tendency to relive the past rather than live one's current life. The "good life" enables the individual to live out his or her unique human potentiality closely following his or her true destiny, that of preserving rather than distorting or blocking out experience, while maintaining feeling contact with oneself, compassion for others, and a deep appreciation of the richness of life. The process of individuation or breaking with the past allows a person to gradually develop his or her capacity to love and be loved and predisposes him or her to pursue activities and goals that imbue life with meaning.

The "good life" represents a natural evolution of Voice Therapy. The dimensions of the lifestyle implied here are based on an understanding of the voice process and the damaging effect of internalized prescriptions for living. The methods of Voice Therapy point toward a style of living that breaks with powerful forces that fracture and distort sensations and emotions, limit personal and vocational successes, and prevent people from fulfilling their natural evolution. Living according to the prescriptions of the voice narrows one's range or life space. The voice predisposes people to reject positive developments over which they have no control and guides them toward negative consequences that are more under their control. Internalized voices restrict life, condemn sexuality, foster prejudice toward others, and turn individuals against themselves.

To the extent that people recover feeling for themselves, they are exposed to a world that is perpetually new. It is a world in which life is open-ended, a real adventure, as contrasted with a manipulative molding of one's interpersonal environment to fit the past. It is as if a person who is well-defended and whose feelings are cut off lives life in a single room. When he or she is emancipated and finally able to fling the doors open, a whole new landscape is revealed.

The essential preconditions for embarking on this adventure are, first, making a wholehearted commitment to life and, second, learning to give oneself value. The process of fully embracing life, to the best of one's ability, regardless of the circumstances in which one finds oneself, ennobles the individual. Taking a stand in relation to this issue lifts people out of the doldrums and routine of everyday life and elevates them to a higher level of existence.

The second precondition, learning to value oneself, is a difficult undertaking because the capacity to see oneself as worthwhile and one's life as having intrinsic value is often seriously damaged during the formative years. For this reason, freeing oneself of one's early programming, separating out conventional, constricted ways of thinking from a nonjudgmental way of perceiving, becomes an important ongoing pursuit. Learning to direct one's gaze outward, rather than looking inward (i.e., perceiving the world through the filter of past distortions) transforms one's perspective on self, others, and the world.

At the same time, one must appreciate that movement toward emotional health and an undefended state temporarily increases one's guilt and fear. It is not an easy task to break with one's initial programming and there can be no growth without anxiety. It takes courage to brave the new world and take the necessary risks involved in deviating from one's original identity within the family.

Guilt reactions associated with increased individuation and the disruption of the fantasy bond with one's family are based on many families' distorted perceptions of independence as rejecting or defiant. Instead of supporting the special priorities of the individual, they perceive them as disloyal and alien. Because of these defensive and condemning reactions, an individual's movement toward autonomy initially leads to intensified voice attacks. The optimistic fact is that when people refuse to submit or alter their behavior based on these attacks and, in a sense, do not "obey" the introjected parent, the attacks will eventually subside.

Most people are imprisoned in the defended state to varying degrees, because they are certain that their anxiety will overwhelm them if they give up their defenses. It is difficult to convince them emotionally of what they themselves know intellectually, that now as adults they have more control over their lives and that their fears could never be of the same magnitude as those that overpowered them as children and originally caused them to become defended. The anticipatory anxiety of stepping out of the self-protective mode becomes more understandable when viewed from this vantage point.

People need courage to live without their customary defenses. It is necessary for them to take risks before they have a chance to live out their destiny as unique individuals. They must throw away their crutches, so to speak, before they can find out if they can walk without them. Living the "good life" involves a complex process of acculturation. Having evolved toward a richer, warmer, more growth-enhancing way of living, an individual must adapt to the vast difference between this new world and the world he or she knew as a child.

As emphasized in the previous chapter, human beings have demonstrated their potential for aggression, greed, and territoriality throughout history, phenomena that led Freud to postulate the death instinct as an explanatory principle. Theorists have tended to deemphasize other qualities that are uniquely and essentially human, such as the capacity for deep feeling, rationality, the ability to use abstract symbols, compassion for self and others, and the compelling search for knowledge, truth, and meaning in life.

The fundamental problem is that these uniquely human attributes are programmed out of the child to varying degrees, while frustration-derived aggression is cultured in. Because of their personal limitations, most parents unwittingly transform an extraordinary creature into an ordinary creature. They offer the gift of life, then take it back. In attempting to socialize their children, they deprive them of their humanity. Despite their best intentions, parents subdue or stamp out the very qualities that distinguish their children from animals.

Regrettably, the socialization process as practiced in most nuclear families categorizes, standardizes, and puts the stamp of conformity on children. It imposes a negative structure, a self-regulating system, that cuts deeply into their feeling reactions and conditions their thoughts and behaviors to meet certain accepted standards. Thereafter, children continue to impose the same structure and programming on themselves in the form of a restrictive, self-punishing voice process. Children imitate their parents' defenses and take on parental prohibitions as their own. To protect themselves from emotional pain and distress, they develop self-nurturing, self-punishing patterns that progressively cut off feeling for themselves and their real experiences in life.

Societies are constantly evolving. Over the millennia, people have created increasingly complex institutions, conventions, belief systems, and sanctions. Each generation has been reared by people whose ancestors were themselves reared by parents who chose to dull their psychological pain and subsequently lived defensively and retreated from investing in their lives. As a result, most adults remain prisoners of their internal programming and pass this on to succeeding generations.

Internalized voices represent the language of parental and cultural restrictions on one's humanness. The patterns of the voice are the key to the defensive processes that lead to self-denial, negative self-attitudes, moralistic, judgmental views, and conformity. Challenging parental prohibitions through Voice Therapy is conducive to maintaining freedom of action in relation to self and others, and reawakens the desire to search for knowledge and meaning in life.

> By understanding how pain and neurosis are passed down from generation to generation, they [people] might decide to break that chain. They could choose to live by an implicit code of morality that . . . doesn't fracture their feelings and experiences or those of others, a morality that enhances their well-being and personal development . . . creating a society that is sensitive to the emotional and psychological fulfillment of its members. (R. Firestone & Catlett, 1989, p. 14)

Those who break the chain are among the unsung heroes throughout the history of humankind.

DIMENSIONS OF THE GOOD LIFE

Each dimension of the good life challenges the way that people impose unnecessary suffering on themselves. Several aspects of this lifestyle can be described. The dimensions are not distinct categories; their manifestations in each area of an individual's life overlap to a considerable extent. However, they can be delineated as follows: (a) autonomy and individuation, (b) affiliation with others, (c) openness and nondefensiveness, (d) the search for meaning and transcendental goals, and (e) spirituality.

Autonomy and Individuation

In the context of the good life, the highest value is placed on the unique self of the individual above any system, whether the couple, the family, religion, the political system, the community, nation, or philosophy. I emphasize movement toward increased individuation and emancipation from destructive ties to family or institutions. Individuation in this sense involves developing a strong sense of self and maintaining distinct boundaries in close relationships.

Autonomy is achieved through the reflective formulation of one's own internal value system rather than a mindless, automatic acceptance of beliefs and values thrust on us by another person, persons, or systems. Only when people are possessed of self, that is, centered in themselves and truly individualistic, are they predisposed to make significant contributions to others and to the community.

Individual freedom and respect for the freedom of others are viewed as congruent, not contradictory values. When people give themselves value and cherish their own experiences, they naturally extend this same appreciation to others and to *their* experiences.

To be close to another person, one has to risk living as a separate person outside one's defense system. No one can become one with another. The closest one can feel to another person is to feel one's separateness, which is an integral part of the sensitive, tender feeling toward the other.

Deep and intimate relationships are fulfilling only when they are not restrictive. In a truly loving couple, each partner recognizes that the motives, desires, and aspirations of the other are as important as his or her own. Loving implies an enjoyment of the other person's emergence as an individual and a sensitivity to his or her wants and motives. Each partner feels congenial toward the other's aspirations and tries not to interfere, intrude, or manipulate to dominate or control the relationship. Marital relationships and other intimate associations that are based on respect for each other's independence and freedom are continually evolving rather than static.

In a healthy relationship, the partners would be nondefensive, open, and self-reliant. The relationship would be inclusive of friends and extended family, rather than an exclusive, closed system. Each partner would possess a strong sense of identity, be nonintrusive, and would not speak for the other. It has been my experience that the more people develop their individuality and give up the false security of a fantasy bond, the greater the opportunity they have for genuine security in relationships built on honest choices and priorities. When they face their real aloneness instead of maintaining illusions of connection, they have a sense of freedom and strength. Most people have known that kind of feeling at one time or another; however, most have rejected it when it became too frightening.

Parents who are committed to nurturing their offspring would attempt to serve their children's best interests rather than try to mold their lives and personalities in a predetermined direction. They would refrain from foisting their interests on their children and would expose them to a wealth of experiences and let them discover their own interests.

Ideally, children would be valued for their uniqueness and emerging individuality. They would be respected and treated as separate human beings, that is, not intruded upon or dealt with as possessions. They need to be "left alone" in the best sense and allowed to feel that they are individuals in their own rights, distinct from others. Their development depends primarily on the strength, independence, and personal integrity of their parents because children learn most readily through imitation.

Parents would support their children's interest in forming friendships outside the family circle. They would avoid promoting a false sense of togetherness and a merged identity that is detrimental to the child's sense of independence. They would encourage their children to speak up, to say what they see, and to ask questions about so-called forbidden subjects. By permitting the child the maximum freedom possible at each age level, parents would be implicitly expressing a belief in his or her inherent potential for making healthy choices and capacity for self-discipline.

Nothing is more conducive to mental health and a true moral position than people seeking the full development of their potential and pursuing their own goals in a direct manner. The attempt to take personal power[1] rather than adopting a victimized, self-denying posture leads to a life of integrity and consequently allows others to pursue their goals without guilt.

There is a definite correlation between individuals seeking personal power and a social order of implicit morality that would be conducive to the personal growth and development of all its members. In a society supportive of the straightforward pursuit of goals, an individual would feel valued for him- or herself, listened to, and recognized for his or her personal attributes. People are capable of handling personal freedom and equality without rampant anarchy or authoritarian rule based on surplus power.

Affiliation With Others

Friendship. The desire and need for social affiliation is a basic human quality; therefore, living in harmony with friends and family in an atmosphere of congeniality and personal communication is preeminent.[2] Close friendship, which stands in opposition to a fantasy bond, has therapeutic value. It provides companionship that is nonintrusive and nonobligatory, qualities that lead to self-awareness and encourage a person to emerge from an inward or isolated posture. Meaningful interaction with a close friend on a daily basis diminishes "voice" attacks and significantly interferes with neurotic tendencies to be self-denying and self-hating. It is important to have a close friend who possesses the qualities to which one aspires. Emulating the qualities of an admirable person and using him or her as an ally is a significant step toward developing one's own sense of values and transcending goals.

---

1 *Personal power,* as distinguished from personal power plays, manipulation, and control of others, refers to taking control of one's life and being direct in the pursuit of one's goals.

2 Findings from recent research in the field of evolutionary psychology emphasize the importance of these positive qualities and potentialities. According to Robert Wright (1995), researchers have noted that since social cooperation increased primitive man's chances of survival, natural selection must have shaped our minds so that we seek friendship, affection, and trust: tendencies referred to by evolutionary psychologists as reciprocal altruism.

Friendships with both men and women are appreciated for what they offer in terms of developing the various dimensions of one's personality. In close associations with members of both sexes, an individual is able to discover aspects of his or her personality that may never have been uncovered in friendships limited to one or the other gender.

Sexuality. The ultimate expression of sexuality is a natural extension of affectionate, friendly feelings rather than an activity isolated from other aspects of a relationship. It is a fulfilling part of life, a gift, a positive offering of pleasure to another and to oneself. Sex plays an important part in the life of the healthy individual, not in the exaggerated sense as conceptualized by a sexually repressive and perverted culture but as a simple human experience. When accompanied by authentic love and tenderness, sex is a high form of expression, approaching a spiritual level. However, interfering with sexuality, attempting to program it out of people's lives, tends to increase frustration and pain, which, in turn, can lead to hostile acting out of aggressive impulses.

In a healthy relationship, the sexual relating is spontaneous and close emotionally, rather than addictive, impersonal, and mechanical. The combination of loving, sexual contact and genuine friendship in a stable, long-lasting relationship is conducive to good mental health and is a highly regarded ideal for most people. The effect of a natural expression of sexuality on one's sense of well-being and overall enjoyment of life cannot be overemphasized. The way people feel about themselves as men and women, the feelings they have about their bodies, and their attitudes toward sex can contribute more to a sense of self and feeling of happiness than any other area of experience.

Openness and Nondefensiveness

Openness and nondefensiveness tend to lead an individual to a deep appreciation of life as a gift, a unique opportunity, an adventure. The only sensible thing to do with this gift of existence is to live a life of integrity and attempt to find one's personal meaning, instead of following prescriptions, belief systems, and dogma imposed from external sources. In living an open and spontaneous life, people are moving toward freedom of choice rather than restricting choice. Movement toward the unknown and unfamiliar is both frightening and exciting as it brings out new dimensions of the personality, but all things considered, it is always alive as contrasted with the deadening effect of nonreflective conventionality.

Within the context of the "good life," an individual is involved in a process of continually *finding* him- or herself rather than *defining* him- or herself. Identity is essentially a flexible and evolving variable rather than a fixed or stable entity. The project of coming to know oneself, discovering one's likes and dislikes, wants and priorities, dreams and fantasies, becomes a fascinating, lifelong enterprise.

The pursuit of self-knowledge presupposes willingness on the part of an individual to come to grips with aspects of his or her personality that may be painful to face. In overcoming their defenses and limitations, it is essential that people gradually modify themselves instead of being critical of their own weaknesses or shortcomings. Thereafter, the task becomes one of representing themselves honestly to others and becoming sensitive and nondefensive about feedback. To achieve this level of personal honesty and integrity, they need to develop an acute awareness of any remnants of falseness or insincerity in themselves. The individual becomes like the musician who, hearing a sour note that grates on his or her nerves, carefully fine-tunes his or her instrument.

In providing the most nurturing environment for their offspring, parents should include other individuals who could be of potential value to the child. An extended family with extended concern for children offers circumstances in which the needs of the child are carefully and conscientiously attended to. An extended family can be defined as consisting of one or more adults in addition to the child's natural parents who maintain consistent contact and interest in the child's well-being over a significant period of time. A close friend, a favorite relative, a godparent, a "Big Brother" or "Big Sister," a teacher or school counselor may fall into this category. Close association with people other than the child's parents or siblings acts to compensate for parents' fears and inadequacies. The extended family situation offers a variety of inputs, points of view different from the parents', that expand the child's world and give him or her an enlarged perspective and a more realistic picture of life. This type of family relationship offers the child an ally, a person in whom he or she can confide, an adult who is relatively unbiased and objective concerning the child's relationship with his or her parents. In addition, children in an extended family setting are generally free of the exaggerated proprietary interest most parents have in their children.

It is of the utmost importance for a child to learn to trust his or her perceptions. This trust can only be achieved in an honest atmosphere. Parents' integrity and truthfulness are necessary for survival in the emotional or psychological sense, just as food and drink are necessary for physical survival. In fulfilling this need, parents would respond as real people to their children rather than role-playing or acting patronizing, strategic, or phony in their interactions with them. Mixed signals and dishonesty disturb the child's reality testing (Bateson et al., 1956/1972).

Children need adults who relate to them directly; they need people who are open with them about their real thoughts and feelings. Children search the faces of their parents and other adults for genuine feeling contact. They have strong needs to feel the humanity of their parents, to see beyond the roles of "Father" and "Mother." When parents dispense with roles and behave in a manner that is natural or personal, they are experienced by their children as human and lovable. Children desperately need to be allowed to feel love *for* their parents; if they are deprived of this opportunity, it causes them unbearable pain.

People need a forum for honest communication, an arena where the opinions of each member, including those of children, are listened to and respected. It is crucial that this encourages the expression of feelings in addition to the verbalization of diverse points of view. Unfortunately, the public display of emotions has been traditionally unacceptable, even in the most open and democratic settings.

With respect to communication between family members, discrepancies between words and actions are capable of creating mental disturbance in children. Lies and illusions can fracture the child's sense of reality, whereas any event or feeling, within reason, can be understood and contended with by most children. When parents are frank, yet sensitive, in talking with their children about taboo subjects, including sexuality, death, "family secrets," and their (own) weaknesses, the results are constructive rather than harmful.

Parents who are honest in their communication with their offspring in relation to their own limitations minimize the tendency that *most* children have to idealize their parents and family to their own detriment. In this situation, children would rarely have to listen to rationalizations such as the familiar, "Your father really loves you, he just has a hard time showing it," or "Your mother only has your best interests at heart," when, in fact, the father is indifferent and the mother controlling.

In contemporary society, it is rare for a person to maintain an adult level of communication with another person, whether child or adult. A respectful dialogue pertaining to real issues without coercion, manipulation, or parent-child role-playing is difficult to come by. When people are strongly defended, adult communication (uncomplicated by phoniness, dishonesty, and efforts to make points) becomes almost impossible.

The Search for Meaning and Transcendental Goals

A fundamental part of the organization of a human being, one that transcends his or her primary needs, is a search for meaning and understanding of life. The unknown, the ambiguous, stimulates our concern, and we have the need to search for meaning beyond our everyday existence. As noted earlier, I agree with Viktor Frankl's (1946/1959) assertion that the direct pursuit of happiness as an end in itself is doomed to failure. Happiness is only attainable incidentally, as a by-product of one's search for meaning and one's commitment to leading an invigorating and significant life. In other words, the search for meaning is primary.

When people are involved in transcendental goals, goals that go beyond their everyday functions, they gain a sense of purpose and of valuing themselves that cannot be achieved by any other means. Thus being generous, compassionate, and concerned with others has a positive effect on mental health in general and leads to a truthful moral philosophy.

Spirituality

Love.

> To love one another, truly, is to walk in the light, to live in truth, to be truly alive, and perfectly free. Otherwise we walk in darkness, live in the lie, are living lies, ignorant, blind, deaf, lame, crooked, diseased, mad, dead, in the body of death, in hell, on earth. Without the grace to love we do not realise this. (Laing, 1989, quoting from *Fürchte deinen Nächsten wie dich Selbs*t by Paul Parin, 1978)

Love is the major force in life that counters existential pain and despair. Loving others helps compensate for the anguish and torment inherent in the human condition. The "good life" is one in which a person gradually develops the capacity to offer and accept love. Loving relationships are characterized by concern and respect for each other's sensibilities and priorities. Real affection involves outward expressions and behaviors as well as positive or tender internal feelings. Many people maintain a fantasy of love (fantasy bond) while their external behavior does not fit any acceptable meaning of the word.

It is more important to love than to be loved. The person who extends him-or herself in love and generosity toward others benefits more from the exchange than the beloved. The lover experiences powerful rewarding reactions to the process of loving another that are purely selfish in a sense, whereas the beloved often suffers from the pain and fear of allowing him- or herself to be loved. Learning to give and receive love, understanding that personal gratification is inherent in simply loving another, rather than looking for some other benefit or reward for one's love, is important in developing and maintaining good relationships. The reward is in the personal feeling; being allowed to love another permits a person to feel good about him- or herself.

Belief system and philosophy. An important emphasis of the good life is placed on searching for and finding one's own faith, that is, developing a personal belief system and inner set of values. In searching for meaning, there is a concern for and understanding of the types of experiences that damage the human spirit. Wherever there is an absence of fact, a person has the right to choose and fully embrace beliefs about the origin and nature of life, the way to live, and issues relating to death or rebirth.

The "good life" involves seeking the "god" within oneself rather than outside oneself. One's belief system or "religion" would not consist of projections of parental images but would deal with how to live one's present life. It would not be prescriptive of any singular way of leading the "good life" but would be suggestive of ways that people could realize their potential as creators of their own philosophy of life.

Finally, it would be a religion open to the mystery of life rather than closed, dogmatic, or disrespectful of human rights. There would be genuine regard and understanding of people with different views or beliefs.

CHARACTERISTICS OF THE UNDEFENDED INDIVIDUAL

I have found that when people become less defended and more open to feeling, important changes are manifested in their overall approach to life. They tend to develop a depth of compassion and a basic trust in others that have a powerful effect on their relationships. The toxic, intrusive behaviors that were acted out previously in close personal interactions are diminished to a remarkable degree. Consequently, they begin to have a positive influence on friends and family, rather than continuing to have a detrimental effect.

The healthy individual is continually evolving in his or her choice of love objects. He or she gradually moves toward selecting a partner who is more willing to accept love and to respond with affection. He or she tends to move away from relationships that are pernicious and that act to shut off his or her loving feelings, and there is corresponding movement toward those people who inspire feelings of tenderness and love. At the same time, the mentally healthy person refrains from acting out any behavior that would control or elicit a response from another person through manipulation of the other's feelings of guilt, anger, pity, sympathy, or remorse.

People living a less defended existence look very different from defended individuals. It is a difference in a positive direction, away from the cultural norm. In society, one can see the defensive posture of most people etched in their faces and bodies. On the other hand, when one is vulnerable and open, one's noticeable attributes such as healthy posture, attractiveness, happiness, generosity, and friendliness show up in one's countenance and expressive movements. People's vitality, energy, and the state of being fully alive are manifested in a warm, friendly glance, softness of expression, a great deal of eye contact and personal relating, and a state of relaxation and calmness, as distinguished from agitation or emotional deadness.

In relation to physical pain, it appears that mentally healthy individuals suffer far less from psychosomatic illness, such as migraine headaches, asthma, or chronic neurasthenia. On the other hand, they may experience a heightened sensitivity to physical pain and generally feel more appropriate concern about their physical health and well-being.

Overall, the psychologically healthy person has a strong emotional investment in living and responds with appropriate affect to both good and bad experiences. Individuals who are connected to their emotions tend to retain their vitality and excitement about living. The capacity for feeling contributes to their spontaneity and creativity and adds dimensions to their personality. By contrast, people who do not have access to their inner experience tend to be more rigid, constricted, and superficial.

An important characteristic in the undefended person's value system is an intolerance of any discrepancy between his or her words and actions. There is also a strong bias against evaluating or judging others, without taking into account their complexity, feeling, or humanness. Any attempt to label, categorize, pigeonhole, or define people, positively or negatively, or to standardize or homogenize personal responses is offensive to the healthy individual. He or she is cognizant that judgments, categorizations, and attributions of goodness and badness to others halt the free flow of feeling between people. Healthy people allow themselves the freedom to take risks in the interpersonal environment, reacting personally and spontaneously, without prejudgment, to significant events and interactions, both positive and negative, in their lives.

People who are relatively undefended are self-directed rather than seeking direction from outside sources. Their commitment is to expanding self-awareness and self-knowledge, to developing an internal system of values, and living a life of integrity according to these values. In developing their own values, they come to know themselves and the many dimensions of their personality. They become progressively more aware of their wants and aspirations and make a concerted effort to direct their actions toward fulfilling their own personal and vocational goals rather than automatically living out parental directives. In pursuing their priorities as well as living by their values, they set the course for their lives rather than remaining passengers on a "rudderless ship."

Self-directed individuals seek a balance between work and their personal lives and consider both to be of equal importance. Similarly, they strive to create an environment for themselves and their loved ones that is optimal for the realization of each person's full potential.

EXISTENTIAL CONCERNS

In remaining vulnerable, people learn to face the fear of death openly without compensation or defenses and to mourn the anticipated loss of self. Their appreciation of life and the human condition gives their lives a poignant meaning in relation to its finality. They have a feeling of compassion and kinship with other people who are undergoing the same experience. Knowing that all human beings face the same fate, they perceive no person as inferior or superior to themselves, no one of greater or lesser status or importance, although others may reflect different cultural, religious, or ethnic backgrounds.

Sadness about one's ultimate loss of self and loved ones is an inescapable part of a feelingful existence, not in the sense of having a morbid preoccupation with dying but with a consciousness of limitation in time. Recognizing and living with these existential truths enhance those precious and irretrievable moments we spend with our loved ones. This awareness can serve to remind us how vital it is *not* to damage the feelings of others, their self-respect, special qualities and desires, and the spirit in which they approach life and invest it with their own personal meaning.

CONCLUSION

Human beings have concerns about their future, curiosity about the mysteries of existence, and a drive for self-expression that matches their basic drive for food or sex. From the beginning of time, they have demonstrated a creative urge that has been expressed through art, music, and science. However, most people have been taught to turn away from the basic strivings that are essential for living the "good life" (Endnote 1). Their curiosity, their quest for self-knowledge, and their desire to search for meaning have been damaged to varying degrees. A materialistic, conformist, hard line has been substituted for a feeling existence. In adopting a defensive lifestyle, most people no longer exhibit the qualities that are uniquely human.

Admittedly, it is difficult to inspire people to take an interest in themselves because they have disconnected from themselves to varying degrees in the process of growing up. Depending on the extent of trauma they suffered, they are content to be indecisive, not to have a clear-cut point of view, not to have a sense of direction in their lives. They have "adjusted" to a life directed by internalized voices (parental prescriptions) and external values, and are content to lead a subhuman existence. Most therapists do not appreciate this painful truth; they are not aware of how deeply their patients have incorporated the defense systems of their parents and how fearful they are of living without these defenses.

Although all forms of psychotherapy challenge defenses to varying degrees, ultimately they are limited by the therapist's own defense system. Often this defense system is supported by the methods, theory, and systems the therapist chooses to apply in his or her practice. (In contrast, it is difficult for the therapist to find refuge in Voice Therapy theory. It appears that fully applying the concepts of the theory to oneself is the ultimate challenge.) Practitioners who place social conformity or social adjustment above the personal interests of their patients perform a great disservice. Therapeutic methodologies that serve to protect the social process that originally caused damage to the patient are perverse and paradoxical.

My therapeutic approach does not attempt to adjust people to a society or social system; rather, its major thrust is to adjust the social process to enhance the individual, that is, people going beyond themselves and structuring a way of life or community that would reflect back in a healthy way on others. My approach supports individuation as a goal, helping human beings to develop their special qualities, to lead an adventurous life within their own priorities and value system.

Voice Therapy focuses on the core issues of interpersonal and existential pain in people's everyday lives. Practitioners of Voice Therapy are deeply concerned with whether individuals are living out *their* lives and fulfilling *their* destinies, or repeating patterns of the past and reliving their parents' lives.

The more people break with negative parental prescriptions for living, the greater the opportunity they have for fulfilling their own destiny. The more they give up their crutches, the soothing mechanisms of their lives, their self-nourishing habits and deadening routines, the more they are able to embrace the "good life." Voice Therapy theory implies a reawakening of an interest in oneself and in one's search for meaning. The methodology suggests ways to lead a better life based on acting against the dictates of internal voices. My associates and I feel that Voice Therapy and Separation Theory represent a major advancement in the field of psychotherapy in that they explain the basic dynamics of resistance in psychotherapy, synthesize psychoanalytic and existential concepts, and reveal the essential truth about defense formation and its detrimental effect on our human experience.

ENDNOTE

1. The following commentary on the problems inherent in the search for the "good life" is excerpted from a literary analysis by Dr. Stuart Boyd (1982), former liberal arts tutor and clinical psychologist, St John's College, Santa Fe:

A 'better life' is clearly a phrase somewhere close to the surface in the sea of human words. . . . Attempts at change in the longed-for direction are directed at the outside socio-political organization, and the inside psychological organization. Change the outside, redistribute equably the goods and resources of the world within a political structure that allows for this, and the human soul will regenerate to harmony and happiness, and there will no longer be a need for a governing or political structure. The problem with this generous and loving idea (so it seems to me) is that it overlooks the corruption and deformity of the human soul which inevitably occurs under the usual conditions of Western upbringing, or expects such deformity to correct itself under the new and freeing conditions. Open the cage and the bird will fly to joyous freedom. Birds raised in cages? Human birds? Would it were so.

Perhaps we could change the outside, not by opening or removing the cage, but by restructuring it so that there is room for all kinds of birds, each functioning in accordance with its proper design and purpose, each doing what it was best designed to do, in a hierarchy with the few wisest birds organizing all from the top, but in such a way that none felt directed, because of the felt justice of doing what one was designed best to do. . . . But the lie is there, and offends.

Again we may change the outside by having the caged creatures choose their leaders within a constitutional framework guaranteeing them life, liberty, and the pursuit of happiness and the freest range to change and climb, or fall, to other levels. Would not perhaps the changing and climbing become identified with or obscure the pursuit of happiness? By the time the quest begins in adult life the damage may have been done and the pressured equality has gone, and the freedom to compete against oneself to become the best self has given way to competition against others.

Bruno Bettelheim (1982) also has written about his beliefs regarding dimensions of the "good life":

> The love for others—the working of eternal Eros—finds its expression in the relations we form with those who are important to us and in what we do to make a better life, a better world for them. The goal is not an impossible utopia. . . . A good life denies neither its real and often painful difficulties nor the dark aspects of our psyche. (p. 110)

Appendix:
Supplemental
Resource Material

AVAILABLE FROM THE GLENDON ASSOCIATION

Supplement to *Combating Destructive Thought Processes: Separation Theory and Voice Therapy* by Robert W. Firestone: A comparative review of the author's theoretical position with respect to psychoanalytic and object relations theory

Documentary Videos
(produced by the Glendon Association and Geoff Parr)

Overall Theoretical Approach:

The Fantasy Bond Video Supplement (1985)

"Inwardness": A Retreat From Feeling (1995)*

Voice Therapy: Theory and Methodology:

Voice Therapy With Dr. Robert Firestone (1984)*

Videotapes for Professional
Training in Voice Therapy Methodology:

Voice Therapy: A Group Session (1986)
"Sonya"—An Individual Session (1992)
Voice Therapy Session: A New Perspective on the Oedipal Complex (1992)
Voice Therapy: A Training Session (1992)

Couple Relationships and Sexuality:

Closeness Without Bonds (1986)*
Bobby and Rosie: Anatomy of a Marriage (1989)*
Sex & Marriage (1990)
Sex & Society: Everyday Abuses to Children's Emerging Sexuality (1989)

Professional Training Videotapes:

Sex & Society: Part II (1990)
Voices in Sex (1990)
Voices About Relationships (1995)

Compassionate Child-Rearing—Resources for Parents:

The Inner Voice in Child Abuse (1986)*
Parental Ambivalence (1987)
Hunger Versus Love: A Perspective on Parent-Child Relations (1987)
The Implicit Pain of Sensitive Child-Rearing (1988)
Children of the Summer (1993)
Invisible Child Abuse (1994)
Teaching Our Children About Feelings (1984)

Professional Training Videotape:

Therapeutic Child-Rearing: An In-Depth Approach to Compassionate Parenting (1987)

Existential Issues:

Defenses Against Death Anxiety (1990)
Life, Death & Denial (1990)

Suicidology:

The Inner Voice in Suicide (1985)*
Microsuicide: A Case Report (1985)*
Teenagers Talk About Suicide (1987)*

Compassionate Child-Rearing:
A Parenting Education Program

Instructors' guidelines, parents' workbooks, videotapes, and in-service training for professionals who offer parent education classes

AVAILABLE FROM THE PSYCHOLOGICAL CORPORATION

The Firestone Assessment of Self-Destructive Thoughts (FAST), a new instrument useful as a screener for persons entering psychological treatment. FAST scores indicate areas in which the client is experiencing the greatest degree of distress, allowing the clinician to focus his or her interventions.

---

*Discussion videotape also available.

References

Abramson, L. Y., Metalsky, G. I., & Alloy, L. B. (1989). Hopelessness depression: A theory-based subtype of depression. *Psychological Review, 96,* 358-372.

Achte, K. A. (1980). The psychopathology of indirect self-destruction. In N. L. Farberow (Ed.), *The many faces of suicide: Indirect self-destructive behavior* (pp. 41-56). New York: McGraw-Hill.

Adams, J. W. (1978). *Psychoanalysis of drug dependence: The understanding and treatment of a particular form of pathological narcissism.* New York: Grune & Stratton.

Adorno, T. W., Frenkel-Brunswik, E., Levinson, D. J., & Sanford, R. N. (with B. Aron, M. H. Levinson, & W. Morrow). (1950). *The authoritarian personality.* New York: Harper.

Ainsworth, M. D. (1963). The development of infant-mother interaction among the Ganda. In B. M. Foss (Ed.), *Determinants of infant behaviour II, Proceedings of the Second Tavistock Seminar on Mother-Infant Interaction* (pp. 67-112). London: Methuen.

Ainsworth, M. D. S., Bell, S. M., & Stayton, D. J. (1972). Individual differences in the development of some attachment behaviors. *Merrill-Palmer Quarterly, 18,* 123-144.

Ainsworth, M. D. S., Blehar, M. C., Waters, E., & Wall, S. (1978). *Patterns of attachment: A psychological study of the strange situation.* Hillsdale, NJ: Lawrence Erlbaum.

Akhtar, S., & Parens, H. (Eds.). (1991). *Beyond the symbiotic orbit: Advances in separation-individuation theory.* Hillsdale, NJ: Analytic Press.

Alexander, F. (1961). *The scope of psychoanalysis 1921-1961: Selected papers of Franz Alexander.* New York: Basic Books.

Alexander, I. E., & Adlerstein, A. M. (1965). Affective responses to the concept of death in a population of children and early adolescents. In R. Fulton (Ed.), *Death and identity* (pp. 111-123). New York: John Wiley. (Original work published 1958)

Altemeier, W. A., Vietze, P. M., Sherrod, K. B., Sandler, H. M., Falsey, S., & O'Connor, S. (1979). Prediction of child maltreatment during pregnancy. *Journal of the American Academy of Child Psychiatry, 18,* 205-218.

Anthony, S. (1971). *The discovery of death in childhood and after.* Harmondsworth, England: Penguin Education.

Ardrey, R. (1966). *The territorial imperative: A personal inquiry into the animal origins of property and nations.* New York: Atheneum.

Arieti, S. (1974). *Interpretation of schizophrenia* (2nd ed.). New York: Basic Books.

Autobiography of a schizophrenic girl. (1951). (G. Rubin-Rabson, Trans.). New York: Grune & Stratton.

Bach, G. R., & Deutsch, R. M. (1979). *Stop! You're driving me crazy.* New York: Berkley.

Bach, G. R., & Torbet, L. (1983). *The inner enemy: How to fight fair with yourself.* New York: William Morrow.

Bachman, J. G., & Johnston, L. D. (1978). *The monitoring the future project: Design and procedures* (Monitoring the Future Occasional Paper 1). Ann Arbor: University of Michigan Institute for Social Research.

Badinter, E. (1981). *Mother love: Myth and reality: Motherhood in modern history.* New York: Macmillan. (Original work published 1980)

Bakan, D. (1971). *Slaughter of the innocents.* San Francisco: Jossey-Bass.

Balint, M. (1985). *Primary love and psycho-analytic technique.* London: Maresfield Library. (Original work published 1952)

Bandura, A. (1971). *Psychological modeling: Conflicting theories.* Chicago: Aldine-Atherton.

Bandura, A., & Walters, R. H. (1963). *Social learning and personality development.* New York: Holt, Rinehart & Winston.

Bateson, G. (1972). *Steps to an ecology of mind.* New York: Ballantine.

Bateson, G., Jackson, D. D., Haley, J., & Weakland, J. H. (1972). Toward a theory of schizophrenia. In G. Bateson, *Steps to an ecology of mind* (pp. 201-227). New York: Ballantine. (Original work published 1956)

Beauvoir, S., de. (1976). Epilogue to a very easy death. In E. S. Shneidman (Ed.), *Death: Current perspectives* (pp. 523-526). Palo Alto, CA: Mayfield. (Original work published 1966)

Beavers, W. R., & Hampson, R. B. (1990). *Successful families: Assessment and intervention.* New York: Norton.

Beck, A. T. (1976). *Cognitive therapy and the emotional disorders.* New York: New American Library.

Beck, A. T. (1978). *Beck Hopelessness Scale.* San Antonio: Psychological Corporation.

Beck, A. T. (1988). *Love is never enough.* New York: Harper & Row.

Beck, A. T., Rush, A. J., Shaw, B. F., & Emery, G. (1979). *Cognitive therapy of depression.* New York: Guilford.

Beck, A. T., Steer, R. A., & Brown, G. (1993). Dysfunctional attitudes and suicidal ideation in psychiatric outpatients. *Suicide and Life-Threatening Behavior, 23,* 11-20.

Becker, E. (1962). *The birth and death of meaning: A perspective in psychiatry and anthropology.* New York: Free Press.

Becker, E. (1964). *The revolution in psychiatry: The new understanding of man.* New York: Free Press.

Becker, E. (1973). *The denial of death.* New York: Free Press.

Becker, E. (1975). *Escape from evil.* New York: Free Press.

Bell, C. M., & Khantzian, E. J. (1991). Contemporary psychodynamic perspectives and the disease concept of addiction: Complementary or competing models? *Psychiatric Annals, 21,* 273-281.

Belsky, J. (1980). Child maltreatment: An ecological integration. *American Psychologist, 35,* 320-335.

Belsky, J., Taylor, D. G., & Rovine, M. (1984). The Pennsylvania infant and family development project, II: The development of reciprocal interaction in the mother-infant dyad. *Child Development, 55,* 706-717.

Benjamin, J. (1988). *The bonds of love: Psychoanalysis, feminism, and the problem of domination.* New York: Pantheon.

Berger, P. L., & Luckman, T. (1967). *The social construction of reality: A treatise on the sociology of knowledge.* Garden City, NY: Anchor.

Berke, J. H. (1988). *The tyranny of malice: Exploring the dark side of character and culture.* New York: Summit.

Berkowitz, L. (1989). Frustration-aggression hypothesis: Examination and reformulation. *Psychological Bulletin, 106,* 59-73.

Berliner, B. (1966). Psychodynamics of the depressive character. *Psychoanalytic Forum, 1,* 244-261.

Bettelheim, B. (1979). Individual and mass behavior in extreme situations. In *Surviving and other essays* (pp. 48-83). New York: Knopf. (Original work published 1943)

Bettelheim, B. (1979). Schizophrenia as a reaction to extreme situations. In *Surviving and other essays* (pp. 112-124). New York: Knopf. (Original work published 1956)

Bettelheim, B. (1979). *Surviving and other essays.* New York: Knopf.

Bettelheim, B. (1982). *Freud and man's soul.* New York: Knopf.

Bettelheim, B. (1983). Afterword. In M. Cardinal, *The words to say it* (pp. 297-308). Cambridge, MA: Van Vactor & Goodheart.

Beutler, L. E. (1995). The germ theory myth and the myth of outcome homogeneity. *Psychotherapy, 32,* 489-494.

Black, C. (1981). *It will never happen to me!* Denver: M.A.C. Printing & Publications Division.

Blanck, G., & Blanck, R. (1974). *Ego psychology: Theory and practice.* New York: Columbia University Press.

Blatt, S. J., McDonald, C., Sugarman, A., & Wilber, C. (1984). Psychodynamic theories of opiate addiction: New directions for research. *Clinical Psychology Review, 4,* 159-189.

Bloch, D. (1978). *"So the witch won't eat me": Fantasy and the child's fear of infanticide.* New York: Grove.

Blum, H. P. (1980). The maternal ego ideal and the regulation of maternal qualities. In S. I. Greenspan & G. H. Pollock (Eds.), *The course of life: Psychoanalytic contributions toward understanding personality development: Vol. 3. Adulthood and the aging process* (pp. 91-114). Washington, DC: U.S. Department of Health and Human Services.

Blumberg, M. L. (1974). Psychopathology of the abusing parent. *American Journal of Psychotherapy, 28,* 21-29.

Bocknek, G., & Perna, F. (1994). Studies in self-representation beyond childhood. In J. M. Masling & R. F. Bornstein (Eds.), *Empirical perspectives on object relations theory* (pp. 29-58). Washington, DC: American Psychological Association.

Bodin, A. M. (1996). Relationship conflict—verbal and physical: Conceptualizing an inventory for assessing process and content. In F. W. Kaslow (Ed.), *Handbook of relational diagnosis and dysfunctional family patterns* (pp. 371-393). New York: John Wiley.

Bolton, F. G., Jr. (1983). *When bonding fails: Clinical assessment of high-risk families.* Beverly Hills, CA: Sage.

Bornstein, R. F. (1993). Parental representations and psychopathology: A critical review of the empirical literature. In J. M. Masling & R. F. Bornstein (Eds.), *Psychoanalytic perspectives on psychopathology* (pp. 1-41). Washington, DC: American Psychological Association.

Boszormenyi-Nagy, I., & Spark, G. M. (1984). *Invisible loyalties: Reciprocity in intergenerational family therapy.* New York: Brunner/Mazel.

Bowen, M. (1978). *Family therapy in clinical practice.* New York: Jason Aronson.

Bowlby, J. (1960). Separation anxiety: A critical review of the literature. *Journal of Child Psychology and Psychiatry, 1,* 251-269.

Bowlby, J. (1969). *Attachment and loss: Vol. 1. Attachment.* New York: Basic Books.

Bowlby, J. (1973). *Attachment and loss: Vol. 2. Separation: Anxiety and anger.* New York: Basic Books.

Bowlby, J. (1988). *A secure base: Parent-child attachment and healthy human development.* New York: Basic Books.

Boyd, S. (1982). [Analysis]. Unpublished manuscript.

Brazelton, T. B., & Cramer, B. G. (1990). *The earliest relationship: Parents, infants, and the drama of early attachment.* Reading, MA: Addison-Wesley.

Brennan, K. A., & Shaver, P. R. (1995). Dimensions of adult attachment, affect regulation, and romantic relationship functioning. *Personality and Social Psychology Bulletin, 21,* 267-283.

Briere, J. N. (1992). *Child abuse trauma: Theory and treatment of the lasting effects.* Newbury Park, CA: Sage.

Briere, J., & Runtz, M. (1987). Post sexual abuse trauma: Data and implications for clinical practice. *Journal of Interpersonal Violence, 2,* 367-379.

Brown, N. O. (1959). *Life against death: The psychoanalytical meaning of history.* Middletown, CT: Wesleyan University Press.

Bugental, D. B. (1986). Unmasking the "polite smile": Situational and personal determinants of managed affect in adult-child interaction. *Personality and Social Psychology Bulletin, 12,* 7-16.

Bugental, J. F. T. (1965). *The search for authenticity: An existential-analytic approach to psychotherapy.* New York: Holt, Rinehart & Winston.

Bugental, J. F. T. (1976). *The search for existential identity.* San Francisco: Jossey-Bass.

Buss, D. M., & Schmitt, D. P. (1993). Sexual strategies theory: An evolutionary perspective on human mating. *Psychological Review, 100,* 204-232.

Byrne, D. (1971). *The attraction paradigm.* New York: Academic Press.

Calderone, M. S. (1977). Eroticism as a norm. In E. S. Morrison & V. Borosage (Eds.), *Human sexuality: Contemporary perspectives* (2nd ed., pp. 39-48). Palo Alto, CA: Mayfield. (Original work published 1974)

Cantor, P. (1989). Intervention strategies: Environmental risk reduction for youth suicide. In M. R. Feinleib (Ed.), *Report of the Secretary's Task Force on Youth Suicide: Vol. 3. Prevention and interventions in youth suicide* (pp. 285-293). Washington, DC: U.S. Department of Health and Human Services.

Centers for Disease Control. (1993). Violence-related attitudes and behaviors of high school students—New York City, 1992. *Morbidity and Mortality Weekly Report, 42*(40) (Washington, DC: U.S. Department of Health and Human Services).

Chasseguet-Smirgel, J. (1985). *The ego ideal: A psychoanalytic essay on the malady of the ideal* (P. Barrows, Trans.). New York: Norton. (Original work published 1975)

Chernin, K. (1985). *The hungry self: Women, eating, and identity.* New York: Times Books.

Choron, J. (1964). *Modern man and mortality.* New York: Macmillan.

Chu, J. A., & Dill, D. L. (1990). Dissociative symptoms in relation to childhood physical and sexual abuse. *American Journal of Psychiatry, 147,* 887-892.

Cialdini, R. B., & Richardson, K. D. (1980). Two indirect tactics of image management: Basking and blasting. *Journal of Personality and Social Psychology, 39,* 406-415.

Cimons, M. (1991, September 20). Study shows a million teen suicide attempts. *Los Angeles Times,* pp. A1, A26.

Cohler, B. J. (1987). Adversity, resilience, and the study of lives. In E. J. Anthony & B. J. Cohler (Eds.), *The invulnerable child* (pp. 363-424). New York: Guilford.

Conte, J. R. (1994). Child sexual abuse: Awareness and backlash. *Future of Children, 4,* 224-232.

Conte, J. R., & Schuerman, J. R. (1987). The effects of sexual abuse on children: A multidimensional view. *Journal of Interpersonal Violence, 2,* 380-390.

Cook, D. R. (1986). *Inventory of Feelings, Problems, and Family Experiences.* Menomonie: University of Wisconsin.

Coopersmith, S. (1975). *Coopersmith Inventory.* Palo Alto, CA: Consulting Psychologists Press.

Cowen, E. L. (1983). Primary prevention in mental health: Past, present, and future. In R. D. Felner, L. A. Jason, J. N. Moritsugu, & S. S. Farber (Eds.), *Preventive psychology: Theory, research and practice* (pp. 11-25). New York: Pergamon.

Cronbach, L. J. (1951). Coefficient alpha and the internal structure of tests. *Psychometrika, 16,* 297-334.

Cull, J. G., & Gill, W. S. (1988). *Suicide Probability Scale (SPS) manual.* Los Angeles: Western Psychological Services.

deMause, L. (Ed.). (1974). *The history of childhood.* New York: Psychohistory Press.

Demos, V. (1986). Crying in early infancy: An illustration of the motivational function of affect. In T. B. Brazelton & M. W. Yogman (Eds.), *Affective development in infancy* (pp. 39-73). Norwood, NJ: Ablex.

Deutscher, S., & Cimbolic, P. (1990). Cognitive processes and their relationship to endogenous and reactive components of depression. *Journal of Nervous and Mental Disease, 178,* 351-359.

Devereux, G. (1953). Why Oedipus killed Laius: A note on the complementary Oedipus complex in Greek drama. *International Journal of Psycho-Analysis, 34,* 132-141.

Devereux, G. (1966). The cannibalistic impulses of parents. *Psychoanalytic Forum, 1,* 114-124.

Dolan, B. (1991, October 7). My own story. *Time,* p. 47.

Dostoyevsky, F. (1958). *The brothers Karamazov* (D. Magarshack, Trans.). London: Penguin. (Original work published 1880)

Drotar, D. (Ed.). (1985). *New directions in failure to thrive: Implications for research and practice.* New York: Plenum.

Drotar, D., Eckerle, D., Satola, J., Pallotta, J., & Wyatt, B. (1990). Maternal interactional behavior with nonorganic failure-to-thrive infants: A case comparison study. *Child Abuse & Neglect, 14,* 41-51.

Duckitt, J. (1992). Psychology and prejudice: A historical analysis and integrative framework. *American Psychologist, 47,* 1182-1193.

Dukas, H., & Hoffmann, B. (Eds.). (1979). *Albert Einstein, the human side: New glimpses from his archives.* Princeton, NJ: Princeton University

Egeland, B., & Sroufe, A. (1981). Developmental sequelae of maltreatment in infancy. *New Directions for Child Development, 11,* 77-92.

Ehrlich, H. J. (1973). *The social psychology of prejudice: A systematic theoretical review and propositional inventory of the American social psychological study of prejudice.* New York: John Wiley.

Ellis, A. (1973). *Humanistic psychotherapy: The rational-emotive approach.* New York: Julian.

Ellis, A., & Harper, R. A. (1975). *A new guide to rational living.* North Hollywood, CA: Wilshire Book Co.

Elson, M. (Ed.). (1987). *The Kohut seminars on self psychology and psychotherapy with adolescents and young adults.* New York: Norton.

Emerson, S., & McBride, M. C. (1986). *A model for group treatment of adults molested as children.* Las Vegas: University of Nevada. (ERIC Document Reproduction Service No. ED 272 814)

Ensink, B. J. (1992). *Confusing realities: A study on child sexual abuse and psychiatric symptoms.* Amsterdam: VU University Press.

Eron, L. D. (1987). The development of aggressive behavior from the perspective of a developing behaviorism. *American Psychologist, 42,* 435-442.

Fairbairn, W. R. D. (1952). *Psychoanalytic studies of the personality.* London: Routledge & Kegan Paul.

Farberow, N. L. (1980). Introduction. In N. L. Farberow (Ed.), *The many faces of suicide: Indirect self-destructive behavior* (pp. 1-12). New York: McGraw-Hill.

Favazza, A. R., & Eppright, T. D. (1986). *Survey on Self-Harm.* Columbia: University of Missouri.

Feinstein, D., & Krippner, S. (1988). *Personal mythology: The psychology of your evolving self.* Los Angeles: Jeremy P. Tarcher.

Feldman, R. S., Devin-Sheehan, L., & Allen, V. L. (1978). Nonverbal cues as indicators of verbal dissembling. *American Educational Research Journal, 15,* 217-231.

Ferenczi, S. (1955). Confusion of tongues between adults and the child. In M. Balint (Ed.), *Final contributions to the problems and methods of psycho-analysis* (E. Mosbacher & others, Trans.) (pp. 156-167). New York: Basic Books. (Original work published 1933)

Feshbach, N. D. (1980). Corporal punishment in the schools: Some paradoxes, some facts, some possible directions. In G. Gerbner, C. J. Ross, & E. Zigler (Eds.), *Child abuse: An agenda for action* (pp. 204-221). New York: Oxford University Press.

Fierman, L. B. (Ed.). (1965). *Effective psychotherapy: The contribution of Hellmuth Kaiser.* New York: Free Press.

Firestone, L. (1991). The Firestone Voice Scale for Self-Destructive Behavior: Investigating the scale's validity and reliability (Doctoral dissertation, California School of Professional Psychology, 1991). *Dissertation Abstracts International, 52,* 3338B.

Firestone, R. W. (1957). *A concept of the schizophrenic process.* Unpublished doctoral dissertation, University of Denver.

Firestone, R. W. (1984). A concept of the primary fantasy bond: A developmental perspective. *Psychotherapy, 21,* 218-225.

Firestone, R. W. (1985). *The fantasy bond: Structure of psychological defenses.* New York: Human Sciences Press.

Firestone, R. W. (1986). The "inner voice" and suicide. *Psychotherapy, 23,* 439-447.

Firestone, R. W. (1987a). Destructive effects of the fantasy bond in couple and family relationships. *Psychotherapy, 24,* 233-239.

Firestone, R. W. (1987b). The "voice": The dual nature of guilt reactions. *American Journal of Psychoanalysis, 47,* 210-229.

Firestone, R. W. (1988). *Voice Therapy: A psychotherapeutic approach to self-destructive behavior.* New York: Human Sciences Press.

Firestone, R. W. (1989). Parenting groups based on Voice Therapy. *Psychotherapy, 26,* 524-529.

Firestone, R. W. (1990a). The bipolar causality of regression. *American Journal of Psychoanalysis, 50,* 121-135.

Firestone, R. W. (1990b). *Compassionate child-rearing: An in-depth approach to optimal parenting.* New York: Plenum.

Firestone, R. W. (1990c). Prescription for psychotherapy. *Psychotherapy, 27,* 627-635.

Firestone, R. W. (1990d). Voice Therapy. In J. Zeig & W. Munion (Eds.), *What is psychotherapy? Contemporary perspectives* (pp. 68-74). San Francisco: Jossey-Bass.

Firestone, R. W. (1993). The psychodynamics of fantasy, addiction, and addictive attachments. *American Journal of Psychoanalysis, 53,* 335-352.

Firestone, R. W. (1994a). A new perspective on the Oedipal complex: A voice therapy session. *Psychotherapy, 31,* 342-351.

Firestone, R. W. (1994b). Psychological defenses against death anxiety. In R. A. Neimeyer (Ed.), *Death anxiety handbook: Research, instrumentation, and application* (pp. 217-241). Washington, DC: Taylor & Francis.

Firestone, R. W., & Catlett, J. (1989). *Psychological defenses in everyday life.* New York: Human Sciences Press.

Firestone, R. W., & Firestone, L. (1996). *Firestone Assessment of Self-Destructive Thoughts.* San Antonio: Psychological Corporation.

Firestone, R. W., & Seiden, R. H. (1987). Microsuicide and suicidal threats of everyday life. *Psychotherapy, 24,* 31-39.

Fontana, V. J. (1983). *Somewhere a child is crying: Maltreatment—causes and prevention* (Rev. ed.). New York: New American Library.

Fraiberg, S., Adelson, E., & Shapiro, V. (1980). Ghosts in the nursery: A psychoanalytic approach to the problems of impaired infant-mother relationships. In S. Fraiberg (Ed.), *Clinical studies in infant mental health: The first year of life* (pp. 164-196). New York: Basic Books. (Original work published 1975)

Frankl, V. E. (1959). *Man's search for meaning* (Rev. ed.). New York: Washington Square Press. (Original work published 1946)

Frankl, V. E. (1967). Group psychotherapeutic experiences in a concentration camp. In V. E. Frankl, *Psychotherapy and existentialism: Selected papers on logotherapy* (pp. 95-105). New York: Simon & Schuster. (Original work published 1954)

Frederick, C. J. (1985). An introduction and overview of youth suicide. In M. L. Peck, N. L. Farberow, & R. E. Litman (Eds.), *Youth suicide* (pp. 1-16). New York: Springer.

Freiberg, P. (1991). Study: Disorders found in 20 percent of children. *APA Monitor, 22,* 36.

Freud, A. (1966). *The ego and the mechanisms of defense* (Rev. ed.). Madison, CT: International Universities Press.

Freud, A., & Burlingham, D. (1944). *Infants without families: The case for and against residential nurseries.* New York: International Universities Press.

Freud, S. (1955). Group psychology and the analysis of the ego. In J. Strachey (Ed. and Trans.), *The standard edition of the complete psychological works of Sigmund Freud* (Vol. 18, pp. 63-143). London: Hogarth. (Original work published 1921)

Freud, S. (1957). On narcissism: An introduction. In J. Strachey (Ed. and Trans.), *The standard edition of the complete psychological works of Sigmund Freud* (Vol. 14, pp. 73-102). London: Hogarth. (Original work published 1914)

Freud, S. (1957). Thoughts for the times on war and death. In J. Strachey (Ed. and Trans.), *The standard edition of the complete psychological works of Sigmund Freud* (Vol. 14, pp. 273-302). London: Hogarth. (Original work published 1915)

Freud, S. (1959). An autobiographical study. In J. Strachey (Ed. and Trans.), *The standard edition of the complete psychological works of Sigmund Freud* (Vol. 20, pp. 7-75). London: Hogarth. (Original work published 1925)

Freud, S. (1959). Inhibitions, symptoms, and anxiety. In J. Strachey (Ed. and Trans.), *The standard edition of the complete psychological works of Sigmund Freud* (Vol. 20, pp. 87-176). London: Hogarth. (Original work published 1926)

Freud, S. (1961). The ego and the id. In J. Strachey (Ed. and Trans.), *The standard edition of the complete psychological works of Sigmund Freud* (Vol. 19, pp. 12-67). London: Hogarth. (Original work published 1923)

Freud, S. (1961). Civilization and its discontents. In J. Strachey (Ed. and Trans.), *The standard edition of the complete psychological works of Sigmund Freud* (Vol. 21, pp. 64-145). London: Hogarth. (Original work published 1930)

Freud, S. (1963). Some thoughts on development and regression—aetiology, Lecture XXII, Introductory lectures on psycho-analysis. In J. Strachey (Ed. and Trans.), *The standard edition of the complete psychological works of Sigmund Freud* (Vol. 16, pp. 339-357). London: Hogarth. (Original work published 1916)

Freud, S. (1964). An outline of psycho-analysis. In J. Strachey (Ed. and Trans.), *The standard edition of the complete psychological works of Sigmund Freud* (Vol. 23, pp. 144-207). London: Hogarth. (Original work published 1940)

Fromm, E. (1941). *Escape from freedom.* New York: Avon.

Fromm, E. (1947). *Man for himself: An inquiry into the psychology of ethics.* New York: Rinehart.

Fromm, E. (1950). *Psychoanalysis and religion.* New Haven, CT: Yale University Press.

Fromm, E. (1955). *The sane society.* New York: Rinehart.

Fromm, E. (1962). *Beyond the chains of illusion: My encounter with Marx and Freud.* New York: Simon & Schuster.

Fromm, E. (1964). *The heart of man: Its genius for good and evil.* New York: Harper & Row.

Fromm, E. (1986). *For the love of life* (R. & R. Kimber, Trans.). New York: Free Press.

Gaddini, R. (1978). Transitional object origins and the psychosomatic symptom. In S. A. Grolnick & L. Barkin (Eds.), *Between reality and fantasy: Transitional objects and phenomena* (pp. 111-131). New York: Jason Aronson.

Garbarino, J., & Gilliam, G. (1980). *Understanding abusive families.* Lexington, MA: Lexington.

Garbarino, J., Guttmann, E., & Seeley, J. W. (1986). *The psychologically battered child.* San Francisco: Jossey-Bass.

Gardner, L. I. (1972). Deprivation dwarfism. *Scientific American, 227,* 76-82.

Garner, D. M., & Olmsted, M. P. (1984). *Eating Disorder Inventory Manual.* Odessa, FL: Psychological Assessment Resources.

Gil, D. G. (1987). Maltreatment as a function of the structure of social systems. In M. R. Brassard, R. Germain, & S. N. Hart (Eds.), *Psychological maltreatment of children and youth* (pp. 159-170). New York: Pergamon.

Gilbert, P. (1989). *Human nature and suffering.* Hove, UK: Lawrence Erlbaum.

Gilpin, A., & Hays, R. D. (1990). *Scalogram analysis program* [Computer program]. Durham, NC: Duke University Press.

Gitlin, T. (1993, Spring). The rise of "identity politics": An examination and a critique. *Dissent,* pp. 172-177.

Glasser, M. (1979). Some aspects of the role of aggression in the perversions. In I. Rosen (Ed.), *Sexual deviation* (2nd ed., pp. 278-305). Oxford, England: Oxford University Press.

Goldberg, C. (1991). *Understanding shame.* Northvale, NJ: Jason Aronson.

Goldberg, C. (1996). *Speaking with the devil: A dialogue with evil.* New York: Penguin.

Goldstein, M., & Davis, E. E. (1972). Race and belief: A further analysis of the social determinants of behavioral intentions. *Journal of Personality and Social Psychology, 22,* 346-355.

Goodall, J. (1986). *The chimpanzees of Gombe: Patterns of behavior.* Cambridge, MA: Belknap.

Gottman, J. M., & Rushe, R. H. (1993). The analysis of change: Issues, fallacies, and new ideas. *Journal of Consulting and Clinical Psychology, 61,* 907-910.

Gove, W. R., & Hughes, M. (1980). Reexamining the ecological fallacy: A study in which aggregate data are critical in investigating the pathological effects of living alone. *Social Forces, 58,* 1157-1177.

Grass, G. (1993, Spring). On loss: The condition of Germany. *Dissent,* pp. 178-188.

Greenberg, J., Pyszczynski, T., Solomon, S., Rosenblatt, A., Veeder, M., Kirkland, S., & Lyon, D. (1990). Evidence for terror management theory II: The effects of mortality salience on reactions to those who threaten or bolster the cultural worldview. *Journal of Personality and Social Psychology, 58,* 308-318.

Greenson, R. R. (1968). Dis-identifying from mother: Its special importance for the boy. *International Journal of Psycho-Analysis, 49,* 370-374.

Greenspan, S. I. (1991). The stages of ego development: Implications for childhood and adult psychopathology. In S. Akhtar & H. Parens (Eds.), *Beyond the symbiotic orbit: Advances in separation-individuation theory* (pp. 85-101). Hillsdale, NJ: Analytic Press.

Grizzle, A. F. (with W. Proctor). (1988). *Mother love, mother hate: Breaking dependent love patterns in family relationships.* New York: Fawcett Columbine.

Guerney, B., Jr., Brock, G., & Coufal, J. (1986). Integrating marital therapy and enrichment: The relationship enhancement approach. In N. S. Jacobson & A. S. Gurman (Eds.), *Clinical handbook of marital therapy* (pp. 151-172). New York: Guilford.

Guidubaldi, J., & Cleminshaw, H. K. (1994). *Parenting Satisfaction Scale.* San Antonio: Psychological Corporation.

Gunderson, M. P., & McCary, J. L. (1979). Sexual guilt and religion. *Family Coordinator, 28,* 353-357.

Guntrip, H. (1961). *Personality structure and human interaction: The developing synthesis of psycho-dynamic theory.* New York: International Universities Press.

Guntrip, H. (1969). *Schizoid phenomena: Object-relations and the self.* New York: International Universities Press.

Hacker, A. (1992). *Two nations: Black and white, separate, hostile, unequal.* New York: Scribner.

Hadas, M. (Ed.). (1967). *The complete plays of Sophocles* (R. C. Jebb, Trans.). New York: Bantam.

Halford, W. K., Sanders, M. R., & Behrens, B. C. (1993). A comparison of the generalization of behavioral marital therapy and enhanced behavioral marital therapy. *Journal of Consulting and Clinical Psychology, 61,* 51-60.

Hall, S. M., Havassy, B. E., & Wasserman, D. A. (1990). Commitment to abstinence and acute stress in relapse to alcohol, opiates, and nicotine. *Journal of Consulting and Clinical Psychology, 58,* 175-181.

Hamilton, D. (1981). Stereotyping and intergroup behavior: Some thoughts on the cognitive approach. In D. Hamilton (Ed.), *Cognitive processes in stereotyping and intergroup behavior* (pp. 333-353). Hillsdale, NJ: Lawrence Erlbaum.

Hamilton, E. W., & Abramson, L. Y. (1983). Cognitive patterns and major depressive disorder: A longitudinal study in a hospital setting. *Journal of Abnormal Psychology, 92,* 173-184.

Hancock, L. (1996, March 18). Mother's little helper. *Newsweek,* pp. 51-56.

Hartmann, H. (1964). *Essays on ego psychology: Selected problems in psychoanalytic theory.* New York: International Universities Press.

Hassler, J. H. (1994). Illnesses, failures, losses: Human misery propelling regression, therapy, and growth. In A. Sugarman (Ed.), *Victims of abuse: The emotional impact of child and adult trauma* (pp. 213-222). Madison, CT: International Universities Press.

Hays, R. D., Hayashi, T., & Stewart, A. L. (1989). A five-item measure of socially desirable response set. *Educational and Psychological Measurement, 49,* 629-636.

Herzog, J. M. (1982). On father hunger: The father's role in the modulation of aggressive drive and fantasy. In S. H. Cath, A. R. Gurwitt, & J. M. Ross (Eds.), *Father and child: Developmental and clinical perspectives* (pp. 163-174). Boston: Little, Brown.

Hewlett, S. A. (1991). *When the bough breaks: The cost of neglecting our children.* New York: Basic Books.

Hinton, J. (1975). The influence of previous personality on reactions to having terminal cancer. *Omega, 6,* 95-111.

Hollon, S. D., Shelton, R. C., & Davis, D. D. (1993). Cognitive therapy for depression: Conceptual issues and clinical efficacy. *Journal of Consulting and Clinical Psychology, 61,* 270-275.

Holt, R. R., & Silverstein, B. (1989). On the psychology of enemy images: Introduction and overview. *Journal of Social Issues, 45,* 1-11.

Hopson, R. E. (1993). A thematic analysis of the addictive experience: Implications for psychotherapy. *Psychotherapy, 30,* 481-494.

Horkheimer, M. (Ed.). (1974). *Studi sull'autoritá e la famiglia.* Torino: UTET. (Originally published 1936).

Horvath, A. O., & Luborsky, L. (1993). The role of the therapeutic alliance in psychotherapy. *Journal of Consulting and Clinical Psychology, 61,* 561-573.

Hughes, R. A. (1990). Psychological perspectives on infanticide in a faith healing sect. *Psychotherapy, 27,* 107-115.

Jackson, D. N. (1970). A sequential system for personality scale development. In C. D. Spielberger (Ed.), *Current topics in clinical and community psychology* (Vol. 2, pp. 61-96). New York: Academic Press.

Jacobson, E. (1964). *The self and the object world.* London: Hogarth.

Jacobson, N. S. (1993). Introduction to special section on couples and couple therapy. *Journal of Consulting and Clinical Psychology, 61,* 5.

Jacobson, N. S., & Addis, M. E. (1993). Research on couples and couple therapy: What do we know? Where are we going? *Journal of Consulting and Clinical Psychology, 61,* 85-93.

Janov, A. (1970). *The primal scream: Primal therapy: The cure for neurosis.* New York: Putnam.

Jaques, E. (1970). *Work, creativity, and social justice.* New York: International Universities Press.

Jason, J., Carpenter, M. M., & Tyler, C. W. (1983). Underrecording of infant homicide in the United States. *American Journal of Public Health, 73,* 195-197.

Joffe, J. (1993). The new Europe: Yesterday's ghosts. *Foreign Affairs, 72,* 29-43.

Jones, E. E. (Ed.). (1993). Special section: Single-case research in psychotherapy. *Journal of Consulting and Clinical Psychology, 61,* 371-430.

Kafka, F. (1977). *The trial* (W. & E. Muir, Trans.). Franklin Center, PA: Franklin Library. (Original work published 1937)

Kahn, C. (1993). The different ways of being a German. *Journal of Psychohistory, 20,* 381-398.

Kaplan, L. J. (1984). *Adolescence: The farewell to childhood.* New York: Simon & Schuster.

Karpel, M. (1976). Individuation: From fusion to dialogue. *Family Process, 15,* 65-82.

Kaslow, F. W. (Ed.). (1996). *Handbook of relational diagnosis and dysfunctional family patterns.* New York: John Wiley.

Kastenbaum, R. (1974, Summer). Childhood: The kingdom where creatures die. *Journal of Clinical Child Psychology,* pp. 11-14.

Kastenbaum, R. (1995). *Death, society, and human experience* (5th ed.). Boston: Allyn & Bacon.

Kaufman, G. (1980). *Shame: The power of caring.* Cambridge, MA: Schenkman.

Kaufman, G., & Raphael, L. (1984). Relating to the self: Changing inner dialogue. *Psychological Reports, 54,* 239-250.

Kaufman, J., & Zigler, E. (1987). Do abused children become abusive parents? *American Journal of Orthopsychiatry, 57,* 186-192.

Keen, S. (1986). *Faces of the enemy: Reflections of the hostile imagination.* San Francisco: Harper & Row.

Kempe, R. S., & Kempe, C. H. (1978). *Child abuse.* Cambridge, MA: Harvard University Press.

Kempe, R. S., & Kempe, C. H. (1984). *The common secret: Sexual abuse of children and adolescents.* New York: Freeman.

Kernberg, O. F. (1980). *Internal world and external reality: Object relations theory applied.* Northvale, NJ: Jason Aronson.

Kerr, M. E., & Bowen, M. (1988). *Family evaluation: An approach based on Bowen theory.* New York: Norton.

Kestenberg, J. S., & Kestenberg, M. (1987). Child killing and child rescuing. In G. G. Neuman (Ed.), *Origins of human aggression: Dynamics and etiology* (pp. 139-154). New York: Human Sciences Press.

Keys, A., Brozek, J., Henschel, A., Mickelsen, O., & Taylor, H. L. (1950). *The biology of human starvation* (Vol. 2). Minneapolis: University of Minnesota Press.

Khan, M. M. (1963). The concept of cumulative trauma. In R. S. Eissler, A. Freud, H. Hartmann, & M. Kris (Eds.), *The psychoanalytic study of the child* (Vol. 18, pp. 286-306). New York: International Universities Press.

Khantzian, E. J., Mack, J. E., & Schatzberg, A. F. (1974). Heroin use as an attempt to cope: Clinical observations. *American Journal of Psychiatry, 131,* 160-164.

Klaus, M. H., & Kennell, J. H. (1976). *Maternal-infant bonding.* St. Louis: C. V. Mosby.

Klein, M. (1964). The importance of symbol-formation in the development of the ego. In M. Klein, *Contributions to psycho-analysis 1921-1945* (pp. 236-250). New York: McGraw-Hill. (Original work published 1930)

Klein, M. (1964). *Contributions to psycho-analysis 1921-1945.* New York: McGraw-Hill. (Original work published 1948)

Kohut, H. (1971). *The analysis of the self* (The Psychoanalytic Study of the Child, Monograph No. 4). New York: International Universities Press.

Kohut, H. (1977). *The restoration of the self.* New York: International Universities Press.

Korbin, J. E. (Ed.). (1981). *Child abuse and neglect: Cross-cultural perspectives.* Berkeley: University of California Press.

Kotelchuck, M. (1980). Nonorganic failure to thrive: The status of interactional and environmental etiologic theories. *Advances in Behavioral Pediatrics, 1,* 29-51.

Kozol, J. (1995). *Amazing grace: The lives of children and the conscience of a nation.* New York: Crown.

Kramer, R. (1995). "The 'bad mother' Freud has never seen": Otto Rank and the birth of object-relations theory. *Journal of the American Academy of Psychoanalysis, 23,* 293-321.

Krystal, H. (1990). An information processing view of object-relations. *Psychoanalytic Inquiry, 10,* 221-251.

Kumin, I. (1996). *Pre-object relatedness: Early attachment and the psychoanalytic situation.* New York: Guilford.

Kunce, L. J., & Shaver, P. R. (1994). An attachment-theoretical approach to caregiving in romantic relationships. In K. Bartholomew & D. Perlman (Eds.), *Advances in personal relationships* (Vol. 5, pp. 205-237). London: Jessica Kingsley.

Laing, R. D. (1961). *Self and others.* Harmondsworth, England: Penguin.

Laing, R. D. (1967). *The politics of experience.* New York: Ballantine.

Laing, R. D. (1969). *The divided self.* London: Penguin. (Original work published 1960)

Laing, R. D. (1972). *The politics of the family and other essays.* New York: Vintage. (Original work published 1969)

Laing, R. D. (1985). Foreword. In R. W. Firestone, *The fantasy bond: Structure of psychological defenses* (pp. 17-20). New York: Human Sciences Press.

Laing, R. D. (1989). *The challenge of love.* Unpublished manuscript.

Laing, R. D. (1990). Foreword. In R. W. Firestone, *Compassionate child-rearing: An in-depth approach to optimal parenting.* New York: Plenum.

Laing, R. D., & Esterson, A. (1970). *Sanity, madness, and the family: Families of schizophrenics.* London: Penguin. (Original work published 1964)

Lambert, W. E., & Klineberg, O. (1967). *Children's views of foreign peoples: A cross-national study.* New York: Appleton-Century-Crofts.

Langs, R. (1982). *Psychotherapy: A basic text.* New York: Jason Aronson.

Lasch, C. (1984). *The minimal self: Psychic survival in troubled times.* New York: Norton.

Lasch, C. (1985). Introduction. In J. Chasseguet-Smirgel, *The ego ideal: A psychoanalytic essay on the malady of the ideal* (pp. ix-xvi). New York: Norton.

Lederer, W. J., & Jackson, D. D. (1968). *The mirages of marriage.* New York: Norton.

Lester, D. (1970). Relation of fear of death in subjects to fear of death in their parents. *Psychological Record, 20,* 541-543.

Levin, A. J. (1951). The fiction of the death instinct. *Psychiatric Quarterly, 25,* 257-281.

Levy, D. M. (1943). *Maternal overprotection.* New York: Columbia University Press.

Lewinsohn, P. M. (1991, August 17). *Depression in older (14-18) adolescents: Summary of results obtained in the Oregon Adolescent Depression Project.* Paper presented at the meeting of the American Psychological Association, San Francisco.

Lewis, H. B. (1971). *Shame and guilt in neurosis.* New York: International Universities Press.

Lewis, M., & Michalson, L. (1984). The socialization of emotional pathology in infancy. *Infant Mental Health Journal, 5,* 125-134.

Lidz, T. (1972). The influence of family studies on the treatment of schizophrenia. In C. J. Sager & H. S. Kaplan (Eds.), *Progress in group and family therapy* (pp. 616-635). New York: Brunner/Mazel. (Original work published 1969)

Lifton, R. J. (1973). *Home from the war: Vietnam veterans: Neither victims nor executioners.* New York: Simon & Schuster.

Lifton, R. J., & Olson, E. (1976). The nuclear age. In E. S. Shneidman (Ed.), *Death: Current perspectives* (pp. 99-109). Palo Alto, CA: Mayfield. (Original work published 1974)

Lifton, R. J., & Olson, E. (1976). The human meaning of total disaster: The Buffalo Creek experience. *Psychiatry, 39,* 1-18.

Linehan, M. M., Goodstein, J. L., Nielsen, S. L., & Chiles, J. A. (1983). Reasons for staying alive when you are thinking of killing yourself: The Reasons for Living Inventory. *Journal of Consulting and Clinical Psychology, 51,* 276-286.

Loewenstein, R. M. (1966). On the theory of the superego: A discussion. In R. M. Loewenstein, L. M. Newman, M. Schur, & A. Solnit (Eds.), *Psychoanalysis—A general psychology: Essays in honor of Heinz Hartmann* (pp. 298-314). New York: International Universities Press.

Lore, R. K., & Schultz, L. A. (1993). Control of human aggression: A comparative perspective. *American Psychologist, 48,* 16-25.

Lorenz, K. (1966). *On aggression* (M. K. Wilson, Trans.). New York: Harcourt, Brace & World. (Original work published 1963)

Loring, M. T. (1994). *Emotional abuse.* New York: Lexington.

Luke, J. L. (1978). Sleeping arrangements of sudden infant death syndrome victims in the District of Columbia: A preliminary report. *Journal of Forensic Sciences, 23,* 379-383.

Lung, C. T., & Daro, D. (1996). *Current trends in child abuse reporting and fatalities: The results of the 1995 Annual Fifty State Survey.* Chicago: National Committee to Prevent Child Abuse.

Maccoby, E. E., & Jacklin, C. N. (1974). *The psychology of sex differences.* Stanford, CA: Stanford University Press.

Macdonald, D. I. (1987). Patterns of alcohol and drug use among adolescents. *Chemical Dependency, 34,* 275-288.

MacNeil-Lehrer Productions, WNET, WETA. (1987, March 12). *Open door policy? Teen suicide: Fall from grace* (Transcript 2989 of the MacNeil/Lehrer NewsHour). New York: Author.

Mahler, M. S. (1974). Symbiosis and individuation: The psychological birth of the human infant. *Psychoanalytic Study of the Child, 29,* 89-106 (New Haven, CT: Yale University Press).

Mahler, M. S. (1979). On sadness and grief in infancy and childhood: Loss and restoration of the symbiotic love object. In *The selected papers of Margaret S. Mahler, M.D.: Vol. 1. Infantile psychosis and early contributions* (pp. 262-279). New York: Jason Aronson. (Original work published 1961)

Mahler, M. S., & McDevitt, J. B. (1968). Observations on adaptation and defense in statu nascendi: Developmental precursors in the first two years of life. *Psychoanalytic Quarterly, 37,* 1-21.

Mahler, M. S., Pine, F., & Bergman, A. (1975). *The psychological birth of the human infant: Symbiosis and individuation.* New York: Basic Books.

Main, M. (1990). Parental aversion to infant-initiated contact is correlated with the parent's own rejecting during childhood: The effects of experience on signals of security with respect to attachment. In K. E. Barnard & T. B. Brazelton (Eds.), *Touch: The foundation of experience* (pp. 461-495). Madison, CT: International Universities Press.

Main, M., Kaplan, N., & Cassidy, J. (1985). Security in infancy, childhood, and adulthood: A move to the level of representation. *Monographs of the Society for Research in Child Development, 50*(1-2, Serial No. 209), 66-104.

Malone, T. P. (1981). Psychopathology as non-experience. *Voices, 17,* 83-91.

Maltsberger, J. T. (1986). *Suicide risk: The formulation of clinical judgment.* New York: New York University Press.

Marcuse, H. (1966). *Eros and civilization: A philosophical inquiry into Freud.* Boston: Beacon. (Original work published 1955)

Margolin, N. L., & Teicher, J. D. (1968). Thirteen adolescent male suicide attempts. *Journal of the American Academy of Child Psychiatry, 7,* 296-315.

Maris, R. W., Berman, A. L., Maltsberger, J. T., & Yufit, R. I. (Eds.). (1992). *Assessment and prediction of suicide.* New York: Guilford.

Maslow, A. H. (1968). *Toward a psychology of being* (2nd ed.). New York: Van Nostrand Reinhold.

Maslow, A. H. (1971). *The farther reaches of human nature.* Harmondsworth, England: Penguin.

Masson, J. M. (1984). *The assault on truth: Freud's suppression of the seduction theory.* New York: Farrar, Straus & Giroux.

Masterson, J. F., & Rinsley, D. B. (1975). The borderline syndrome: The role of the mother in the genesis and psychic structure of the borderline personality. *International Journal of Psycho-Analysis, 56,* 163-177.

May, D. S., & Solomon, M. (Producers). (1984). *Theoretical aspects of attachment* [Video]. Los Angeles: UCLA Neuropsychiatric Institute and Hospital.

May, R. (1958). Contributions of existential psychotherapy. In R. May, E. Angel, & H. F. Ellenberger (Eds.), *Existence: A new dimension in psychiatry and psychology* (pp. 37-91). New York: Basic Books.

May, R. (1983). *The discovery of being: Writings in existential psychology.* New York: Norton.

McCarthy, J. B. (1980). *Death anxiety: The loss of the self.* New York: Gardner.

McCullers, C. (1940). *The heart is a lonely hunter.* New York: Bantam.

McIntire, M. S., Angle, C. R., & Struempler, L. J. (1972). The concept of death in midwestern children and youth. *American Journal of Diseases of Children, 123,* 527-532.

Mead, M. (1960). One vote for this age of anxiety. In C. A. Glasrud (Ed.), *The age of anxiety* (pp. 174-177). Boston: Houghton Mifflin. (Original work published 1956)

Meindl, J. R., & Lerner, M. J. (1984). Exacerbation of extreme responses to an out-group. *Journal of Personality and Social Psychology, 47,* 71-84.

Meyer, J. E. (1975). *Death and neurosis* (M. Nunberg, Trans.). New York: International Universities Press.

Meyer, M. (1991, December 16). Be kinder to your 'kinder.' *Newsweek,* p. 43.

Milgram, S. (1974). *Obedience to authority: An experimental view.* London: Tavistock.

Miller, A. (1981). *Prisoners of childhood: The drama of the gifted child and the search for the true self* (R. Ward, Trans.). New York: Basic Books. (Original work published 1979)

Miller, A. (1984). *For your own good: Hidden cruelty in child-rearing and the roots of violence* (H. & H. Hannum, Trans.) (2nd ed.). New York: Farrar, Straus & Giroux. (Original work published 1980)

Miller, A. (1984). *Thou shalt not be aware: Society's betrayal of the child* (H. & H. Hannum, Trans.). New York: Farrar, Straus & Giroux. (Original work published 1981)

Miller, A. (1991). *Breaking down the wall of silence: The liberating experience of facing painful truth* (S. Worrall, Trans.). New York: Dutton. (Original work published 1990)

Miller, H. (1947). *Remember to remember.* New York: New Directions.

Miller, N. E., & Dollard, J. (1941). *Social learning and imitation.* New Haven, CT: Yale University Press.

Miranda, J., & Persons, J. B. (1988). Dysfunctional attitudes are mood-state dependent. *Journal of Abnormal Psychology, 97,* 76-79.

Moe, J. L., Nacoste, R. W., & Insko, C. A. (1981). Belief versus race as determinants of discrimination: A study of southern adolescents in 1966 and 1979. *Journal of Personality and Social Psychology, 41,* 1031-1050.

Morgenstern, J., & Leeds, J. (1993). Contemporary psychoanalytic theories of substance abuse: A disorder in search of a paradigm. *Psychotherapy, 30,* 194-206.

Morrison, A. P. (1989). *Shame: The underside of narcissism.* Hillsdale, NJ: Jason Aronson.

Mowrer, O. H. (1953). *Psychotherapy: Theory and research.* New York: Ronald Press.

Moynihan, D. P. (1993). *Pandaemonium: Ethnicity in international politics.* New York: Oxford University Press.

Mumford, L. (1966). *The myth of the machine: Technics and human development.* New York: Harcourt, Brace & World.

Nachman, P. A. (1991). Contemporary infant research and the separation-individuation theory of Margaret S. Mahler. In S. Akhtar & H. Parens (Eds.), *Beyond the symbiotic orbit: Advances in separation-individuation theory* (pp. 121-149). Hillsdale, NJ: Analytic Press.

Nagy, M. H. (1959). The child's view of death. In H. Feifel (Ed.), *The meaning of death* (pp. 79-98). New York: McGraw-Hill. (Original work published 1948)

National Center for Health Statistics. (1996). [Deaths for 282 selected causes by 5-year age groups, color, and sex: United States, 1979-93]. Unpublished data.

Newlands, M., & Emery, J. S. (1991). Child abuse and cot deaths. *Child Abuse & Neglect, 15,* 275-278.

Niebuhr, R. (1944). *The children of light and the children of darkness: A vindication of democracy and a critique of its traditional defense.* New York: Scribner.

Novey, S. (1955). The role of the superego and ego-ideal in character formation. *International Journal of Psycho-Analysis, 36,* 254-259.

Noyes, R., Hoenk, P. R., Kuperman, S., & Slymen, D. J. (1977). Depersonalization in accident victims and psychiatric patients. *Journal of Nervous and Mental Disease, 164,* 401-407.

Oaklander, V. (1978). *Windows to our children: A Gestalt therapy approach to children and adolescents.* Moab, UT: Real People Press.

Okey, J. L. (1992). Human aggression: The etiology of individual differences. *Journal of Humanistic Psychology, 32,* 51-64.

Orbach, I. (1988). *Children who don't want to live: Understanding and treating the suicidal child.* San Francisco: Jossey-Bass.

Orlinsky, D. E., Geller, J. D., Tarragona, M., & Farber, B. (1993). Patients' representations of psychotherapy: A new focus for psychodynamic research. *Journal of Consulting and Clinical Psychology, 61,* 596-610.

Owen, D. (1993). The future of the Balkans: An interview with David Owen. *Foreign Affairs, 72,* 1-9.

Pagels, E. (1988). *Adam, Eve, and the serpent.* New York: Random House.

Parens, H. (1991). Separation-individuation theory and psychosexual theory. In S. Akhtar & H. Parens (Eds.), *Beyond the symbiotic orbit: Advances in separation-individuation theory* (pp. 3-34). Hillsdale, NJ: Analytic Press.

Parker, B. L., & Drummond-Reeves, S. J. (1993). The death of a dyad: Relational autopsy, analysis, and aftermath. *Journal of Divorce & Remarriage, 21,* 95-119.

Parin, P. (1978). *Fürchte deinen Nächsten wie dich Selbst.* Frankfurt: Suhrkamp.

Parker, G. (1983). *Parental overprotection: A risk factor in psychosocial development.* New York: Grune & Stratton.

Parr, G. (Producer). (1986). *The inner voice in child abuse* [Video]. Santa Barbara, CA: Glendon Association.

Parr, G. (Producer). (1989). *Bobby and Rosie: Anatomy of a marriage* [Videotape]. Santa Barbara, CA: Glendon Association.

Parr, G. (Producer). (1995a). *Invisible child abuse* [Videotape]. Santa Barbara, CA: Glendon Association.

Parr, G. (Producer). (1995b). *Inwardness: A retreat from feeling* [Videotape]. Santa Barbara, CA: Glendon Association.

Patterson, G. R., DeBaryshe, B. D., & Ramsey, E. (1989). A developmental perspective on antisocial behavior. *American Psychologist, 44,* 329-335.

Peck, M. S. (1983). *People of the lie: The hope for healing human evil.* New York: Simon & Schuster.

Pinar, W. F. (1996). Parenting in the promised land. In J. L. Kincheloe, S. R. Steinberg, & A. D. Gresson III (Eds.), *Measured lies: The bell curve examined* (pp. 227-236). New York: St. Martin's.

Plomin, R. (1989). Environment and genes: Determinants of behavior. *American Psychologist, 44,* 105-111.

Pollitt, E., Gilmore, M., & Valcarcel, M. (1978). Early mother-infant interaction and somatic growth. *Early Human Development, 1-4,* 325-336.

Puhar, A. (1993). Childhood origins of the war in Yugoslavia: I. Infant mortality. *Journal of Psychohistory, 20,* 373-379.

Putnam, F. W., Guroff, J. J., Silberman, E. K., Barban, L., & Post, R. M. (1986). The clinical phenomenology of multiple personality disorder: Review of 100 recent cases. *Journal of Clinical Psychiatry, 47,* 285-293.

Radloff, L. S. (1977). The CES-D Scale: A self-report depression scale for research in the general population. *Applied Psychological Measurement, 1,* 385-401.

Rado, S. (1933). The psychoanalysis of pharmacothymia (drug addiction). *Psychoanalytic Quarterly, 2,* 1-23.

Rado, S. (1958). Narcotic bondage: A general theory of the dependence on narcotic drugs. In P. H. Hoch & J. Zubin (Eds.), *Problems of addiction and habituation* (pp. 27-36). New York: Grune & Stratton.

Rank, O. (1941). *Beyond psychology.* New York: Dover.

Rank, O. (1972). *Will therapy and truth and reality* (J. Taft, Trans.). New York: Knopf. (Original work published 1936)

Rascovsky, A. (1995). *Filicide: The murder, humiliation, mutilation, denigration, and abandonment of children by parents* (S. H. Rogers, Trans.). Northvale, NJ: Jason Aronson.

Rascovsky, A., & Rascovsky, M. (1968). On the genesis of acting out and psychopathic behaviour in Sophocles' Oedipus: Notes on filicide. *International Journal of Psycho-Analysis, 49,* 390-394.

Reik, T. (1941). *Masochism in modern man* (M. H. Beigel & G. M. Kurth, Trans.). New York: Farrar, Straus.

Rheingold, J. C. (1964). *The fear of being a woman: A theory of maternal destructiveness.* New York: Grune & Stratton.

Rheingold, J. C. (1967). *The mother, anxiety, and death: The catastrophic death complex.* Boston: Little, Brown.

Richman, J. (1986). *Family therapy for suicidal people.* New York: Springer.

Roazen, P. (1973). Introduction: Sigmund Freud. In P. Roazen (Ed.), *Makers of modern social science: Sigmund Freud* (pp. 1-21). Englewood Cliffs, NJ: Prentice Hall.

Rochlin, G. (1967). How younger children view death and themselves. In E. A. Grollman (Ed.), *Explaining death to children* (pp. 51-85). Boston: Beacon.

Rogers, C. R. (1951). *Client-centered therapy: Its current practice, implications, and theory.* Boston: Houghton Mifflin.

Rohner, R. P. (1986). *The warmth dimension: Foundations of parental acceptance-rejection theory.* Newbury Park, CA: Sage.

Rohner, R. P. (1991). *Handbook for the study of parental acceptance and rejection.* Storrs: University of Connecticut.

Rose, D. T., & Abramson, L. Y. (1992). Developmental predictors of depressive cognitive style: Research and theory. In D. Ciochetti & S. L. Toth (Eds.), *Rochester Symposium on Developmental Psychopathology: Vol. 4. Developmental perspectives on depression* (pp. 325-349). Rochester, NY: University of Rochester Press.

Rose, D. T., Abramson, L. Y., Hodulik, C. J., Halberstadt, L., & Leff, G. (1994). Heterogeneity of cognitive style among depressed inpatients. *Journal of Abnormal Psychology, 103,* 419-429.

Rosen, J. N. (1953). *Direct analysis: Selected papers.* New York: Grune & Stratton.

Rosen, K. S., & Rothbaum, F. (1993). Quality of parental caregiving and security of attachment. *Developmental Psychology, 29,* 358-367.

Rosen, T. S., & Johnson, H. L. (1988). Drug-addicted mothers, their infants, and SIDS. In P. J. Schwartz, D. P. Southall, & M. Valdes-Dapena (Eds.), *Annals of the New York Academy of Sciences: Vol. 533. The sudden infant death syndrome: Cardiac and respiratory mechanisms and interventions* (pp. 89-95). New York: New York Academy of Sciences.

Rosenbaum, M., & Richman, J. (1970). Suicide: The role of hostility and death wishes from the family and significant others. *American Journal of Psychiatry, 126,* 1652-1655.

Rosenblatt, A., Greenberg, J., Solomon, S., Pyszczynski, T., & Lyon, D. (1989). Evidence for terror management theory: I. The effects of mortality salience on reactions to those who violate or uphold cultural values. *Journal of Personality and Social Psychology, 57,* 681-690.

Rosenfeld, A. (1978, April 1). The "elastic mind" movement: Rationalizing child neglect? *Saturday Review,* pp. 26-28.

Ross, C. A., Miller, S. D., Reagor, P., Bjornson, L., Fraser, G. A., & Anderson, G. (1990). Structured interview data on 102 cases of multiple personality disorder from four centers. *American Journal of Psychiatry, 147,* 596-601.

Rubin, T. I. (with E. Rubin). (1975). *Compassion and self-hate: An alternative to despair.* New York: David McKay.

Rutter, M. (1981). *Maternal deprivation reassessed* (2nd ed.). Harmondsworth, England: Penguin.

Sabbath, J. C. (1969). The suicidal adolescent: The expendable child. *Journal of the American Academy of Child Psychiatry, 8,* 272-289.

Sager, C. J., & Hunt, B. (1979). *Intimate partners: Hidden patterns in love relationships.* New York: McGraw-Hill.

St. Clair, M. (1986). *Object relations and self psychology: An introduction.* Monterey, CA: Brooks/Cole.

Sanders, B., & Giolas, M. H. (1991). Dissociation and childhood trauma in psychologically disturbed adolescents. *American Journal of Psychiatry, 148,* 50-54.

Sandler, J. (1987). The concept of the superego. In J. Sandler (Ed.), *From safety to superego: Selected papers of Joseph Sandler* (pp. 17-44). London: Karnac. (Original work published 1960)

Schakel, J. A. (1987). Emotional neglect and stimulus deprivation. In M. R. Brassard, R. Germain, & S. N. Hart (Eds.), *Psychological maltreatment of children and youth* (pp. 100-109). New York: Pergamon.

Scharff, D. E., & Scharff, J. S. (1991). *Object relations couple therapy.* Northvale, NJ: Jason Aronson.

Schlesinger, A. M., Jr. (1991). *The disuniting of America.* New York: Norton.

Schmemann, S. (1992, May 24). Ethnic battles flaring in former Soviet fringe. *New York Times,* p. 7.

Schnarch, D. M. (1991). *Constructing the sexual crucible: An integration of sexual and marital therapy.* New York: Norton.

Schneer, H. I., Kay, P., & Brozovsky, M. (1961). Events and conscious ideation leading to suicidal behavior in adolescence. *Psychiatric Quarterly, 35,* 507-515.

Schoenewolf, G. (1989). *Sexual animosity between men and women.* Northvale, NJ: Jason Aronson.

Searles, H. F. (1961). Schizophrenia and the inevitability of death. *Psychiatric Quarterly, 35,* 631-665.

Searles, H. F. (1965a). Problems of psycho-analytic supervision. In H. F. Searles, *Collected papers on schizophrenia and related subjects* (pp. 584-604). London: Hogarth. (Original work published 1962)

Searles, H. F. (1965b). Scorn, disillusionment and adoration in the psychotherapy of schizophrenia. In H. F. Searles, *Collected papers on schizophrenia and related subjects* (pp. 605-625). London: Hogarth. (Original work published 1962)

Sechehaye, M. A. (1951). *Symbolic realization: A new method of psychotherapy applied to a case of schizophrenia* (B. Wursten & H. Wursten, Trans.). New York: International Universities Press.

Secunda, V. (1990). *When you and your mother can't be friends: Resolving the most complicated relationship of your life.* New York: Delacorte.

Seiden, R. H. (1965). Salutary effects of maternal separation. *Social Work, 10,* 25-29.

Seiden, R. H. (1966). Campus tragedy: A study of student suicide. *Journal of Abnormal Psychology, 71,* 389-399.

Seiden, R. H. (1984). Death in the West: A regional analysis of the youthful suicide rate. *Western Journal of Medicine, 140,* 969-973.

Seixas, J. S., & Youcha, G. (1985). *Children of alcoholism: A survivor's manual.* New York: Harper & Row.

Seligman, M. E. P. (1975). *Helplessness: On depression, development, and death.* New York: Freeman.

Seligman, M. E. P. (1995). The effectiveness of psychotherapy: The *Consumer Reports* study. *American Psychologist, 50,* 965-974.

Shaver, P. R., & Clark, C. L. (1994). The psychodynamics of adult romantic attachment. In J. M. Masling & R. F. Bornstein (Eds.), *Empirical perspectives on object relations theory* (pp. 105-156). Washington, DC: American Psychological Association.

Shaver, P. R., & Hazan, C. (1993). Adult romantic attachment: Theory and evidence. In D. Perlman & W. Jones (Eds.), *Advances in personal relationships* (Vol. 4, pp. 29-70). London: Jessica Kingsley.

Shearer, S. L., & Herbert, C. A. (1987). Long-term effects of unresolved sexual trauma. *American Family Physician, 36,* 169-175.

Shengold, L. (1989). *Soul murder: The effects of childhood abuse and deprivation.* New Haven, CT: Yale University Press.

Shengold, L. (1991). A variety of narcissistic pathology stemming from parental weakness. *Psychoanalytic Quarterly, 60,* 86-92.

Shirer, W. L. (1960). *The rise and fall of the Third Reich: A history of Nazi Germany.* New York: Simon & Schuster.

Shneidman, E. S. (1989). Overview: A multidimensional approach to suicide. In D. Jacobs & H. N. Brown (Eds.), *Suicide: Understanding and responding* (pp. 1-30). Madison, CT: International Universities Press.

Silverman, L. H., Lachmann, F. M., & Milich, R. H. (1982). *The search for oneness.* New York: International Universities Press.

Silverstein, B. (1989). Enemy images: The psychology of U.S. attitudes and cognitions regarding the Soviet Union. *American Psychologist, 44,* 903-913.

Solomon, M. F. (1989). *Narcissism and intimacy.* New York: Norton.

Solomon, S. (1986, June). *Isms make schisms: Can we have peace and culture also?* Paper presented at the meeting of the International Society of Political Psychology, Amsterdam, Holland.

Solomon, S., Greenberg, J., & Pyszczynski, T. (1991). A terror management theory of social behavior: The psychological functions of self-esteem and cultural worldviews. *Advances in Experimental Social Psychology, 24,* 93-159.

Spitz, R. A. (1945). Hospitalism: An inquiry into the genesis of psychiatric conditions in early childhood. *Psychoanalytic Study of the Child 1,* 53-74 (New York: International Universities Press).

Spitz, R. A. (1946a). *Grief: A peril in infancy* [Film]. New York: New York University Film Library.

Spitz, R. A. (1946b). Hospitalism: A follow-up report on investigation described in Volume I, 1945. *Psychoanalytic Study of the Child, 2,* 113-117 (New York: International Universities Press).

Sroufe, L. A., & Ward, M. J. (1980). Seductive behavior of mothers of toddlers: Occurrence, correlates, and family origins. *Child Development, 51,* 1222-1229.

Steele, B. F. (1970). Parental abuse of infants and small children. In E. J. Anthony & T. Benedek (Eds.), *Parenthood: Its psychology and psychopathology* (pp. 449-477). Boston: Little, Brown.

Steele, B. F. (1990). Some sequelae of the sexual maltreatment of children. In H. B. Levine (Ed.), *Adult analysis and childhood sexual abuse* (pp. 21-34). Hillsdale, NJ: Analytic Press.

Stern, D. N. (1985). *The interpersonal world of the infant: A view from psychoanalysis and developmental psychology.* New York: Basic Books.

Stern, M. M. (1968). Fear of death and neurosis. *Journal of the American Psychoanalytic Association, 16,* 3-31.

Stern, M. M. (1972). Trauma, death anxiety and fear of death. *Psyche, 26,* 901-928.

Stiles, W. B., Shapiro, D. A., & Elliott, R. (1986). "Are all psychotherapies equivalent?" *American Psychologist, 41,* 165-180.

Stolorow, R. D., Brandchaft, B., & Atwood, G. E. (1987). *Psychoanalytic treatment: An intersubjective approach.* Hillsdale, NJ: Analytic Press.

Straus, M. A. (with D. A. Donnelly). (1994). *Beating the devil out of them: Corporal punishment in American families.* New York: Lexington.

Straus, M. A., & Gelles, R. J. (1986). Societal change and change in family violence from 1975 to 1985 as revealed by two national surveys. *Journal of Marriage and the Family, 48,* 465-479.

Strunk, R. C., Mrazek, D. A., Fuhrmann, G. S., & LaBrecque, J. F. (1985). Physiologic and psychological characteristics associated with deaths due to asthma in childhood. *Journal of the American Medical Association, 254,* 1193-1198.

Strupp, H. H. (1989). Psychotherapy: Can the practitioner learn from the researcher? *American Psychologist, 44,* 717-724.

Suzuki, D. T., Fromm, E., & DeMartino, R. (1960). *Zen Buddhism and psychoanalysis.* New York: Harper.

Symonds, M. (1975). Victims of violence: Psychological effects and aftereffects. *American Journal of Psychoanalysis, 35,* 19-26.

Szalai, A. (Ed.). (1972). *The use of time: Daily activities of urban and suburban populations in twelve countries.* The Hague, Netherlands: Mouton.

Szasz, T. S. (1961). *The myth of mental illness: Foundations of a theory of personal conduct.* New York: Hoeber-Harper.

Szasz, T. S. (1963). *Law, liberty, and psychiatry: An inquiry into the social uses of mental health practices.* New York: Collier.

Szasz, T. S. (1975). *Ceremonial chemistry: Ritual persecution of drug addicts and pushers.* Garden City, NY: Doubleday.

Szasz, T. (1978). *The myth of psychotherapy: Mental healing as religion, rhetoric, and repression.* Garden City, NY: Anchor.

Taft, J. (1958). *Otto Rank.* New York: Julian.

Tesser, A. (1988). Toward a self-evaluation maintenance model of social behavior. *Advances in Experimental Social Psychology, 21,* 181-227.

Tolpin, M. (1971). On the beginnings of a cohesive self: An application of the concept of transmuting internalization to the study of the transitional object and signal anxiety. *Psychoanalytic Study of the Child, 26,* 316-352 (New York: Quadrangle).

Toth, J. (1992, January 1). Foster care to streets: A beaten path, study finds. *Los Angeles Times,* p. A5.

Toynbee, A. (1968a). Changing attitudes towards death in the modern Western world. In A. Toynbee, A. K. Mant, N. Smart, J. Hinton, S. Yudkin, E. Rhode, R. Heywood, & H. H. Price (Eds.), *Man's concern with death* (pp. 122-132). London: Hodder and Stoughton.

Toynbee, A. (1968b). Death in war. In A. Toynbee, A. K. Mant, N. Smart, J. Hinton, S. Yudkin, E. Rhode, R. Heywood, & H. H. Price (Eds.), *Man's concern with death* (pp. 145-152). London: Hodder and Stoughton.

Tronick, E. (1980). Infant communicative intent. In A. P. Reilly (Ed.), *The communication game: Perspectives on the development of speech, language and non-verbal communication skills* (pp. 4-9). Skillman, NJ: Johnson & Johnson Baby Products Co.

Tronick, E. Z., Cohn, J., & Shea, E. (1986). The transfer of affect between mothers and infants. In T. B. Brazelton & M. W. Yogman (Eds.), *Affective development in infancy* (pp. 11-25). Norwood, NJ: Ablex.

Turner, J. (1978). Social categorization and social discrimination in the minimal group paradigm. In H. Tajfel (Ed.), *Differentiation between social groups: Studies in the social psychology of intergroup relations.* London: Academic Press.

Vergote, A. (1988). *Guilt and desire: Religious attitudes and their pathological derivatives* (M. H. Wood, Trans.). New Haven, CT: Yale University Press. (Original work published 1978)

von Gebsattel, V. E. (1951). Anthropology of anxiety. *Hochland, 43,* 352-364.

Watts, A. W. (1961). *Psychotherapy East and West.* New York: Pantheon.

Weisz, J. R., Weiss, B., & Donenberg, G. R. (1992). The lab versus the clinic: Effects of child and adolescent psychotherapy. *American Psychologist, 47,* 1578-1585.

Welldon, E. V. (1988). *Mother, madonna, whore: The idealization and denigration of motherhood.* London: Free Association Books.

Wexler, J., & Steidl, J. (1978). Marriage and the capacity to be alone. *Psychiatry, 41,* 72-82.

Whitaker, C. A., & Malone, T. P. (1981). *The roots of psychotherapy.* New York: Brunner/Mazel.

Whitfield, C. L. (1995). *Memory and abuse: Remembering and healing the effects of trauma.* Deerfield Beach, FL: Health Communications.

Willi, J. (1982). *Couples in collusion: The unconscious dimension in partner relationships* (W. Inayat-Khan & M. Tchorek, Trans.). Claremont, CA: Hunter House. (Original work published 1975)

Winnicott, D. W. (1958). *Collected papers: Through paediatrics to psycho-analysis.* London: Tavistock.

Winnicott, D. W. (1965a). Ego distortion in terms of true and false self. In D. W. Winnicott, *The maturational processes and the facilitating environment: Studies in the theory of emotional development* (pp. 140-152). Madison, CT: International Universities Press. (Original work published 1960)

Winnicott, D. W. (1965b). The theory of the parent-infant relationship. In D. W. Winnicott, *The maturational processes and the facilitating environment: Studies in the theory of emotional development* (pp. 37-55). Madison, CT: International Universities Press. (Original work published 1960)

Wolberg, L. R. (1954). *The technique of psychotherapy.* New York: Grune & Stratton.

Wolfe, T. (1983). *The right stuff.* New York: Farrar, Straus & Giroux.

Wolman, T. (1991). Mahler and Winnicott: Some parallels in their lives and work. In S. Akhtar & H. Parens (Eds.), *Beyond the symbiotic orbit: Advances in separation-individuation theory* (pp. 35-60). Hillsdale, NJ: Analytic Press.

Wright, R. (1994, August 15). Our cheating hearts. *Time,* pp. 36-44.

Wright, R. (1995, August 28). The evolution of despair. *Time,* pp. 50-54, 56-57.

Wurmser, L., & Zients, A. (1982). The return of the denied superego. *Psychoanalytic Inquiry, 2,* 539-580.

Wynne, L. C. (1972). Communication disorders and the quest for relatedness in families of schizophrenics. In C. J. Sager & H. S. Kaplan (Eds.), *Progress in group and family therapy* (pp. 595-615). New York: Brunner/Mazel.

Yalom, I. D. (1980). *Existential psychotherapy.* New York: Basic Books.

Zeig, J. K., & Munion, W. M. (Eds.). (1990). *What is psychotherapy? Contemporary perspectives.* San Francisco: Jossey-Bass.

Zilboorg, G. (1932). Sidelights on parent-child antagonism. *American Journal of Orthopsychiatry, 2,* 35-43.

Zilboorg, G. (1943). Fear of death. *Psychoanalytic Quarterly, 12,* 465-475.

Zuckerman, M. (1959). Reversed scales to control acquiescence response set in the Parental Attitude Research Instrument. *Child Development, 30,* 523-532.

Name Index

Berger, P. L., 278
Bergman, A., 91n.4, 226
Berke, J. H., 40, 271, 284, 290n.8
Berkowitz, L., 279, 289n.2
Berliner, B., 202n.3
Berman, A. L., 202n.2
Bettelheim, B., 58, 60, 220, 222n.4, 290n.4, 307n.1
Beutler, L. E., 252n.1
Bjornson, L., 35
Black, C., 43
Blanck, G., 26n.3
Blanck, R., 26n.3
Blatt, S. J., 225
Blehar, M. C., 10, 12n.4, 19, 78
Bloch, D., 63
Blum, H. P., 91n.4
Blumberg, M. L., 20
Bocknek, G., 71n.1
Bodin, A. M., 103, 108n.4
Bolton, F. G., Jr., 79, 91-92n.5
Bornstein, R. F., 72n.1
Boszormenyi-Nagy, I., 107n.1
Bowen, M., 48, 107n.1, 167n.3, 182n.2, 290n.9
Bowlby, J., 10, 12n.4, 23, 26n.2, 35, 53-54, 77, 78, 210
Boyd, S., 306-307n.1
Brandchaft, B., 226
Brazelton, T. B., 38, 48
Brennan, K. A., 12n.4
Briere, J., 35
Briere, J. N., 20
Brock, G., 182n.3, 188
Brozek, J., 239n.2
Brozovsky, M., 44n.4
Bugental, D. B., 27n.7
Bugental, J. F. T., 26n.3
Burlingham, D., 23, 28n.10
Byrne, D., 281

Calderone, M. S., 40, 271
Cantor, P., 26n.2
Carpenter, M. M., 44n.2
Cassidy, J., 10, 12n.4, 78
Catlett, J., 296
Chasseguet-Smirgel, J., 148n.1, 280, 290n.3
Chernin, K., 230
Chiles, J. A., 200

Choron, J., 250, 261
Chu, J. A., 35
Cialdini, R. B., 281
Cimbolic, P., 188
Cimons, M., 22
Clark, C. L., 10, 12n.4
Cleminshaw, H. K., 56n.4
Cohler, B. J., 40
Cohn, J., 26n.4
Conte, J. R., 20, 25
Cook, D. R., 200
Coopersmith, S., 56n.4
Coufal, J., 182n.3
Cowen, E. L., 183n.4
Cramer, B. G., 38, 48
Cronbach, L. J., 199
Cull, J. G., 190, 200

Daro, D., 27n.5
Davis, D. D., 253n.1
Davis, E. E., 281
DeBaryshe, B. D., 22
DeMartino, R., 270
deMause, L., 22
Demos, V., 226
Deutsch, R. M., 87
Deutscher, S., 188
Devereux, G., 202n.3
Devin-Sheehan, L., 27n.7
Dill, D. L., 35
Dolan, B., 15
Dollard, J., 279
Donenberg, G. R., 253n.1
Dostoyevsky, F., 270
Drotar, D., 36
Drummond-Reeves, S., 108n.4
Duckitt, J., 281

Eckerle, D., 36
Egeland, B., 44n.5
Ehrlich, H. J., 285
Einstein, A., 287
Elliott, R., 242
Ellis, A., 148n.2, 188
Elson, M., 92n.6
Emerson, S., 20
Emery, G., 148n.2
Emery, J. S., 44n.2

Subject Index

About the Author

ౘ

Robert W. Firestone, Ph.D., has been affiliated with the Glendon Association in Santa Barbara, a nonprofit organization dedicated to the development and dissemination of concepts and practices in psychotherapy since 1979. From 1957 to 1979, Dr. Firestone was engaged in the private practice of psychotherapy as a clinical psychologist, working with a wide range of patients, amplifying his original ideas on schizophrenia, and applying these concepts to a comprehensive theory of neurosis. His major works include, *The Fantasy Bond: Structure of Psychological Defenses,* and *Compassionate Child-Rearing: An In-Depth Approach to Optimal Parenting,* which describe how couples form destructive bonds that impair their psychological functioning and have a damaging effect on their child-rearing practices. His studies of negative thought processes and their associated affect have led to the development of a therapeutic methodology to uncover and contend with aspects of destructive cognition, elucidated in *Voice Therapy: A Psychotherapeutic Approach to Self-Destructive Behavior.* In recent years, he has applied his concepts to empirical research and to developing the *Firestone Assessment of Self-Destructive Thoughts* (FAST), a scale that assesses suicide potential. He is currently completing a book on suicide, *Voices in Suicide,* and is involved in research to develop a scale to assess family violence. His ideas related to psychotherapy, couple and family relationships, suicide, child abuse, and existential issues have been disseminated to mental health professionals and the general public through a series of film and video documentaries. In addition to his contributions to the mental health community, Dr. Firestone serves as a consultant to several large corporations.

THESE THINGS AIN'T
GONNA SMOKE THEMSELVES

BY THE SAME AUTHOR

LULU EIGHTBALL

THESE THINGS AIN'T GONNA SMOKE THEMSELVES

A ~~LOVE~~ ~~HATE~~ ~~LOVE~~ ~~HATE~~ ~~LOVE~~ LETTER TO A VERY BAD HABIT

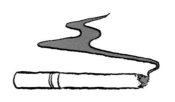

EMILY FLAKE

BLOOMSBURY

PUBLISHED BY BLOOMSBURY USA, NEW YORK
DISTRIBUTED TO THE TRADE BY HOLTZBRINCK PUBLISHERS

ALL PAPERS USED BY BLOOMSBURY USA ARE
NATURAL, RECYCLABLE PRODUCTS MADE FROM WOOD
GROWN IN WELL-MANAGED FORESTS. THE
MANUFACTURING PROCESSES CONFORM TO THE
ENVIRONMENTAL REGULATIONS OF THE
COUNTRY OF ORIGIN.

LIBRARY OF CONGRESS CATALOGING-IN-PUBLICATION DATA

FLAKE, EMILY, 1977-
THESE THINGS AIN'T GONNA SMOKE THEMSELVES:
A LETTER TO A VERY BAD HABIT/EMILY FLAKE.
P. CM.
ISBN-13: 978-1-59691-328-8
ISBN-10: 1-59691-328-2

1. SMOKING- COMIC BOOKS, STRIPS, ETC. 2. TOBACCO USE-
COMIC BOOKS, STRIPS, ETC. I. TITLE.
RC567. F53 2007
616. 86'5 - dc22
2006047992

FIRST U.S. EDITION 2007
1 3 5 7 9 10 8 6 4 2

PRINTED IN CHINA BY SOUTH CHINA PRINTING CO.

FOR DLJ

INTRODUCTION

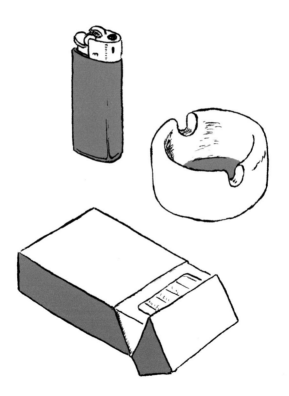

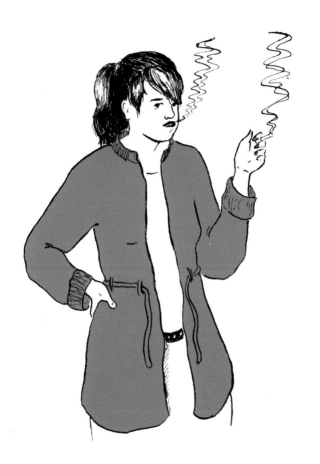

MAYBE YOU SMOKE.

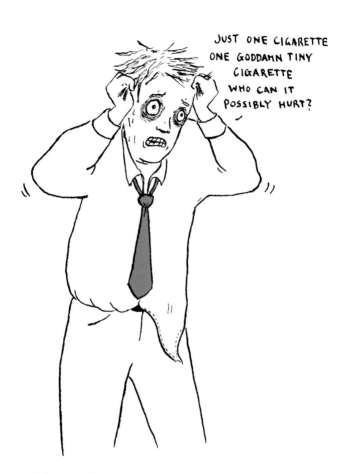

MAYBE YOU JUST QUIT AND YOU'RE
CLIMBING THE WALLS IN AGONY.

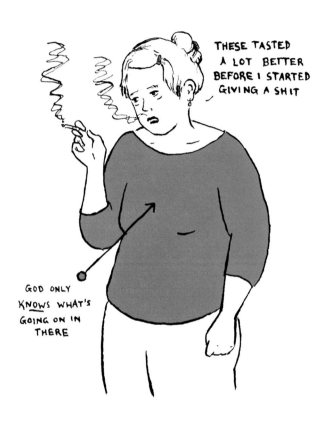

OR MAYBE, LIKE ME, YOU SMOKE BUT
YOU'RE STARTING TO FEEL INCREASINGLY
GUILTY ABOUT IT, OR WORRIED, OR JUST
NOT AS, ERM, HEALTHY AS YOU MIGHT LIKE.

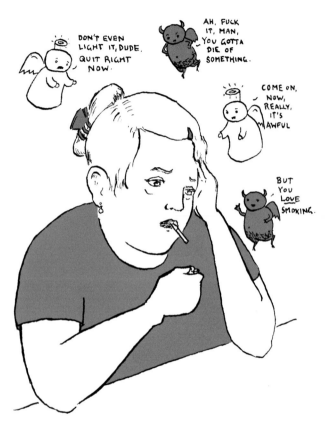

WHEREVER YOU'RE AT, CHANCES ARE YOU'RE
GRAPPLING WITH THE SAME THING AS ME—
THE LOVE OF A TERRIBLE HABIT, SORROW AT
THE THOUGHT OF GIVING IT UP, AND FEAR
OF THE FACT THAT IT'LL PROBABLY KILL YOU.

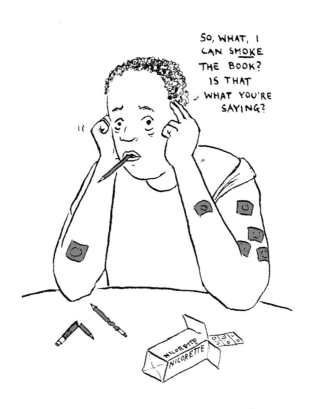

SO MAYBE, JUST MAYBE, THIS BOOK WILL HELP YOU. OR AT LEAST MAKE YOU FEEL LIKE YOU'RE NOT ALONE.

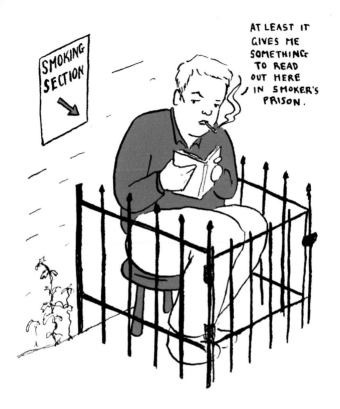

HALF VALENTINE, HALF DEAR JOHN
LETTER, IT'S A PERSONAL HISTORY OF A
DIFFICULT RELATIONSHIP WITH A VICE
IN ITS WANING DAYS OF POPULARITY.

ENJOY IT IN GOOD HEALTH.

BACK IN THE DAY

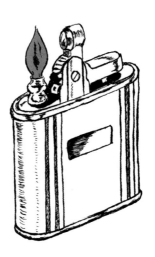

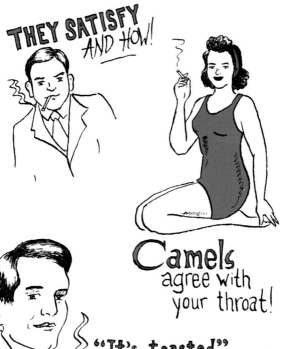

ONCE UPON A TIME, CIGARETTES
WEREN'T BAD FOR YOU.

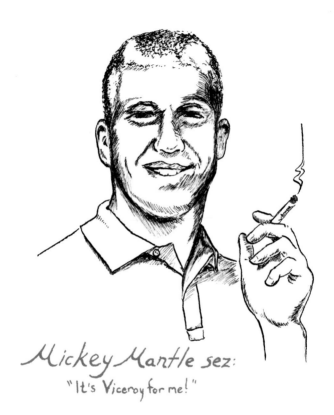

Mickey Mantle sez:

"It's Viceroy for me!"

POPULAR CROONERS SANG THE PRAISES
OF LUCKIES. MOVIE STARS WOULD WALK
A MILE FOR A CAMEL. AND THOUGH
IT DEFIES ALL LOGIC, EVEN PRO
ATHLETES PLAYED THE SHILL.

AND NOW- CHESTERFIELD FIRST TO GIVE YOU SCIENTIFIC FACTS IN FAVOR OF SMOKING

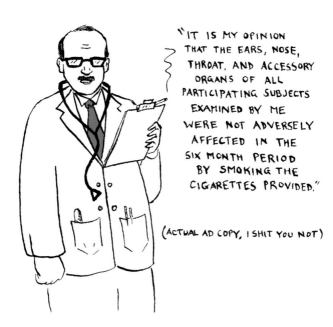

"IT IS MY OPINION THAT THE EARS, NOSE, THROAT, AND ACCESSORY ORGANS OF ALL PARTICIPATING SUBJECTS EXAMINED BY ME WERE NOT ADVERSELY AFFECTED IN THE SIX MONTH PERIOD BY SMOKING THE CIGARETTES PROVIDED."

(ACTUAL AD COPY, I SHIT YOU NOT)

DOCTORS- DOCTORS!- GOT ON BOARD, TOUTING THE RELATIVE BENEVOLENCE OF THIS BRAND OR THAT.

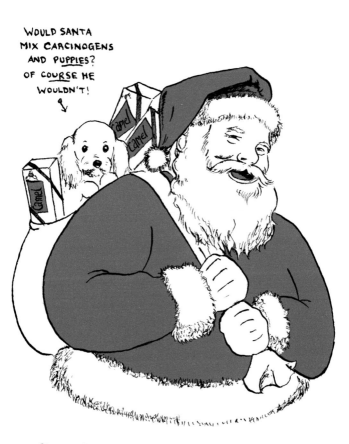

EVEN SANTA CLAUS WAS IN ON THE ACTION. WHAT STUFFS A STOCKING BETTER THAN A CARTON OF CAMELS?

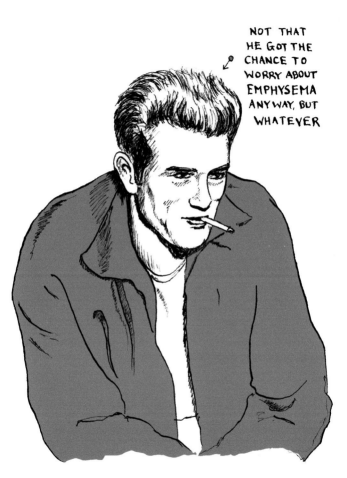

SMOKING WAS ADULT, GLAMOROUS, AND IRREFUTABLY COOL.

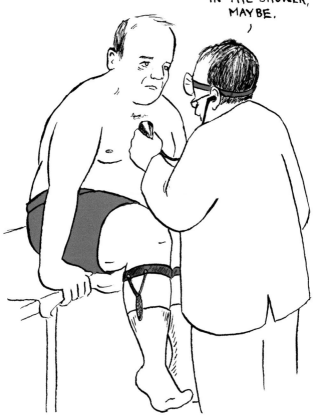

WHEN THE FIRST RUMBLINGS OF A CANCER
LINK STARTED TO MAKE THEMSELVES HEARD,
DOCTORS ADVISED SMOKERS TO LIMIT
THEMSELVES TO A SPARTAN PACK A DAY.

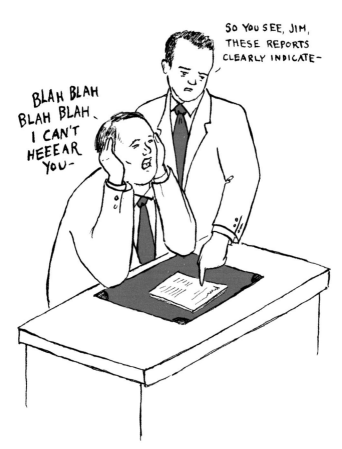

THE BAD NEWS KEPT ROLLING IN, DESPITE THE BEST EFFORTS ON THE PART OF THE INDUSTRY TO QUELL IT.

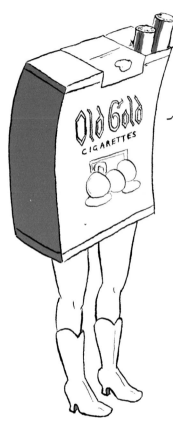

TELEVISION ADVERTISING WAS BANNED.
THE OLD GOLD DANCING CIGARETTE
PACKS PRANCED OFFSTAGE FOREVER.

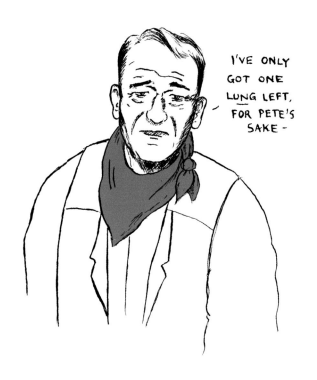

I'VE ONLY GOT ONE LUNG LEFT, FOR PETE'S SAKE -

SOON ENOUGH, THOSE GLAMOROUS DAYS LOOKED IMPOSSIBLY NAIVE. AND SOME OF THOSE GLAMOROUS CELEBRITIES, SICK AND REPENTANT, PLEADED WITH THE PUBLIC TO GIVE THE HABIT UP.

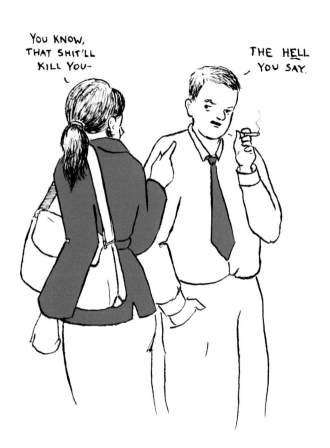

IT SEEMED LIKE A GOOD IDEA AT THE TIME

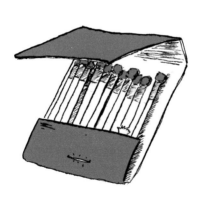

HOW I TOOK UP SMOKING

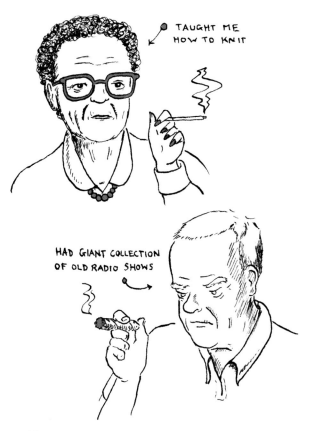

TAUGHT ME
HOW TO KNIT

HAD GIANT COLLECTION
OF OLD RADIO SHOWS

AS A KID, I HAD A PAIR OF SURROGATE
GRANDPARENTS NAMED CHARLIE AND MARGARET,
WHO LIVED ACROSS THE STREET. CHARLIE SMOKED
CIGARS. MARGARET SMOKED LONG, SKINNY MORES.

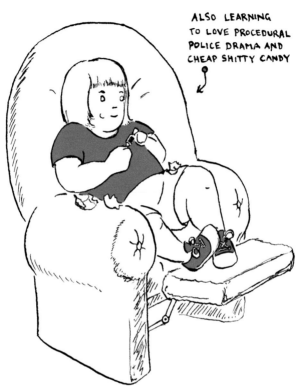

ALSO LEARNING TO LOVE PROCEDURAL POLICE DRAMA AND CHEAP SHITTY CANDY

I SPENT A LOT OF TIME OVER THERE, WATCHING "MATLOCK" AND EATING TOOTSIE ROLLS. MY PARENTS HATED HOW I'D COME HOME FULL OF SMOKE- BUT I LEARNED TO LOVE THE SMELL. SMELLED LIKE SAFETY AND THE PROMISE OF TOOTSIE ROLLS.

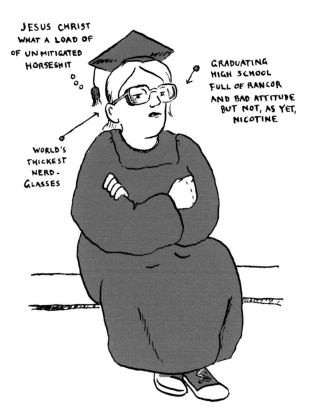

I STARTED SMOKING MYSELF WHEN I
WAS PLENTY OLD ENOUGH TO KNOW BETTER.
I HAD PLENTY OF SMOKER FRIENDS AS A
TEENAGER, BUT IT NEVER OCCURRED
TO ME TO START UP.

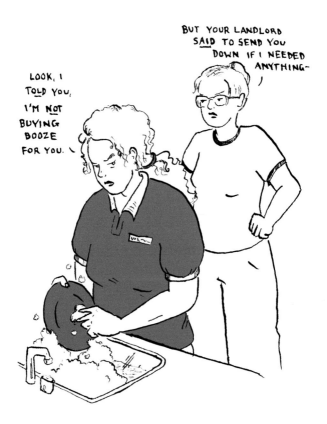

I DIDN'T GET AROUND TO IT TILL THE
SUMMER BETWEEN MY FRESHMAN AND
SOPHOMORE YEAR IN COLLEGE, WHEN I LIVED
WITH MY SISTER ABOVE A LIQUOR STORE.

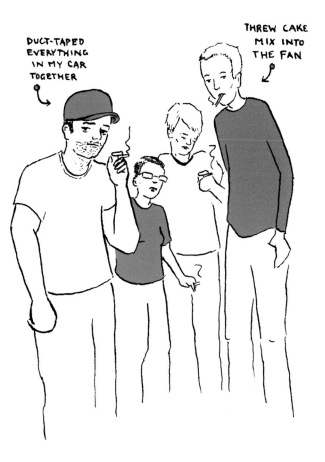

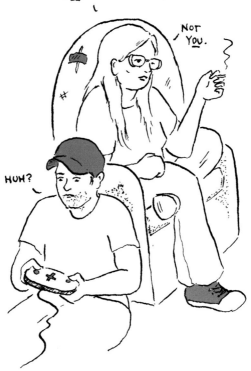

ONE DAY OUT OF PURE BOREDOM,
I FINALLY GAVE IT A SHOT.
AND TOOK TO IT IMMEDIATELY.

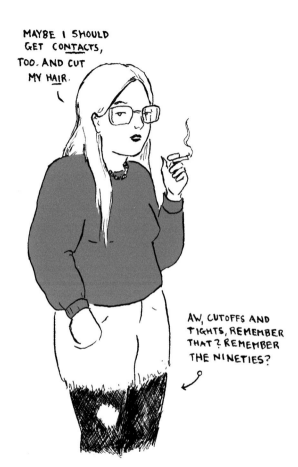

I RETURNED TO SCHOOL WITH A FULL-FLEDGED
SMOKING HABIT AND A VAGUE NOTION THAT
I SEEMED COOLER. TOUGHER. MORE INTERESTING.

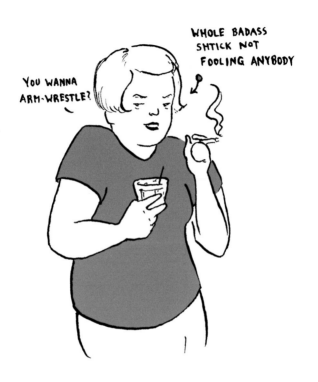

IT WAS THE START OF A WHOLE NEW ME.

I'VE HAD THE NOTION FOR A LONG TIME
THAT I WOULD QUIT WHEN I WAS 29.
THE REASONING BEHIND THAT'S PRETTY
ARBITRARY- I WAS SITTING IN THE
COFFEE/CIGARETTE STORE WHERE I
WORKED WHEN A LADY PICKED UP
MY PACK OF SMOKES, PARLIAMENTS
AT THE TIME. "AWW, I USED TO
SMOKE THESE," SHE SAID. SHE
TOOK A LONG, APPRAISING LOOK
AT ME. "QUIT WHEN YOU'RE 29,"
SHE SAID IN A DECISIVE TONE.
"YES MA'AM," I REPLIED.

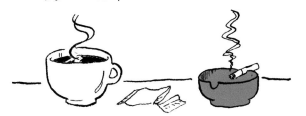

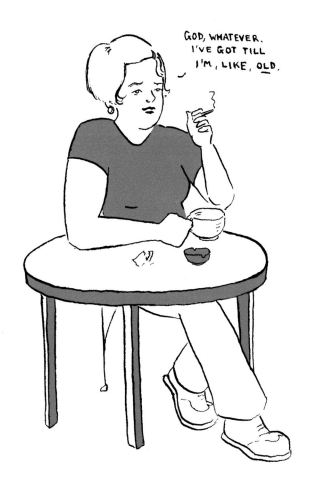

I WAS 21. I HAD OCEANS OF TIME.

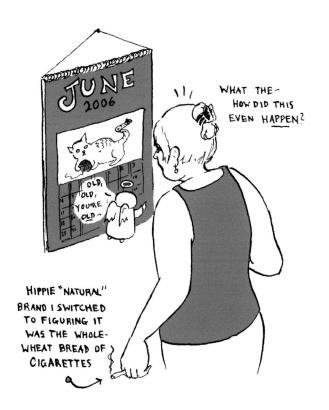

EXCEPT NOW, OF COURSE, I DON'T.
I WAS BORN ON JUNE 16TH, 1977.
THOSE OCEANS OF TIME DRIED
UP INCREDIBLY FAST.

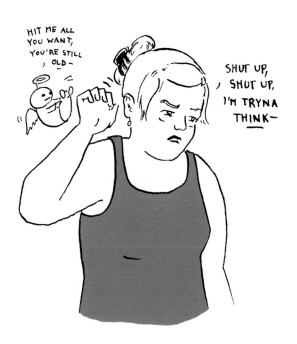

AS MY BIRTHDAY APPROACHED, I FOUND MYSELF WONDERING: DID I MEAN I'D QUIT, LIKE, THE MINUTE I TURNED 29? OR JUST, YOU KNOW, SOMETIME THAT YEAR?

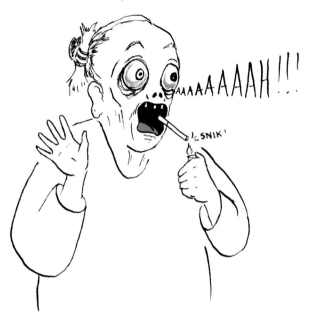

AND I DON'T T<u>HIN</u>K THAT LADY
WAS A GYPSY, BUT WHAT IF SHE WAS?
DID SHE TO<u>UC</u>H ME? DO I HAVE
TO WORRY ABOUT G<u>YP</u>SY CURSES IF
I FAIL TO COMPLY? I MEAN, THAT'S
SILLY, RIGHT? RIGHT???

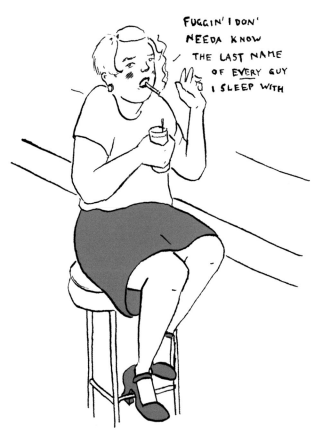

GYPSY CURSES ASIDE, 29 IS 29. IT'S NOT
20, WHEN YOU FEEL INDESTRUCTIBLE, THE
NOTION OF THINGS LIKE AN UNPLEASANT
DEATH FAR FROM YOUR MIND.

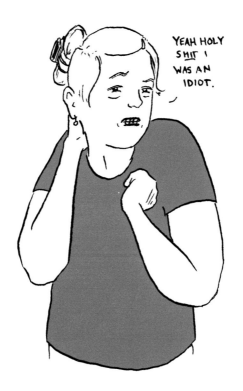

SOMETHING ABOUT SHADING INTO YOUR
30's PUTS THE THOUGHT IN YOUR HEAD
THAT BAD HABITS ACTUALLY CA_N TAKE
A TOLL, AND THAT MAYBE GYPSY
CURSES ARE THE LEAST OF YOUR PROBLEMS.

THEY JUST DON'T UNDERSTAND

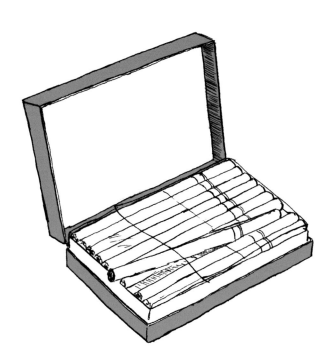

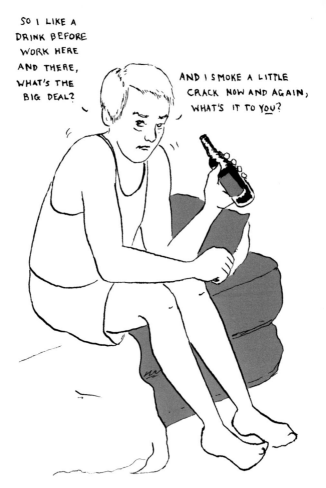

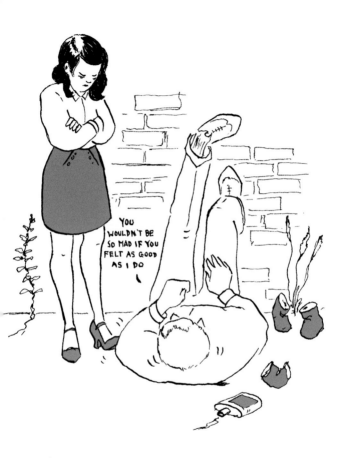

JUSTIFYING THEM TO PEOPLE WHO
DON'T SHARE THEM IS A WHOLE
OTHER BALL OF WAX.

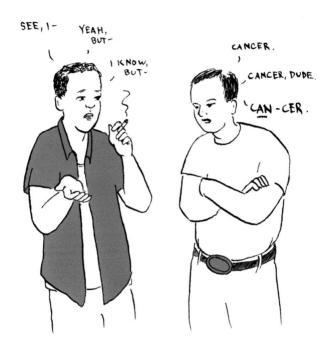

SMOKING'S A TOUGH ONE TO JUSTIFY
ON ACCOUNT OF IT MAKES NO SENSE.
THERE'S REALLY NOTHING YOU CAN SAY
THAT MAKES IT ANYTHING LESS THAN
A HORRIBLE, DESTRUCTIVE HABIT.

AND YET...

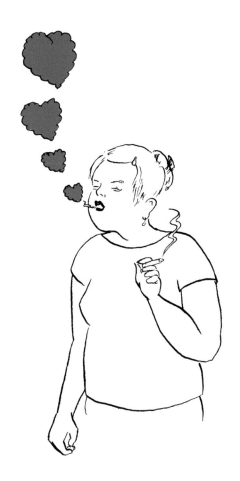

AND YET, I LOVE TO SMOKE. YEAH,
I KNOW THAT'S A FUCKED-UP THING
TO SAY. BUT FUCK IT, IT'S TRUE.

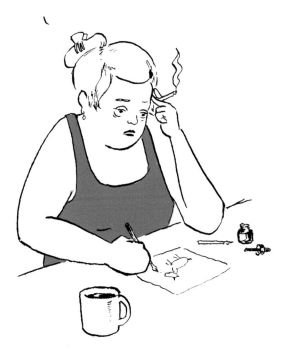

OVER A LONG NIGHT'S WORK, A
CIGARETTE CAN BE YOUR BEST FRIEND
IN THE WORLD, FOCUSING YOUR
THOUGHTS, KEEPING YOU AWAKE.

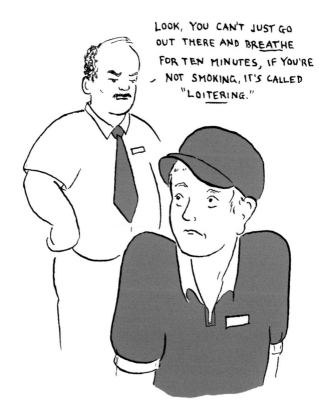

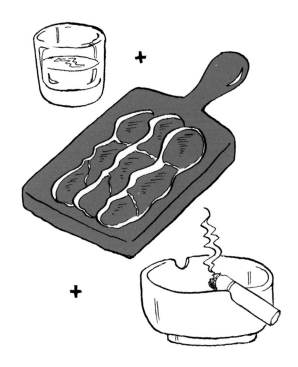

AND HERE'S A MAGICAL VICE
TRIFECTA: QUALITY BOURBON, FINE
PROSCIUTTO, AND A CIGARETTE. ENJOY
TOGETHER AND IT'S LIKE ANGELS ARE
THROWING A PARTY IN YOUR MOUTH.

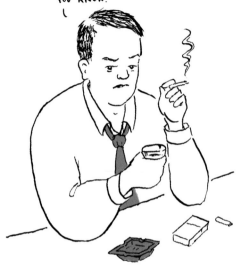

IF YOU'RE ALONE IN A BAR, CIGARETTES
KEEP YOU COMPANY. YOU'RE NOT JUST
SITTING THERE HOPING A FRIEND
WILL SHOW UP OR THAT SOMEONE
WILL TALK TO YOU, YOU'RE TENDING
TO IMPORTANT SMOKING DUTIES.

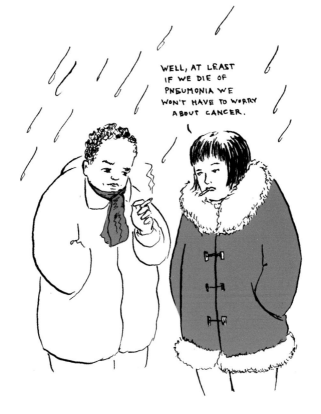

IF YOU LIVE IN A PLACE WHERE
THEY DON'T ALLOW SMOKING IN BARS,
CIGARETTES CAN HELP YOU MAKE
NEW FRIENDS, OR AT LEAST GIVE
YOU SOMETHING TO BITCH ABOUT
WITH YOUR OLD ONES.

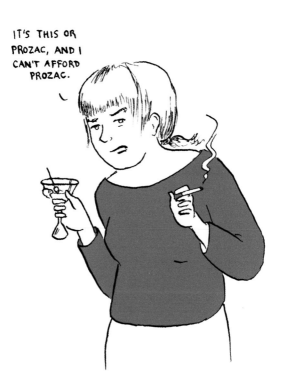

IT'S TOO BAD, THOUGH, THAT THEY'VE SEPARATED THE TWO BEST-FRIEND VICES – THE MENTAL HEALTH BENEFITS OF THE SMOKE-DRINK COMBO ARE UNDENIABLE. TO SMOKERS, ANYWAY.

AND, ERM, DRINKERS.

IF YOU ARE THE ENGINE, CIGARETTE SMOKE IS YOUR EXHAUST. SMOKING PUNCTUATES YOUR LIFE. IT PROVIDES COUNTERPOINT TO CONVERSATIONS DULL OR LIVELY, UNCOMFORTABLE OR INTENSE. IT'S A VERY SOCIABLE HABIT, A SOCIAL LUBRICANT, A SHARED EXPERIENCE THAT FORMS A TINY, TEMPORARY COMMUNITY. THE LITTLE BURN, THE CONSTRICTION WHEN IT HITS YOUR THROAT- WELL, IT JUST KIND OF REMINDS YOU YOU'RE ALIVE. IT IS, FOR ALL INTENTS AND PURPOSES, AN INTENSELY PLEASURABLE AND SATISFYING ACTIVITY.

OL' CRISPY LUNG

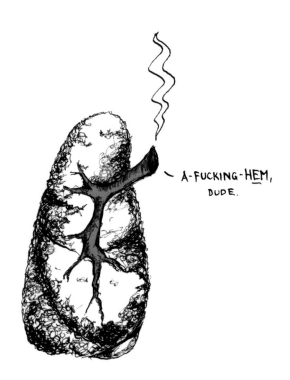

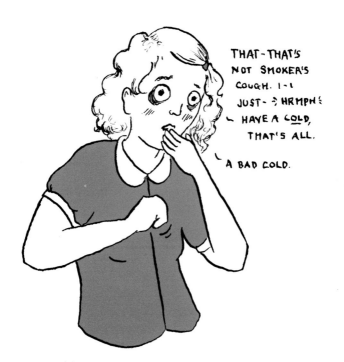

YOU DON'T NEED ME TO TELL
YOU THERE'S A REAL DARK SIDE
TO THIS ROMANCE, THOUGH. LET'S
NOT PRETEND YOUR LOVER
DOESN'T BEAT YOU.

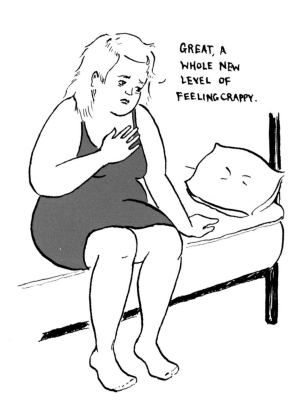

WHILE DELIGHTFUL WHEN PAIRED
WITH BOOZE, CIGARETTES ARE A
MAGICAL HANGOVER BOOSTER.

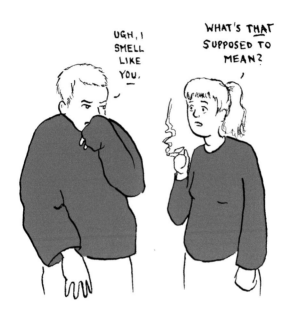

THE SMOKE STANKS UP YOUR
CLOTHES. AND WORSE, THE
CLOTHES OF YOUR NON-
SMOKING FRIENDS.

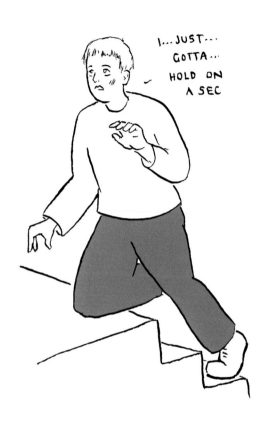

GETTING WINDED GOING UP
A FLIGHT OF STAIRS IS
SORT OF EMBARRASSING.

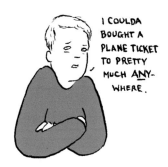

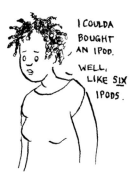

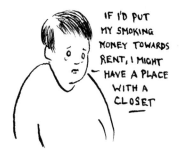

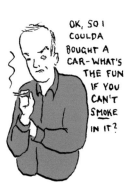

IT COSTS A FAINTLY RIDICULOUS AMOUNT OF MONEY, ESPECIALLY IF YOU TOTAL IT UP BY THE YEAR.

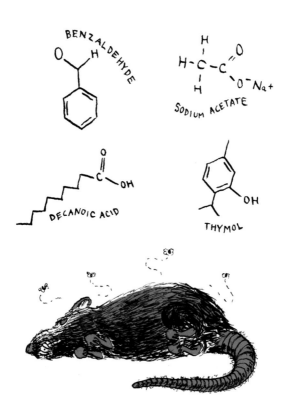

THERE'S A GALAXY OF CHEMICALS
AND ADDITIVES AND WEIRD SHIT IN
EVERY DRAG. IF IT CAN KILL RATS
OR STRIP PAINT OR WHATEVER
YOU PROLLY SHOULDN'T SMOKE IT.

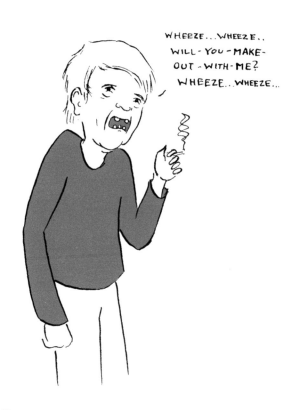

EMPHYSEMA, RECEDING GUMS, FERTILITY
PROBLEMS, STROKE-ALL SHIT YOU
CAN GET FROM SMOKING.

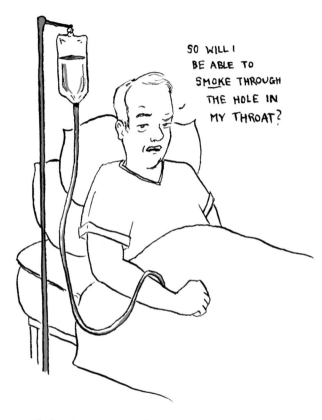

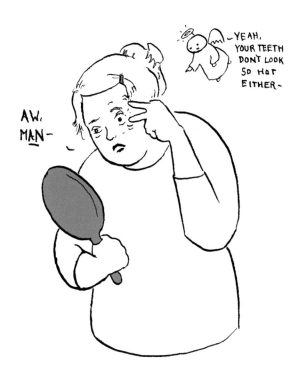

AND AS FOR ME, BECAUSE I AM SO VAIN, I WORRY THE MOST ABOUT THE EFFECTS ON THE SKIN.

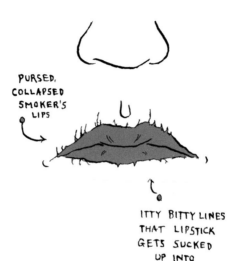

PURSED,
COLLAPSED
SMOKER'S
LIPS

ITTY BITTY LINES
THAT LIPSTICK
GETS SUCKED
UP INTO

LUNGS, SCHMUNGS, IT'S THE CROW'S
FEET AND FARRAH FAWCETT LINES
THAT PUT THE FEAR OF GOD INTO
ME. AND THEN TOO: IF I CAN SEE
SOMETHING HAPPENING TO MY
FACE, SURELY DIRTY THINGS ARE
GOING ON IN THE REST OF ME.

WISH I COULD QUIT YOU

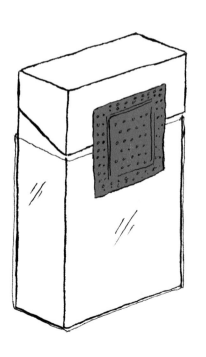

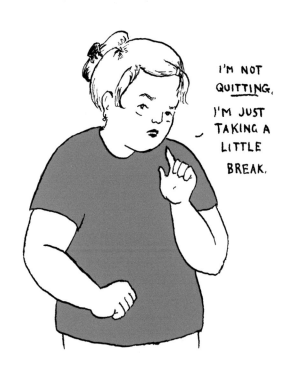

ONCE, JUST AS A LITTLE
EXPERIMENT, I DECIDED NOT
TO SMOKE FOR A FEW DAYS.

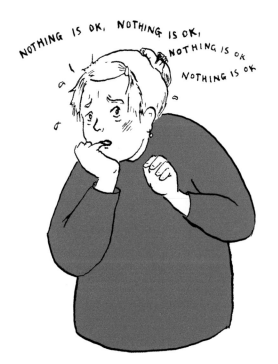

IT WAS FUCKING AWFUL. I FELT
LIKE I'D BEEN DUMPED: WEEPY,
ANXIOUS, AND OBSESSED WITH
THE THING I COULDN'T HAVE.

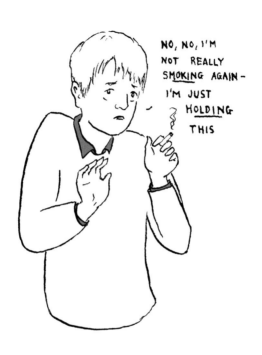

SUPPOSEDLY THAT FEELING
WANES, BUT WE ALL KNOW PEOPLE
WHO'VE QUIT-FOR YEARS,
EVEN- AND FALLEN RIGHT
BACK OFF THE WAGON.

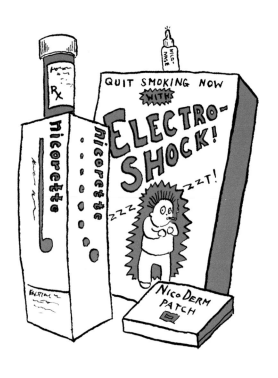

THAT'S WHY THE MARKET
OFFERS AN ARRAY OF PRODUCTS
TO HELP THE WHOLE QUIT
THING TAKE.

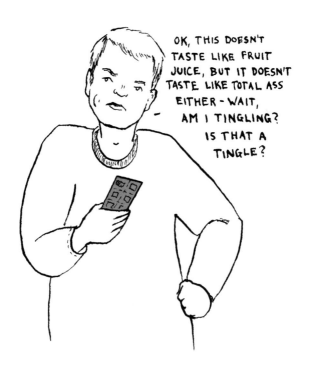

NICORETTE, SURPRISINGLY, DOESN'T
TASTE AS BAD AS YOU MIGHT THINK.
IT IS, HOWEVER, AN EXTREMELY WEIRD
GUM EXPERIENCE. YOU HAVE TO ENGAGE
IN SOME BIZARRO "CHEW TILL IT TINGLES,
THEN STOP, THEN CHEW AGAIN" RITUAL.

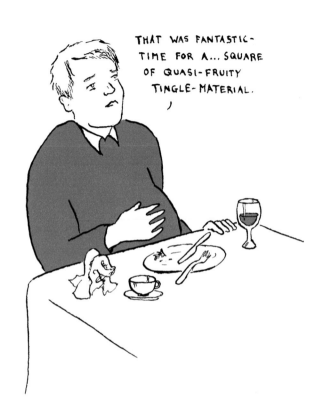

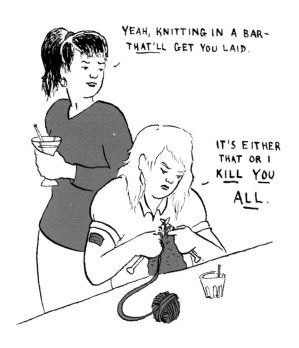

THE PATCH'LL GET SOME DRUGS
TO YOUR BRAIN, TOO, BUT IF YOU
DON'T GIVE YOUR HANDS SOMETHING
TO DO, YOU'RE PRETTY WELL SCREWED.

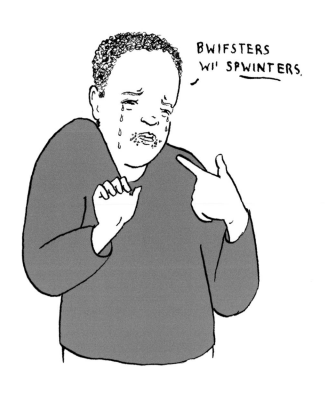

THOSE LITTLE TEA-TREE OIL PEPPERMINT
TOOTHPICKS ARE ACTUALLY PRETTY DELIGHTFUL,
UNTIL YOU CHEW SO MANY THAT
YOUR MOUTH BREAKS OUT IN BLISTERS.

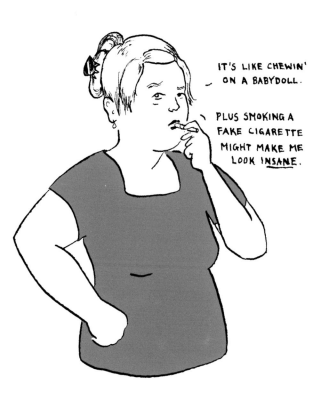

IT'S LIKE CHEWIN' ON A BABYDOLL.

PLUS SMOKING A FAKE CIGARETTE MIGHT MAKE ME LOOK INSANE.

I ALSO SENT AWAY FOR A LITTLE DEVICE THAT WAS SHAPED LIKE A CIGARETTE AND FEATURED AN ADJUST-ABLE DRAW. IT MIGHT'VE HELPED, IF IT HADN'T TASTED SO MUCH OF CHEAP PLASTIC.

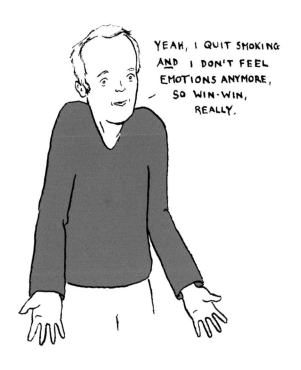

AND THEN THERE'S WELLBUTRIN,
A HAPPY-DRUG THAT SOME GENIUS
FIGURED OUT HELPS CURB THE
URGE TO SMOKE. TAKE THAT, PAXIL!

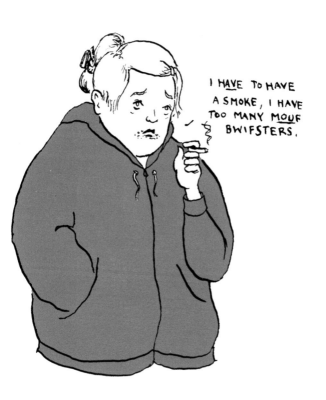

BUT, LIKE SO MUCH IN LIFE, DIFFERENT
THINGS WORK - OR DON'T - FOR DIFFERENT
PEOPLE. AS I UNDERSTAND IT, THE TRICK
IS TO KEEP TRYING. AND TO NOT
   GIVE UP. OR SOMETHING.

THE HOLE IN A GRATEFUL HEART

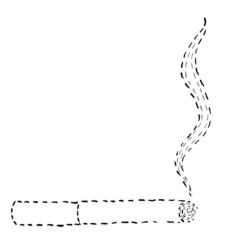

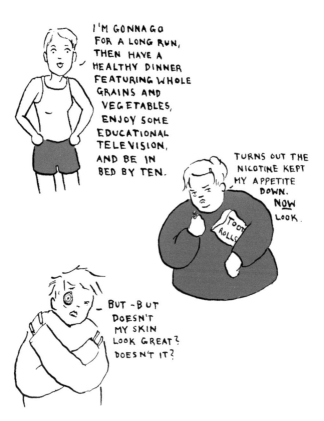

SO THEN THERE'S THIS, AND I
THINK IT'S A BIGGER CONSIDERATION
THAN MOST SMOKERS LET ON:
WHO WILL I <u>BE</u> IF I QUIT SMOKING?

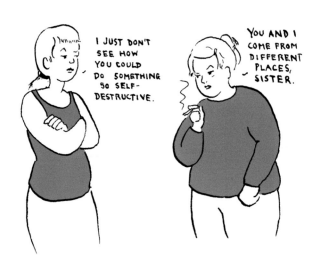

IT'S IRRATIONAL IN THE EXTREME, BUT DEEP DOWN I FEEL JUST A TINGE OF DISTRUST FOR NON-SMOKERS.

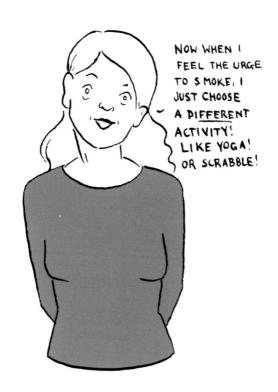

AND SOME OF THE DORKWADS
ON THE QUIT-SMOKING SITES—THAT'S
JUST NOT KOOL-AID I WANT TO DRINK.

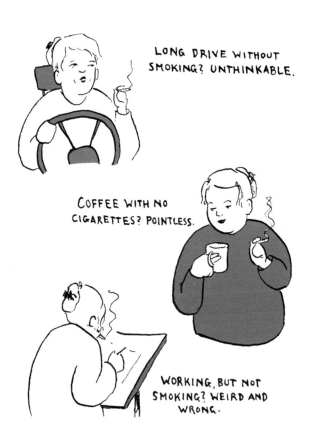

LONG DRIVE WITHOUT SMOKING? UNTHINKABLE.

COFFEE WITH NO CIGARETTES? POINTLESS.

WORKING, BUT NOT SMOKING? WEIRD AND WRONG.

IT DOESN'T SAY GREAT THINGS ABOUT ME, BUT SMOKING HAS BEEN A CONSTANT PRESENCE IN MY LIFE FOR A LONG TIME - AND I DON'T REMEMBER WHAT I USED TO DO - OR HOW I USED TO BE - WITHOUT IT.

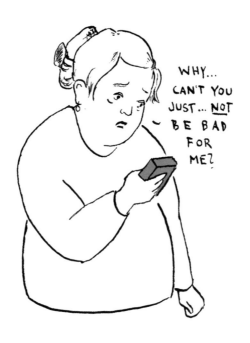

CALL IT A CRUTCH, 'CAUSE THAT'S WHAT IT IS – BUT THE WORRY REMAINS. BUT THEN, HERE WE ARE AGAIN AT BAD SKIN AND CRISPY LUNGS AND TERRIBLE INCURABLE DISEASES. WHO WINS?

SO... WHAT NOW?

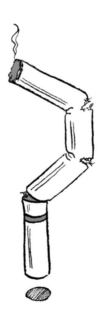

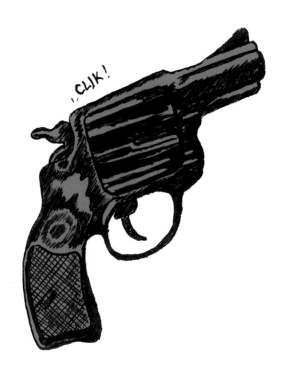

ALL OF THIS, ALL MY LOVE AND
YOUR LOVE AND DESIRES AND ADDICTIONS
AND WHATNOT, WOULD BE RENDERED
COMPLETELY IRRELEVANT SHOULD
THE RUSSIAN ROULETTE GAME BE LOST.

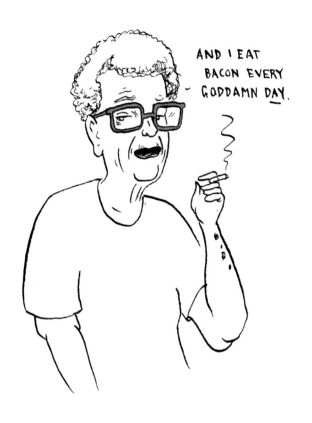

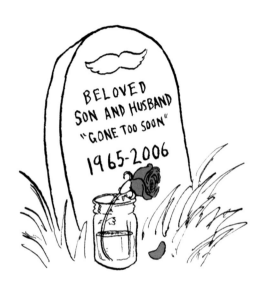

A LOT OF PEOPLE DON'T.

IF YOU PLAY THOSE CHANCES
AND DO GET SICK, IMAGINE
THE DEPTHS OF YOUR REGRET
THEN. IT'LL BE AWFULLY HARD
TO ASK FOR SYMPATHY ON
YOUR DEATHBED IF YOU PLANNED,
BUILT, AND PAVED YOUR OWN
SUPERHIGHWAY THERE IN
THE FIRST PLACE. KIND OF
LIKE HOW NOBODY HAS A
LOT OF SYMPATHY FOR
YOUR HANGOVER, BUT TIMES
LIKE A MILLION.

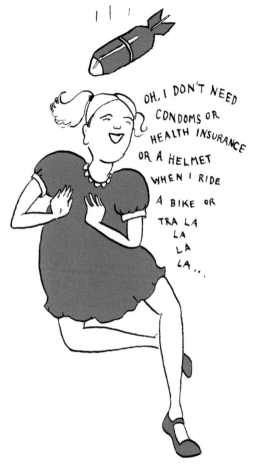

AND THERE'S THE RUB. THE TRUE WEIGHT OF ANY AWFULNESS IS PRETTY ABSTRACT UNTIL SOMETHING ACTUALLY HAPPENS.

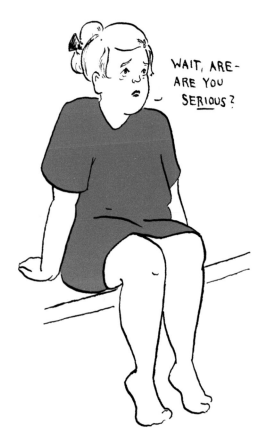

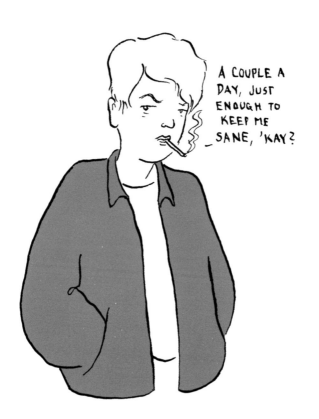

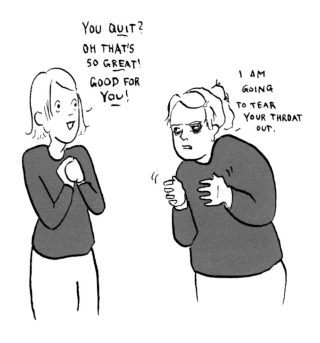

MY PLAN FOR WHEN (IF? AAAAAGH WHEN)
I DO QUIT HINGES ON THIS: THE LAST
THING YOU WANT TO HEAR WHEN
YOU'RE FEELING THAT ROTTEN IS
"CONGRATULATIONS." YOU'RE IN HELL.

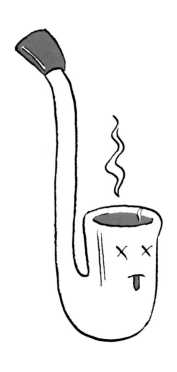

PAUL THEROUX HAD A GREAT LINE
FOR HAVING TO GIVE UP HIS PIPE:
"I MISS IT LIKE A DEAD FRIEND," HE
SAID. SO I THINK IT'LL BE BEST TO
HAVE A LITTLE FUNERAL.

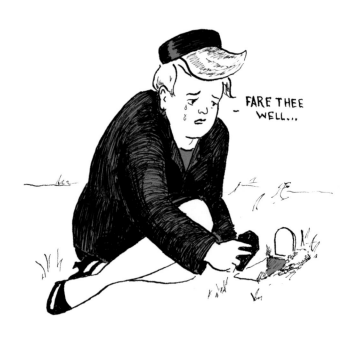

I'LL TAKE THE LAST CIGARETTE
OF THE PACK. I'LL FASHION A LITTLE
COFFIN AND DRESS IN MOURNING
CLOTHES. I MAY EVEN CRY-OF COURSE
I'LL BE SAD, MY FRIEND IS DEAD!

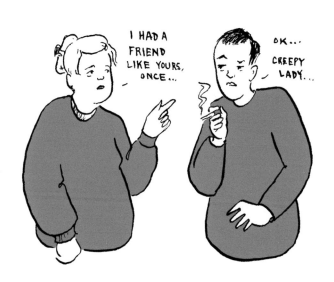

I'LL SEE OTHER PEOPLE
SMOKE, OF COURSE, AFTER THIS,
BUT THAT'S JUST THEM TALKING
TO THEIR FRIEND.

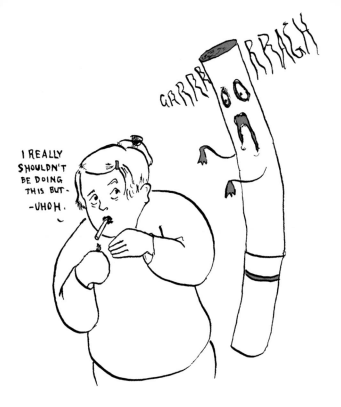

AND IF MY FRIEND COMES BACK
TO LIFE, WELL, THAT MEANS I
HAVE A ≩ZOMBIE PROBLEM≩
AND I MUST TAKE CARE OF IT
≩IMMEDIATELY.≩

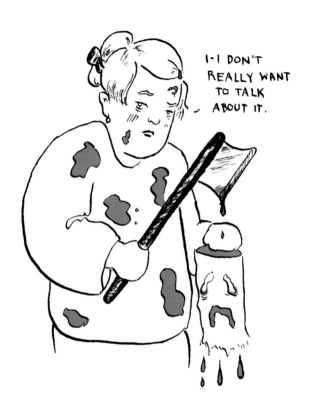

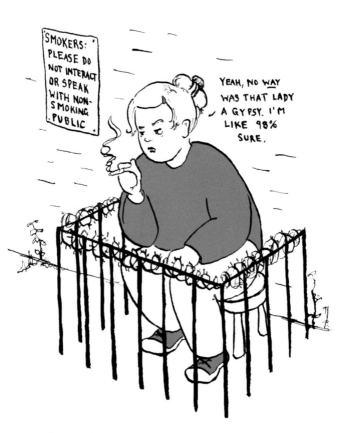

BUT UNTIL THEN, I'LL BE OUTSIDE,
TAKING DRAG AFTER GUILTY DRAG AND
THINKING HARD ABOUT THE FUTURE.

ACKNOWLEDGMENTS

MY DEEPEST THANKS TO JAMI ATTENBERG; TO ERIN HOSIER; TO BLOOMSBURY USA, IN PARTICULAR COLIN, MILES, GREG, AMY, AND ALONA; TO ED, ANGELINA, AND TIM FOR THEIR EYEBALLS AND ADVICE; AND TO JOHN "MR. FATTY" PASTORE, WHO DOES NOT SMOKE.

A NOTE ON THE AUTHOR

EMILY FLAKE IS A CRITICALLY ACCLAIMED ILLUSTRATOR AND CARTOONIST WHOSE WORK HAS APPEARED IN *McSWEENEY'S*, THE *NATION*, *NICKELODEON MAGAZINE*, AND THE *WALL STREET JOURNAL*, AMONG OTHERS. HER WEEKLY STRIP, *LULU EIGHTBALL*, RUNS IN TEN ALTERNATIVE NEWSWEEKLIES AND WAS COLLECTED INTO A BOOK, ALSO ENTITLED *LULU EIGHTBALL*.